2014
The Year Book of ENDOCRINOLOGY®

Editor-in-Chief
Matthias Schott, MD, PhD
Professor for Endocrinology, Head, Division for Specific Endocrinology, University Hospital Düsseldorf, Düsseldorf, Germany

ELSEVIER
MOSBY

ELSEVIER
MOSBY

Vice President, Global Medical Reference: Mary E. Gatsch
Editor: Jessica McCool
Developmental Editor: Barbara Cohen-Kligerman
Production Supervisor, Electronic Year Books: Donna M. Skelton
Electronic Article Manager: Mike Sheets
Senior Illustrations and Permissions Coordinator: Dawn Vohsen

2014 EDITION

Composition by TNQ Books and Journals Pvt Ltd, India

Editorial Office:
Elsevier
Suite 1800
1600 John F. Kennedy Blvd
Philadelphia, PA 19103-2899

International Standard Serial Number: 0084-3741
International Standard Book Number: 978-0-323-26495-2

Associate Editors

Bart L. Clarke, MD

Associate Professor of Medicine, Mayo Clinic College of Medicine; Consultant, St. Mary's Hospital; Consultant, Rochester Methodist Hospital, Rochester, Minnesota

Erica A. Eugster, MD

Professor of Pediatrics, Director, Section of Pediatric Endocrinology/ Diabetology, Riley Hospital for Children, Indiana University School of Medicine, Indianapolis, Indiana

Lalita Khaodhiar, MD

Assistant Professor of Medicine, Section of Endocrinology, Diabetes and Nutrition, Boston University Medical Center, Boston, Massachusetts

A. Wayne Meikle, MD

Professor of Endocrinology, University of Utah School of Medicine; Medical Director of Endocrine Testing, ARUP Laboratories, The University of Utah Hospitals, Salt Lake City, Utah

Elke Oetjen, MD

Professor of Pharmacology, Institute of Clinical Pharmacology and Toxicology, University Medical Center Hamburg-Eppendorf, Hamburg, Germany

Stephan Petersenn, MD

Professor, ENDOC Center for Endocrine Tumors, Hamburg, Germany

Peter P. Toth, MD, PhD, FAAFP, FNLA, FCCP, FAHA, FACC

Director of Preventative Cardiology, CGH Medical Center, Sterling, Illinois; Professor of Clinical Family and Community Medicine, University of Illinois College of Medicine, Peoria, Illinois; Professor of Clinical Medicine, Michigan State University College of Osteopathic Medicine, East Lansing, Michigan; Adjunct Associate Professor of Medicine, Johns Hopkins University School of Medicine, Baltimore, Maryland

Holger S. Willenberg, MD, PhD

Professor of Endocrinology, Head, Division of Endocrinology and Metabolism, Rostock University Medical Center, Rostock, Germany

Contributing Editor

Margret Ehlers, PhD

Division for Specific Endocrinology, University Hospital Duesseldorf, Duesseldorf, Germany

Table of Contents

Journals Represented

Journals represented in this Year Book are listed below.

American Heart Journal
American Journal of Cardiology
American Journal of Medicine
American Journal of Transplantation
Annals of Internal Medicine
Cancer
Cancer Research
Cell
Cell Reports
Circulation
Clinical Cancer Research
Clinical Endocrinology
Clinical Neurology and Neurosurgery
Contraception
Diabetes
Diabetes Care
Drugs
Endocrinology
European Heart Journal
European Journal of Endocrinology
Fertility and Sterility
Heart
Hypertension
International Journal of Cardiology
Journal of Bone Mineral Research
Journal of Clinical Investigation
Journal of Immunology
Journal of Internal Medicine
Journal of Pediatrics
Journal of the American College of Cardiology
Journal of the American College of Surgeons
Journal of the American Medical Association
Journal of the American Medical Association Pediatrics
Lancet
Nature
Nature Genetics
Nature Medicine
New England Journal of Medicine
Osteoporosis International
Pediatrics
Proceedings of the National Academy of Sciences of the United States of America

The Journal of Clinical Endocrinology and Metabolism
The Lancet Diabetes & Endocrinology

Standard Abbreviations

The following terms are abbreviated in this edition: acquired immunodeficiency syndrome (AIDS); adrenocorticotropin hormone (ACTH); cardiopulmonary resuscitation (CPR); central nervous system (CNS); cerebrospinal fluid (CSF); computed tomography (CT); corticotropin-releasing hormone (CRH); deoxyribonucleic acid (DNA); electrocardiography (ECG); follicle-stimulating hormone (FSH); gonadotropin-releasing hormone (GnRH); growth hormone (GH); health maintenance organization (HMO); high-density lipoprotein (HDL); human immunodeficiency virus (HIV); insulin-dependent diabetes mellitus (IDDM); insulin-like growth factor I (IGF-I); intensive care unit (ICU); intermediate-density lipoprotein (IDL); intramuscular (IM); intravenous (IV); low-density lipoprotein (LDL); luteinizing hormone (LH); magnetic resonance (MR) imaging (MRI); multiple endocrine neoplasia (MEN); non-insulin-dependent diabetes mellitus (NIDDM); parathyroid hormone (PTH); prolactin (PRL); releasing hormone (RH); ribonucleic acid (RNA); thyrotropin-releasing hormone (TRH); thyroid-stimulating hormone or thyrotropin (TSH); thyroxine (T_4); triiodothyronine (T_3); ultrasound (US); and very-low-density lipoprotein (VLDL).

Note

The Year Book of Endocrinology is a literature survey service providing abstracts of articles published in the professional literature. Every effort is made to assure the accuracy of the information presented in these pages. Neither the editor nor the publisher of the Year Book of Endocrinology can be responsible for errors in the original materials. The editors' comments are their own opinions. Mention of specific products within this publication does not constitute endorsement.

To facilitate the use of the Year Book of Endocrinology as a reference tool, all illustrations and tables included in this publication are now identified as they appear in the original article. This change is meant to help the reader recognize that any illustration or table appearing in the Year Book of Endocrinology may be only one of many in the original article. For this reason, figure and table numbers appear to be out of sequence within the Year Book of Endocrinology.

Introduction

The number of scientific articles worldwide is largely increasing every year. Before I started to write this introduction, I again performed a PubMed search for keywords such as "thyroid." The search yielded about 6836 articles. For "osteoporosis," the search yielded about 4004 articles. When entering the keyword "diabetes mellitus," the results were even more impressive, with 19 767 articles showing up on the computer screen. Because of the extremely high number of papers also published in 2013, it is not possible for the editorial team to review "all" articles in order to select the best articles from all fields of endocrinology, including thyroid, bone, adrenal, pituitary, etc. Although there is the potential for bias in the process of selecting articles to review, the editorial team has done its best to avoid bias and select the best papers published in 2013.

From my point of view, one of the best articles in the last year is the study by Bath et al that was published in *The Lancet*.[1] The aim of this study was to investigate whether women with low iodine status in early pregnancy have children with poorer cognitive outcomes than those of women with higher iodine status. A previous Avon Longitudinal Study of Parents and Children (ALSPAC) showed a positive association between maternal seafood consumption and child intelligence quotient (IQ), which the authors suggest could have been driven at least partly by the high iodine content of seafood. The study by Bath et al observed a significant difference in the verbal and the total IQ in children of iodine-deficient mothers compared to children of mothers with normal iodine intake. This study is in line with former studies showing a lower IQ in children of mothers with (subclinical) hypothyroidism during pregnancy compared to children of euthyroid mothers. Because of this and other studies, the World Health Organization has made a clear recommendation to supplement iodine in iodine-deficient areas and especially in pregnant woman.

Another very important study dealing with the question of fracture risk was published by Compston and coworkers.[2] The study reports that body weight, height, and body mass index (BMI) predicted differential fracture risk at different skeletal sites in a large international clinical practice cohort, the Global Longitudinal Study of Osteoporosis in Women. Of 52 939 women in the cohort, 3628 (6.9%) reported incidents of clinical fractures during the 3-year follow-up period. Linear modelling of BMI showed a significant inverse association with hip, clinical spine, and wrist fractures, with linear modelling of weight positively associated with ankle fractures, and linear modelling of height positively associated with upper arm/shoulder and clavicular fractures. Nonlinear modelling of BMI or weight predicted pelvis or rib fractures, with inverse associations at low BMI/weight and positive associations at higher values. These findings indicate that the relationships between fracture and body weight, height, and BMI are site-specific.

These are only two of many excellent papers published in 2013. The editors of the Year Book of Endocrinology 2014 hope that all selected articles and their accompanying editorial comments provide our readers fresh insight into endocrine problems encountered in everyday practice. In the name of all editors ...

Matthias Schott, MD, PhD

References

1. Bath SC, Steer CD, Golding J, Emmett P, Rayman MP. Effect of inadequate iodine status in UK pregnant women on cognitive outcomes in their children: results from the Avon Longitudinal Study of Parents and Children (ALSPAC). *Lancet*. 2013; 382:331-337.
2. Compston JE, Flahive J, Hosmer DW, et al. Relationship of weight, height, and body mass index with fracture risk at different sites in postmenopausal women: the Global Longitudinal study of Osteoporosis in Women (GLOW). *J Bone Miner Res*. 2014;29:487-493.

1 Diabetes

Introduction

The adequate treatment of diabetes mellitus in order to prevent long-term complications remains challenging in areas such as cardiovascular diseases, kidney insufficiency, and blindness. Drugs targeting the incretin system, either acting as agonist for the GLP-1 receptor or enhancing endogenous levels of GLP-1 and GIP by inhibiting the incretin degrading enzyme dipeptidyl peptidase IV seemed to be a good choice, since these drugs do not induce hypoglycemia and are reported to protect beta-cell mass or even to promote beta-cell proliferation. No serious adverse effects have been reported so far. This has changed within the last years. The debate about the beneficial and the adverse effects of GLP-1 and DPP IV inhibitors will certainly continue. In addition, the debate about potential protective effects on the cardiovascular system will continue. Ever since the realization that a subacute chronic inflammation might provide the link between obesity and diabetes, either old anti-inflammatory drugs such as salsalate have been re-evaluated or new targets for drugs ameliorating the inflammation have been investigated. In 2013 several studies were published investigating the efficiency of salsalate. Several studies were published on potential new antidiabetic drugs such as the inhibitors of the 11-beta hydroxysteroid dehydrogenase and a novel inhibitor of the hepatic glucokinase. The question whether treatment of and education about diabetes improves outcome is addressed as well, with somewhat disappointing results.

Elke Oetjen, MD

Complications

Glucose Levels and Risk of Dementia

Crane PK, Walker R, Hubbard RA, et al (Univ of Washington, Seattle; Group Health Res Inst, Seattle, WA)

N Engl J Med 369:540-548, 2013

Background.—Diabetes is a risk factor for dementia. It is unknown whether higher glucose levels increase the risk of dementia in people without diabetes.

Methods.—We used 35,264 clinical measurements of glucose levels and 10,208 measurements of glycated hemoglobin levels from 2067 participants without dementia to examine the relationship between glucose levels and the risk of dementia. Participants were from the Adult Changes in Thought study and included 839 men and 1228 women whose mean age at baseline was 76 years; 232 participants had diabetes, and 1835 did not. We fit Cox regression models, stratified according to diabetes status and adjusted for age, sex, study cohort, educational level, level of exercise, blood pressure, and status with respect to coronary and cerebrovascular diseases, atrial fibrillation, smoking, and treatment for hypertension.

Results.—During a median follow-up of 6.8 years, dementia developed in 524 participants (74 with diabetes and 450 without). Among participants without diabetes, higher average glucose levels within the preceding 5 years were related to an increased risk of dementia ($P = 0.01$); with a glucose level of 115 mg per deciliter (6.4 mmol per liter) as compared with 100 mg per deciliter (5.5 mmol per liter), the adjusted hazard ratio for dementia was 1.18 (95% confidence interval [CI], 1.04 to 1.33). Among participants with diabetes, higher average glucose levels were also related to an increased risk of dementia ($P = 0.002$); with a glucose level of 190 mg per deciliter (10.5 mmol per liter) as compared with 160 mg per deciliter (8.9 mmol per liter), the adjusted hazard ratio was 1.40 (95% CI, 1.12 to 1.76).

Conclusions.—Our results suggest that higher glucose levels may be a risk factor for dementia, even among persons without diabetes. (Funded by the National Institutes of Health.)

▶ Because of demographic changes that have resulted in an increasing number of older people, the incidence of dementia is increasing. Diabetes is a known risk factor for dementia; however, the underlying mechanisms are poorly understood. In addition, dementia is caused by multiple diverse etiologies. Identification of risk factors for the development of diabetes is desirable. Using sophisticated statistical models, this prospective, community-based cohort study found that elevated glucose levels are associated with dementia in populations with and without diabetes. The type of dementia was not specified. The threshold glucose level is higher in the diabetic population than the nondiabetic population, suggesting that diabetes and glucose levels might be independent risk factors. This study sheds light on the association between dementia and diabetes/prediabetes, with elevated glucose levels playing a role.

E. Oetjen, MD

An association between gestational diabetes mellitus and long-term maternal cardiovascular morbidity

Kessous R, Shoham-Vardi I, Pariente G, et al (Ben-Gurion Univ of the Negev, Beer-Sheva, Israel)

Heart 99:1118-1121, 2013

Objective.—To investigate whether a diagnosis of gestational diabetes mellitus (GDM) is a risk factor for subsequent long-term cardiovascular morbidity.

Design.—A population-based study.

Setting.—Soroka University Medical Center, a tertiary centre in the southern region of Israel.

Patients.—A cohort of women with and without a diagnosis of GDM who delivered during the years 1988–1999 with a follow-up period until 2010.

Interventions.—A comparison of the incidence of cardiovascular morbidity.

Results.—Of 47 909 deliveries that met the inclusion criteria, 4928 (10.3%) occurred in patients who were diagnosed with GDM. During a follow-up period of more than 10 years, compared with women who gave birth at the same time period, after adjustment for age and ethnicity, patients with GDM had higher rates of cardiovascular morbidity including non-invasive cardiac diagnostic procedures (OR = 1.8; 95% CI 1.4 to 2.2), simple cardiovascular events (OR = 2.7; 95% CI 2.4 to 3.1) and total cardiovascular hospitalisations (OR = 2.3; 95% CI 2.0 to 2.5). In a Cox proportional hazards model, adjusted for comorbidities such as pre-eclampsia and obesity, GDM was independently associated with cardiovascular hospitalisations (adjusted HR 2.6, 95% CI 2.3 to 3).

Conclusions.—GDM is an independent risk factor for long-term cardiovascular morbidity in a follow-up period of more than a decade.

▶ Gestational diabetes mellitus is defined as glucose intolerance that begins with or is often first recognized during pregnancy. It is often reversible but predisposes to gestational diabetes in later pregnancies and the development of the metabolic syndrome and diabetes type 2 in later years. It can be assumed that gestational diabetes is a risk factor for cardiovascular diseases as well. This is not well documented. The authors of this population-based 1-center study remedy this and show that gestational diabetes is independently associated with hospitalizations for cardiovascular events. The study was undertaken in 1 medical center; in terms of follow-up, this is a strength because this study site is the only hospital in that large area; however, it might be a disadvantage as well, because only a selected population visits this hospital. Nevertheless, the finding is quite interesting and puts gestational diabetes, the most frequently occurring complication in pregnancy, into focus.

E. Oetjen, MD

Combined Angiotensin Inhibition for the Treatment of Diabetic Nephropathy

Fried LF, for the VA NEPHRON-D Investigators (Veterans Affairs (VA) Pittsburgh Healthcare System and Univ of Pittsburgh School of Medicine, PA; et al)

N Engl J Med 369:1892-1903, 2013

Background.—Combination therapy with angiotensin-converting–enzyme (ACE) inhibitors and angiotensin-receptor blockers (ARBs) decreases proteinuria; however, its safety and effect on the progression of kidney disease are uncertain.

Methods.—We provided losartan (at a dose of 100 mg per day) to patients with type 2 diabetes, a urinary albumin-to-creatinine ratio (with albumin measured in milligrams and creatinine measured in grams) of at least 300, and an estimated glomerular filtration rate (GFR) of 30.0 to 89.9 ml per minute per 1.73 m^2 of body-surface area and then randomly assigned them to receive lisinopril (at a dose of 10 to 40 mg per day) or placebo. The primary end point was the first occurrence of a change in the estimated GFR (a decline of $\geq$30 ml per minute per 1.73 m^2 if the initial estimated GFR was $\geq$60 ml per minute per 1.73 m^2 or a decline of $\geq$50% if the initial estimated GFR was <60 ml per minute per 1.73 m^2), end-stage renal disease (ESRD), or death. The secondary renal end point was the first occurrence of a decline in the estimated GFR or ESRD. Safety outcomes included mortality, hyperkalemia, and acute kidney injury.

Results.—The study was stopped early owing to safety concerns. Among 1448 randomly assigned patients with a median follow-up of 2.2 years, there were 152 primary end-point events in the monotherapy group and 132 in the combination-therapy group (hazard ratio with combination therapy, 0.88; 95% confidence interval [CI], 0.70 to 1.12; $P = 0.30$). A trend toward a benefit from combination therapy with respect to the secondary end point (hazard ratio, 0.78; 95% CI, 0.58 to 1.05; $P = 0.10$) decreased with time ($P = 0.02$ for nonproportionality). There was no benefit with respect to mortality (hazard ratio for death, 1.04; 95% CI, 0.73 to 1.49; $P = 0.75$) or cardiovascular events. Combination therapy increased the risk of hyperkalemia (6.3 events per 100 person-years, vs. 2.6 events per 100 person-years with monotherapy; $P < 0.001$) and acute kidney injury (12.2 vs. 6.7 events per 100 person-years, $P < 0.001$).

Conclusions.—Combination therapy with an ACE inhibitor and an ARB was associated with an increased risk of adverse events among patients with diabetic nephropathy. (Funded by the Cooperative Studies Program of the Department of Veterans Affairs Office of Research and Development; VA NEPHRON-D ClinicalTrials.gov number, NCT00555217.)

▶ Nephropathy leading to kidney insufficiency requiring dialysis is an often-observed complication of diabetes. To ameliorate this complication is a desirable goal. Proteinuria and the reduction of the glomerular filtration rate (GFR) are symptoms of nephropathy in which the degree of reduction in proteinuria correlates with the extent to which the decrease in GFR is slowed. Both blockers of the renin—angiotensin system, inhibitors of the angiotensin-converting enzyme (ACE inhibitors) and angiotensin-II-receptor blockers (ARBs), reduce proteinuria, and their combination results in a greater decrease in proteinuria than monotherapy with either an ACE inhibitor or ARB alone. The present study investigates whether the combination of an ACE inhibitor with ARB is more effective in slowing the progression of proteinuric diabetic nephropathy than therapy with an ACE inhibitor alone and whether this combination therapy is safe. This trial was stopped because of safety concerns, with acute kidney injury being the main serious adverse event. Hence the promise of the combination of 2 blockers of the renin-angiotensin system to effectively prevent end-stage renal disease in patients with proteinuric diabetic nephropathy was not fulfilled.

E. Oetjen, MD

Diabetic hyperglycaemia activates CaMKII and arrhythmias by *O*-linked glycosylation

Erickson JR, Pereira L, Wang L, et al (Univ of California, Davis, Davis; et al)

Nature 502:372-376, 2013

Ca^{2+}/calmodulin-dependent protein kinase II (CaMKII) is an enzyme with important regulatory functions in the heart and brain, and its chronic activation can be pathological. CaMKII activation is seen in heart failure, and can directly induce pathological changes in ion channels, Ca^{2+} handling and gene transcription. Here, in human, rat and mouse, we identify a novel mechanism linking CaMKII and hyperglycaemic signalling in diabetes mellitus, which is a key risk factor for heart and neurodegenerative diseases. Acute hyperglycaemia causes covalent modification of CaMKII by O-linked *N*-acetylglucosamine (O-GlcNAc). O-GlcNAc modification of CaMKII at Ser 279 activates CaMKII autonomously, creating molecular memory even after Ca^{2+} concentration declines. O-GlcNAc-modified CaMKII is increased in the heart and brain of diabetic humans and rats. In cardiomyocytes, increased glucose concentration significantly enhances CaMKII-dependent activation of spontaneous sarcoplasmic reticulum Ca^{2+} release events that can contribute to cardiac mechanical dysfunction and arrhythmias. These effects were prevented by pharmacological inhibition of O-GlcNAc signalling or genetic ablation of CaMKIIδ. In intact perfused hearts, arrhythmias were aggravated by increased glucose concentration through O-GlcNAc- and CaMKII-dependent pathways. In diabetic animals, acute blockade of O-GlcNAc inhibited arrhythmogenesis. Thus, O-GlcNAc modification of CaMKII is a novel signalling event in pathways that may contribute critically to cardiac and neuronal pathophysiology in diabetes and other diseases.

▶ Diabetes is a major risk factor for the development of cardiovascular diseases, and more than 60% of type 2 diabetic patients die from myocardial infarction or stroke. Although the deleterious effects of diabetes on the micro- and macrovascular system are undoubted, it is still elusive how diabetes directly affects the heart. The study by Erickson et al provides an interesting explanation of how hyperglycemia might affect cardiomyocyte function. The authors show that *O*-linked glycosylation of CaMKII renders this kinase constitutively active. This posttranslational modification is triggered by high glucose in cell culture and by hyperglycemia in humans and in rats. Activation of CaMKII in the heart can be pathological. Unfortunately, the authors do not state clearly whether they use a well-established rat diabetes model like Zucker diabetic fatty rats or a transgenic that overexpressed human amylin in β-cells. Although CaMKII is presumably not the only dysregulated enzyme in diabetic cardiomyopathy, this study provides an interesting link between diabetes and cardiac dysfunction.

E. Oetjen, MD

Changing Impact of Modifiable Risk Factors on the Incidence of Major Outcomes of Type 1 Diabetes: The Pittsburgh Epidemiology of Diabetes Complications Study

Miller RG, Secrest AM, Ellis D, et al (Univ of Pittsburgh, PA)
Diabetes Care 36:3999-4006, 2013

Objective.—The incidence of type 1 diabetes complications appears to be decreasing, but relative contributions of risk factors are unclear. We thus estimated the effect of modifiable risk factors on the incidence of a composite end point, major outcomes of diabetes (MOD).

Research Design and Methods.—The Pittsburgh Epidemiology of Diabetes Complications (EDC) Study was used to derive two cohorts based on diabetes diagnosis year (1960–1969 and 1970–1980). Baseline exam data in the current analysis for the 1960s group were collected in 1986–1988 and for the 1970s in 1996–1998. Each group was followed for 8 years for MOD incidence (diabetes-related death, myocardial infarction, revascularization procedure/blockage ≥50%, stroke, end-stage renal disease, blindness, and amputation). Assessed risk factors include the following: HbA_{1c}, hypertension, microalbuminuria, BMI, hypercholesterolemia, and smoking. Accelerated failure time models were used to estimate the acceleration factor.

Results.—MOD incidence decreased in the 1970s cohort (15.8% [95% CI 11.6–21.4]) compared with the 1960s (22.6% [17.0–29.1]) over the 8-year follow-up ($P = 0.06$). Hypertension and microalbuminuria were associated with significantly accelerated MOD incidence in both cohorts ($P < 0.01$ for both). High HbA_{1c} ($P = 0.0005$), hypercholesterolemia ($P = 0.01$), and current smoking ($P = 0.003$) significantly accelerated the incidence of MOD in the 1960s but not 1970s cohort. BMI was not associated with MOD in either cohort.

Conclusions.—These results suggest that hypertension and microalbuminuria remain important predictors of complications that are not being adequately addressed.

▶ It is tempting to speculate that the incidence of type 1 diabetes complications is decreasing because of better medical treatment and thereby a reduction of risk factors that might predict these diabetic complications. But no data are available. The retrospective study of Miller et al tries to remedy this. From The Pittsburg Epidemiology of Diabetes Complications Study, 2 cohorts were derived, one in which diabetes was diagnosed in the years from 1960 to 1969, the other one from 1970 to 1980. The incidence of major outcomes in diabetes decreased, but the risk factors, hypertension and microalbuminuria, still remain important predictors of major outcomes in diabetes. This suggests that these 2 risk factors are not adequately addressed and urges to put more attention to the treatment of these 2 symptoms.

E. Oetjen, MD

Glycemic Control

Biguanides suppress hepatic glucagon signalling by decreasing production of cyclic AMP

Miller RA, Chu Q, Xie J, et al (Univ of Pennsylvania, Philadelphia; Cell Signaling Technology, Inc, Danvers, MA; et al)

Nature 494:256-260, 2013

Glucose production by the liver is essential for providing a substrate for the brain during fasting. The inability of insulin to suppress hepatic glucose output is a major aetiological factor in the hyperglycaemia of type-2 diabetes mellitus and other diseases of insulin resistance. For fifty years, one of the few classes of therapeutics effective in reducing glucose production has been the biguanides, which include phenformin and metformin, the latter the most frequently prescribed drug for type-2 diabetes. Nonetheless, the mechanism of action of biguanides remains imperfectly understood. The suggestion a decade ago that metformin reduces glucose synthesis through activation of the enzyme AMP-activated protein kinase (AMPK) has recently been challenged by genetic loss-of-function experiments. Here we provide a novel mechanism by which metformin antagonizes the action of glucagon, thus reducing fasting glucose levels. In mouse hepatocytes, metformin leads to the accumulation of AMP and related nucleotides, which inhibit adenylate cyclase, reduce levels of cyclic AMP and protein kinase A (PKA) activity, abrogate phosphorylation of critical protein targets of PKA, and block glucagon-dependent glucose output from hepatocytes. These data support a mechanism of action for metformin involving antagonism of glucagon, and suggest an approach for the development of antidiabetic drugs.

▶ Biguanides and especially metformin have been used for more than 50 years in the treatment of diabetes mellitus type 2, and metformin is now the first-line treatment. However, metformin's mechanisms of action are still not completely understood. It was generally assumed that metformin, through inhibition of mitochondrial complex 1 leading to increased intracellular concentrations of adenosine monophosphate (AMP), activates AMP kinase, which accounts for the reduction of hepatic glucose output. This hypothesis was recently challenged by Foretz et al,[1] who demonstrated that metformin inhibits hepatic gluconeogenesis independent of AMP kinase. This hypothesis is supported by Miller et al, who show that metformin blocks adenylate cyclase. Considering the glucagon receptor is a Gs-protein-coupled receptor, the inhibition of adenylate cyclase prevents hepatic glucagon action. Thus, the glucose-lowering effect of metformin depends not only on the activation of AMP kinase but also on suppression of glucagon action.

E. Oetjen, MD

Reference

1. Foretz M, Hébrard S, leclerc J, et al. Metformin inhibits gluconeogenesis in mice independently of the LKB1/AMPK pathway via a decrease in hepatic energy state. *J Clin Invest*. 2010;120:2355-2369.

Liver-Derived Systemic Factors Drive β Cell Hyperplasia in Insulin-Resistant States

El Ouaamari A, Kawamori D, Dirice E, et al (Joslin Diabetes Ctr and Harvard Med School, Boston, MA; et al)
Cell Rep 3:401-410, 2013

Integrative organ crosstalk regulates key aspects of energy homeostasis, and its dysregulation may underlie metabolic disorders such as obesity and diabetes. To test the hypothesis that crosstalk between the liver and pancreatic islets modulates β cell growth in response to insulin resistance, we used the liver-specific insulin receptor knockout (LIRKO) mouse, a unique model that exhibits dramatic islet hyperplasia. Using complementary in vivo parabiosis and transplantation assays, as well as in vitro islet culture approaches, we demonstrate that humoral, nonneural, non-cell-autonomous factor(s) induces β cell proliferation in LIRKO mice. Furthermore, we report that a hepatocyte-derived factor(s) stimulates mouse and human β cell proliferation in ex vivo assays, independent of ambient glucose and insulin levels. These data implicate the liver as a critical source of β cell growth factor(s) in insulin-resistant states.

▶ Guided by their observations that mice in which the insulin receptor is deleted in the liver exhibit dramatic islet hyperplasia to compensate for the insulin resistance, the authors further elucidated the underlying mechanism. In demanding animal experimentation, they show specifically that β-cell proliferation is induced by factor(s) that are presumably secreted from the insulin-resistant hepatocytes. Insulin-resistant hepatocyte conditioned medium induced proliferation of islet β-cells from type 2 diabetic donors. The factor(s) themselves were not identified. This study provides an explanation for the observed β-cell hyperplasia in the insulin-resistant state and gives another example of the crosstalk between organs. Given that the decline in functional β-cell mass seems to be the critical step in the pathogenesis of diabetes, these factor(s) might become a novel class of antidiabetic drugs. However, is it really sufficient only to increase β-cell mass in the face of obesity-induced diabetes with the additional metabolic deteriorations?

E. Oetjen, MD

11β-HSD1 Inhibitors for the Treatment of Type 2 Diabetes and Cardiovascular Disease

Anderson A, Walker BR (Univ of Edinburgh, Scotland, UK)
Drugs 73:1385-1393, 2013

Inhibition of the enzyme 11β-hydroxysteroid dehydrogenase type 1 (11β-HSD1) has been proposed as a novel therapeutic target for the treatment of type 2 diabetes mellitus. Over 170 new compounds targeting 11β-HSD1 have been developed. This article reviews the current published literature on compounds that have reached phase II clinical trials in patients with type 2 diabetes, and summarises the preclinical evidence that such agents may be useful for associated conditions, including peripheral vascular disease, coronary artery disease and cognitive decline. In clinical trials, 11β-HSD1 inhibitors have been well tolerated and have improved glycaemic control, lipid profile and blood pressure, and induced modest weight loss. The magnitude of the effects are small relative to other agents, so that further development of 11β-HSD1 inhibitors for the primary therapeutic indication of type 2 diabetes has stalled. Ongoing programmes are focused on additional benefits for cognitive function and other cardiovascular risk factors.

▶ Increased plasma cortisol levels as in Cushing's syndrome lead to central obesity, glucose dysregulation, dyslipidemia, and hypertension, symptoms that resemble those of the metabolic syndrome. This observation lead to the idea that increased cortisol action might contribute to the development of the metabolic syndrome. Cortisol production is regulated by the central hypothalamic-pituitary-adrenal axis and locally by 2 11β-hydroxysteroid dehydrogenases (11β-HSD), whereby 11β-HSD type 2 converts cortisol into the inactive cortisone, and 11β-HSD type 1 promotes the reduction of cortisone to cortisol and the reverse reaction, depending on substrate and cofactor availability. Mice deficient in 11β-HSD type 1 or treated with specific 11β-HSD type 1 inhibitors show improved glucose tolerance, reduced insulin resistance, and decreases in body weight.[1-3] Hence, drugs inhibiting 11β-HSD type 1 might be beneficial in the treatment of diabetes mellitus. So far, a superior glucose-lowering effect of the 11β-HSD type 1 inhibitors is lacking (and drugs inhibiting both 11β-HSD type 1 and type 2 even result in hypertension), but this novel class might have additional beneficial effects. In this review, several 11β-HSD type 1 inhibitors and their effects are reported, giving a thorough overview of this fascinating field.

E. Oetjen, MD

References

1. Morgan SA, Sherlock M, Gathercole LL, et al. 11beta-Hydroxysteroid dehydrogenase type 1 regulates glucocorticoid-induced insulin resistance in skeletal muscle. *Diabetes*. 2009;58:2506-2515.
2. Tahrani AA, Bailey CJ, Del Prato S, Barnett AH. Management of type 2 diabetes: new and future developments in treatment. *Lancet*. 2011;378:182-197.
3. Anagnostis P, Katsiski N, Adamidou F, et al. 11beta-Hydroxysteroid dehydrogenase type 1 inhibitors: novel agents for the treatment of metabolic syndrome and obesity-related disorders? *Metabolism*. 2013;62:21-33.

Antidiabetic effects of glucokinase regulatory protein small-molecule disruptors

Lloyd DJ, St Jean DJ Jr, Kurzeja RJM, et al (Dept of Metabolic Disorders, Thousand Oaks, CA; Dept of Therapeutic Discovery, Thousand Oaks, CA; et al)
Nature 504:437-440, 2013

Glucose homeostasis is a vital and complex process, and its disruption can cause hyperglycaemia and type II diabetes mellitus. Glucokinase (GK), a key enzyme that regulates glucose homeostasis, converts glucose to glucose-6-phosphate in pancreatic β-cells, liver hepatocytes, specific hypothalamic neurons, and gut enterocytes. In hepatocytes, GK regulates glucose uptake and glycogen synthesis, suppresses glucose production, and is subject to the endogenous inhibitor GK regulatory protein (GKRP). During fasting, GKRP binds, inactivates and sequesters GK in the nucleus, which removes GK from the gluconeogenic process and prevents a futile cycle of glucose phosphorylation. Compounds that directly hyperactivate GK (GK activators) lower blood glucose levels and are being evaluated clinically as potential therapeutics for the treatment of type II diabetes mellitus. However, initial reports indicate that an increased risk of hypoglycaemia is associated with some GK activators. To mitigate the risk of hypoglycaemia, we sought to increase GK activity by blocking GKRP. Here we describe the identification of two potent small-molecule GK–GKRP disruptors (AMG-1694 and AMG-3969) that normalized blood glucose levels in several rodent models of diabetes. These compounds potently reversed the inhibitory effect of GKRP on GK activity and promoted GK translocation both *in vitro* (isolated hepatocytes) and *in vivo* (liver). A co-crystal structure of full-length human GKRP in complex with AMG-1694 revealed a previously unknown binding pocket in GKRP distinct from that of the phosphofructose-binding site. Furthermore, with AMG-1694 and AMG-3969 (but not GK activators), blood glucose lowering was restricted to diabetic and not normoglycaemic animals. These findings exploit a new cellular mechanism for lowering blood glucose levels with reduced potential for hypoglycaemic risk in patients with type II diabetes mellitus.

▶ Glucokinase is an important enzyme in the maintenance of glucose homeostasis. In pancreatic β-cells, it acts as a glucose sensor and by phosphorylation of glucose triggers glucose oxidation, insulin biosynthesis, and finally insulin secretion. In the hepatocytes, this enzyme enhances glucose uptake, glycolysis, glycogen synthesis, and lipogenesis. Hence, activators of glucokinase effectively lower blood glucose levels. However, in a phase II trial, hypoglycemic events occurred, limiting the use of this glucokinase activator.[1] In this study, small molecules that specifically activate hepatic glucokinase are described. Lloyd et al take advantage of the hepatic regulation of glucokinase in which, in the fasting state, the endogenous glucokinase regulatory protein (GKRP) interacts with glucokinase and retains it in the nucleus. Upon the rise of glucose levels, the interaction between GKRP and the enzyme is disrupted; glucokinase translocates to the cytoplasm and phosphorylates glucose. Thus, disruptors of the glucokinase-GKRP complex specifically activate hepatic glucokinase and lower blood glucose levels without increasing insulin secretion, thereby attenuating the risk of hypoglycemia. The long-term effects of these novel small molecule glucokinase-GKRP disruptors on hepatic steatosis and the potential loss of efficacy as observed with other glucokinase activators remain to be seen.[1,2]

E. Oetjen, MD

References

1. Meininger GE, Scott R, Alba M, et al. Effects of MK-0941, a novel glucokinase activator, on glycemic control in insulin-treated patients with type 2 diabetes. *Diabetes Care*. 2011;34:2560-2566.
2. De Ceuninck F, Kargar C, Charton Y, et al. 50131 and S 51434, two novel small molecule glucokinase activators, lack chronic efficacy despite potent acute antihyperglycaemic activity in diabetic mice. *Br J Pharmacol*. 2013; 168:999-1010.

Evaluation of the dual peroxisome proliferator–activated receptor α/γ agonist aleglitazar to reduce cardiovascular events in patients with acute coronary syndrome and type 2 diabetes mellitus: Rationale and design of the AleCardio trial

Lincoff AM, Tardif J-C, Neal B, et al (Cleveland Clinic Coordinating Ctr for Clinical Res (C5Res), OH; Université de Montréal, Quebec, Canada; Univ of Sydney, Australia; et al)

Am Heart J 166:429-434.e1, 2013

Background.—Peroxisome proliferator–activated receptors (PPARs) regulate transcription of genes involved in glucose uptake, lipid metabolism, and inflammation. Aleglitazar is a potent dual PPAR agonist with insulin-sensitizing and glucoselowering actions and favorable effects on lipid profiles and biomarkers of cardiovascular risk. The AleCardio trial examines whether the addition of aleglitazar to standard medical therapy reduces the risk of cardiovascular morbidity and mortality in patients with type 2 diabetes mellitus and recent acute coronary syndrome.

Study Design.—AleCardio is a phase 3, multicenter, randomized, double-blind, placebo-controlled trial. A total of 7,228 patients were randomized to aleglitazar 150 μg or placebo daily in addition to standard medical therapy. The primary efficacy end point is time to the first event of cardiovascular death, myocardial infarction, or stroke. Principal safety end points are hospitalization due to heart failure and changes in renal function. Treatment will continue until 7,000 patients are followed up for at least 2.5 years and 950 primary end point events are adjudicated.

Conclusions.—AleCardio will establish whether the PPAR-α/γ agonist aleglitazar improves cardiovascular outcomes in patients with diabetes and high-risk coronary disease.

▶ Agonists of the peroxisome proliferator–activated receptor (PPAR)-α, like the fibrates, effectively lower plasma lipid levels; agonists of PPAR-γ, like the glitazones, increase insulin sensitivity, lower blood glucose levels, and exert anti-inflammatory actions. A combination of these drugs (ie, dual agonists of PPAR-α and PPAR-γ) promises both beneficial effects for the cardiovascular system and antidiabetic action. Hence, these dual agonists, called glitazars, might be ideal to treat diabetes and prevent cardiovascular events in patients with diabetes. With this in mind, the phase 3 trial AleCardio was started to investigate whether aleglitazar improves cardiovascular outcome. In addition to the combined desired effects such dual agonists might exert, combined adverse effects include osteoporosis, renal fluid retention, and rhabdomyolysis. Indeed, in July 2013, a press release by Roche stated that the AleCardio trial and all other trials involving aleglitazar were stopped because of safety concerns.

E. Oetjen, MD

An inhibitor of the protein kinases TBK1 and IKK-ϵ improves obesity-related metabolic dysfunctions in mice

Reilly SM, Chiang S-H, Decker SJ, et al (Univ of Michigan, Ann Arbor; et al)
Nat Med 19:313-321, 2013

Emerging evidence suggests that inflammation provides a link between obesity and insulin resistance. The noncanonical IκB kinases IKK-ϵ and TANK-binding kinase 1 (TBK1) are induced in liver and fat by NF-κB activation upon high-fat diet feeding and in turn initiate a program of counter-inflammation that preserves energy storage. Here we report that amlexanox, an approved small-molecule therapeutic presently used in the clinic to treat aphthous ulcers and asthma, is an inhibitor of these kinases. Treatment of obese mice with amlexanox elevates energy expenditure through increased thermogenesis, producing weight loss, improved insulin sensitivity and decreased steatosis. Because of its record of safety in patients, amlexanox may be an interesting candidate for clinical evaluation in the treatment of obesity and related disorders.

► The realization that low-grade inflammation provides the link between obesity and insulin resistance stimulated research to elucidate the underlying molecular mechanism. Two protein kinases were detected that might initiate a counterinflammatory program to preserve energy storage despite insulin resistance. The present study shows that these kinases are inhibited by amlexanox, used to treat aphthous ulcers and asthma, without knowing its precise mechanism of action. Amlexanox reduced the weight and insulin resistance in 3 murine obesity models, presumably by increasing energy expenditure. Translated to everyday life, this would mean that people take amlexanox and stick to their calorie-rich diets, without becoming obese and insulin resistant. However, the increased drug-induced energy expenditure might be dangerous. Depending on the dose, it might deteriorate mitochondrial function and ultimately result in cell death.

E. Oetjen, MD

Salicylate (Salsalate) in Patients With Type 2 Diabetes: A Randomized Trial

Goldfine AB, for the Targeting Inflammation Using Salsalate in Type 2 Diabetes Study Team (Joslin Diabetes Ctr and Harvard Med School, Boston, MA; et al)

Ann Intern Med 159:1-12, 2013

Background.—Short-duration studies show that salsalate improves glycemia in type 2 diabetes mellitus (T2DM).

Objective.—To assess 1-year efficacy and safety of salsalate in T2DM.

Design.—Placebo-controlled, parallel trial; computerized randomization and centralized allocation, with patients, providers, and researchers blinded to assignment. (ClinicalTrials.gov: NCT00799643)

Setting.—3 private practices and 18 academic centers in the United States.

Patients.—Persons aged 18 to 75 years with fasting glucose levels of 12.5 mmol/L or less (≤225 mg/dL) and hemoglobin A_{1c} (HbA_{1c}) levels of 7.0% to 9.5% who were treated for diabetes.

Intervention.—286 participants were randomly assigned (between January 2009 and July 2011) to 48 weeks of placebo ($n = 140$) or salsalate, 3.5 g/d ($n = 146$), in addition to current therapies, and 283 participants were analyzed (placebo, $n = 137$; salsalate, $n = 146$).

Measurements.—Change in hemoglobin A_{1c} level (primary outcome) and safety and efficacy measures.

Results.—The mean HbA_{1c} level over 48 weeks was 0.37% lower in the salsalate group than in the placebo group (95% CI, −0.53% to −0.21%; $P < 0.001$). Glycemia improved despite more reductions in concomitant diabetes medications in salsalate recipients than in placebo recipients.

Lower circulating leukocyte, neutrophil, and lymphocyte counts show the anti-inflammatory effects of salsalate. Adiponectin and hematocrit levels increased more and fasting glucose, uric acid, and triglyceride levels decreased with salsalate, but weight and low-density lipoprotein cholesterol levels also increased. Urinary albumin levels increased but reversed on discontinuation; estimated glomerular filtration rates were unchanged.

Limitation.—Trial duration and number of patients studied were insufficient to determine long-term risk–benefit of salsalate in T2DM.

Conclusion.—Salsalate improves glycemia in patients with T2DM and decreases inflammatory mediators. Continued evaluation of mixed cardiorenal signals is warranted.

▶ Already in 1876, Ebstein proposed that salicylic acid, natron, should be used to treat diabetes.[1] With the realization of insulin resistance and diabetes as a chronic inflammatory disease, salicylate as an anti-inflammatory drug was re-evaluated in the treatment of diabetes. Patients with type 2 diabetes treated with 7 g/d of salicylic acid exhibited reduced fasting glucose levels and hepatic glucose output and improved insulin-stimulated peripheral glucose uptake.[2] Because of the adverse effects of acetyl salicylic acid (ie, anti-thrombotic action and irritation of the gastrointestinal tract) the dimer of salicylic acid, salsalate, was used. A randomized 1-year trial in patients with type 2 diabetes with inadequate glucose control showed improved HbA_{1c} levels and decreased inflammatory parameters. An additional 12-week trial in patients at risk for diabetes showed lowered fasting glucose levels.[3] Thus, salsalate might indeed be an old but novel drug for the treatment of diabetes.

E. Oetjen, MD

References

1. Ebstein W. Zur Therapie des Diabetes mellitus, insbesondere über Anwendung des salicylsauren Natrons bei demselben. *Berl Klin Wochenschr.* 1876;13:337-340.
2. Hundal RS, Petersen KF, Mayerson AB, et al. Mechanism by which high-dose aspirin improves metabolism in type 2 diabetes. *J Clin Invest.* 2002;109:1321-1326.
3. Goldfine AB, Conlin PR, Halperin F, et al. A randomised trial of salsalate for insulin resistance and cardiovascular risk factors in persons with abnormal glucose tolerance. *Diabetologia.* 2013;56:714-723.

Saxagliptin and Cardiovascular Outcomes in Patients with Type 2 Diabetes Mellitus

Scirica BM, for the SAVOR-TIMI 53 Steering Committee and Investigators (Brigham and Women's Hosp, Boston, MA; et al)

N Engl J Med 369:1317-1326, 2013

Background.—The cardiovascular safety and efficacy of many current antihyperglycemic agents, including saxagliptin, a dipeptidyl peptidase 4 (DPP-4) inhibitor, are unclear.

Methods.—We randomly assigned 16,492 patients with type 2 diabetes who had a history of, or were at risk for, cardiovascular events to receive saxagliptin or placebo and followed them for a median of 2.1 years. Physicians were permitted to adjust other medications, including antihyperglycemic agents. The primary end point was a composite of cardiovascular death, myocardial infarction, or ischemic stroke.

Results.—A primary end-point event occurred in 613 patients in the saxagliptin group and in 609 patients in the placebo group (7.3% and 7.2%, respectively, according to 2-year Kaplan—Meier estimates; hazard ratio with saxagliptin, 1.00; 95% confidence interval [CI], 0.89 to 1.12; $P = 0.99$ for superiority; $P < 0.001$ for noninferiority); the results were similar in the "on-treatment" analysis (hazard ratio, 1.03; 95% CI, 0.91 to 1.17). The major secondary end point of a composite of cardiovascular death, myocardial infarction, stroke, hospitalization for unstable angina, coronary revascularization, or heart failure occurred in 1059 patients in the saxagliptin group and in 1034 patients in the placebo group (12.8% and 12.4%, respectively, according to 2-year Kaplan—Meier estimates; hazard ratio, 1.02; 95% CI, 0.94 to 1.11; $P = 0.66$). More patients in the saxagliptin group than in the placebo group were hospitalized for heart failure (3.5% vs. 2.8%; hazard ratio, 1.27; 95% CI, 1.07 to 1.51; $P = 0.007$). Rates of adjudicated cases of acute and chronic pancreatitis were similar in the two groups (acute pancreatitis, 0.3% in the saxagliptin group and 0.2% in the placebo group; chronic pancreatitis, <0.1% and 0.1% in the two groups, respectively).

Conclusions.—DPP-4 inhibition with saxagliptin did not increase or decrease the rate of ischemic events, though the rate of hospitalization for heart failure was increased. Although saxagliptin improves glycemic control, other approaches are necessary to reduce cardiovascular risk in patients with diabetes. (Funded by AstraZeneca and Bristol-Myers Squibb; SAVOR-TIMI 53 ClinicalTrials.gov number, NCT01107886.)

▶ Since 2008, the Food and Drug Administration and the European Medicines Agency require a demonstration of cardiovascular safety for all new glucose-lowering therapies for their approval processes. In phase 2 and 3 studies, the dipeptidyl peptidase IV inhibitor saxagliptin improved glycemic control and reduced the risk of major cardiovascular events (Frederich R, Alexander JH, Fiedorek, 2010), but long-term data on the safety and efficacy of this drug in diabetic patients at risk for cardiovascular were still missing. In the present study, saxagliptin did not protect against cardiovascular events but increased the risk of hospitalization for heart failure and the risk of hypoglycemic events. These findings are disappointing, but in comparison to the UK Prospective Diabetes Study, the follow-up with a median of 2.1 years was rather short. Of note, cases of chronic or acute pancreatitis were similar in the saxagliptin and placebo groups.

E. Oetjen, MD

Alogliptin after Acute Coronary Syndrome in Patients with Type 2 Diabetes

White WB, for the EXAMINE Investigators (Univ of Connecticut School of Medicine, Farmington; et al)

N Engl J Med 369:1327-1335, 2013

Background.—To assess potentially elevated cardiovascular risk related to new antihyperglycemic drugs in patients with type 2 diabetes, regulatory agencies require a comprehensive evaluation of the cardiovascular safety profile of new antidiabetic therapies. We assessed cardiovascular outcomes with alogliptin, a new inhibitor of dipeptidyl peptidase 4 (DPP-4), as compared with placebo in patients with type 2 diabetes who had had a recent acute coronary syndrome.

Methods.—We randomly assigned patients with type 2 diabetes and either an acute myocardial infarction or unstable angina requiring hospitalization within the previous 15 to 90 days to receive alogliptin or placebo in addition to existing antihyperglycemic and cardiovascular drug therapy. The study design was a double-blind, noninferiority trial with a prespecified noninferiority margin of 1.3 for the hazard ratio for the primary end point of a composite of death from cardiovascular causes, nonfatal myocardial infarction, or nonfatal stroke.

Results.—A total of 5380 patients underwent randomization and were followed for up to 40 months (median, 18 months). A primary endpoint event occurred in 305 patients assigned to alogliptin (11.3%) and in 316 patients assigned to placebo (11.8%) (hazard ratio, 0.96; upper boundary of the one-sided repeated confidence interval, 1.16; $P < 0.001$ for noninferiority). Glycated hemoglobin levels were significantly lower with alogliptin than with placebo (mean difference, −0.36 percentage points; $P < 0.001$). Incidences of hypoglycemia, cancer, pancreatitis, and initiation of dialysis were similar with alogliptin and placebo.

Conclusions.—Among patients with type 2 diabetes who had had a recent acute coronary syndrome, the rates of major adverse cardiovascular events were not increased with the DPP-4 inhibitor alogliptin as compared with placebo. (Funded by Takeda Development Center Americas; EXAMINE ClinicalTrials.gov number, NCT00968708.)

▶ In addition to concerns about incretin-based therapy's compliance with the requirements of regulatory agencies, its protective effects on the cardiovascular system are a matter of debate. The protective effects have been described in diverse animal models and in some pilot studies in humans. The aim of this study was to investigate whether alogliptin was superior to placebo in type 2 diabetic patients after acute coronary syndrome. The median follow-up of 18 months was rather short. Alogliptin was neither inferior nor superior to placebo. Hence, more studies with longer follow-up times are needed to determine whether incretin-based therapy has a protective effect on the cardiovascular system. Of note, in this study the incidence of hypoglycemia and pancreatitis was not enhanced by alogliptin treatment.

E. Oetjen, MD

Linagliptin for patients aged 70 years or older with type 2 diabetes inadequately controlled with common antidiabetes treatments: a randomised, double-blind, placebo-controlled trial

Barnett AH, Huisman H, Jones R, et al (Heart of England NHS Foundation Trust, Birmingham, UK; Boehringer Ingelheim, Alkmaar, Netherlands; Boehringer Ingelheim, Bracknell, UK; et al)

Lancet 382:1413-1423, 2013

Background.—A substantial proportion of patients with type 2 diabetes are elderly (≥65 years) but this group has been largely excluded from clinical studies of glucose-lowering drugs. We aimed to assess the effectiveness of linagliptin, a dipeptidyl peptidase-4 inhibitor, in elderly patients with type 2 diabetes.

Methods.—In this randomised, double-blind, parallel-group, multinational phase 3 study, patients aged 70 years or older with type 2 diabetes, glycated haemoglobin A_{1c} (HbA_{1c}) of 7·0% or more, receiving metformin, sulfonylureas, or basal insulin, or combinations of these drugs, were randomised (by computer-generated randomisation sequence, concealed with a voice—response system, stratified by HbA_{1c} level [<8·5% *vs* ≥8·5%] and insulin use [yes *vs* no], block size four) in a 2:1 ratio to once-daily oral treatment with linagliptin 5 mg or matching placebo for 24 weeks. Investigators and participants were masked to assignment throughout the study. The primary endpoint was change in HbA_{1c} from baseline to week 24. This trial is registered with ClinicalTrials.gov, number NCT01084005.

Findings.—241 community-living outpatients were randomised (162 linagliptin, 79 placebo). Mean age was 74·9 years (SD 4·3). Mean HbA_{1c} was 7·8% (SD 0·8). At week 24, placebo-adjusted mean change in HbA_{1c} with linagliptin was −0·64% (95% CI −0·81 to −0·48, $p < 0·0001$). Overall safety and tolerability were much the same between the linagliptin and placebo groups; 75·9% of patients in both groups had an adverse event (linagliptin n = 123, placebo n = 60). No deaths occurred. Serious adverse events occurred in 8·6% (14) of patients in the linagliptin group and 6·3% (five) patients in the placebo group; none were deemed related to study drug. Hypoglycaemia was the most common adverse event in both groups, but did not differ between groups (24·1% [39] in the linagliptin group, 16·5% [13] in the placebo group; odds ratio 1·58, 95% CI 0·78–3·78, $p = 0·2083$).

Interpretation.—In elderly patients with type 2 diabetes linagliptin was efficacious in lowering glucose with a safety profile similar to placebo. These findings could inform treatment decisions for achieving individualised glycaemic goals with minimal risk in this important population of patients.

▶ Because of improved medical care, individuals with type 2 diabetes become older than ever. With increasing age, β-cell function further declines, which might result in inadequately controlled diabetes despite antidiabetic therapy. Elderly people have declined renal function, thereby prolonging the elimination of drugs or even aggravating adverse drug effects. However, in most clinical studies, people aged older than 65 years are excluded. The present study was specifically designed to investigate whether the dipeptidyl peptidase (DPP) IV inhibitor linagliptin was efficient in lowering blood glucose levels as an add on to existing antidiabetic therapy without causing undesired effects. To date, linagliptin is the only DPP IV inhibitor that is eliminated by the kidney only to a very small extent, making it suitable for use in elderly and in patients with impaired renal function without dose adjustment. The results of this study suggest that linagliptin, because of its favorable pharmacokinetic, could be used in elderly patients as well without increasing the risk of adverse drug effects.

E. Oetjen, MD

Marked Expansion of Exocrine and Endocrine Pancreas with Incretin Therapy in Humans with Increased Exocrine Pancreas Dysplasia and the Potential for Glucagon-Producing Neuroendocrine Tumors

Butler AE, Campbell-Thompson M, Gurlo T, et al (Univ of California Los Angeles; Univ of Florida, Gainesville)
Diabetes 62:2595-2604, 2013

Controversy exists regarding the potential regenerative influences of incretin therapy on pancreatic β cells versus possible adverse pancreatic proliferative effects. Examination of pancreata from age matched organ donors with type 2 diabetes (DM) treated by incretin therapy (n = 8) or other therapy (n = 12) and non diabetic controls (n = 14) reveals a ~40% increased pancreatic mass in DM treated with incretin therapy with both increased exocrine cell proliferation ($P < 0.0001$) and dysplasia (increased pancreatic intraepithelia neoplasia, $P < 0.01$). Pancreas in DM treated with incretin therapy was notable for α cell hyperplasia and glucagon expressing microadenomas (3/8) and a neuroendocrine tumor. β cell mass was reduced by approximately 60% in those with DM, yet a 6 fold increase was observed in incretin treated subjects although diabetes persists. Endocrine cells co-staining for insulin and glucagon were increased in DM compared to non diabetic controls ($P < 0.05$) and markedly further increased by incretin therapy ($P < 0.05$). In conclusion, in humans, incretin therapy resulted in a marked expansion of the exocrine and endocrine pancreatic compartments, the former being accompanied by increased proliferation and dysplasia, the latter by α cell hyperplasia with the potential for evolution into neuroendocrine tumors.

► Glucagon-like peptide-1 (GLP-1) receptor agonists and inhibitors of the dipeptidylpeptidase IV (gliptines), enhancing the endogenous levels of GLP-1, are important drugs in antidiabetic therapy. They effectively lower blood glucose levels and prevent postprandial glucose peaks without causing hypoglycemia and weight gain. At least in rodents, GLP-1 agonists preserve beta-cell function and mass, thus making them nearly ideal drugs for the treatment of diabetes. This view was challenged by a report of Butler et al, however. This postmortem analysis shows increased beta-cell mass in diabetics treated with incretin therapy. In addition, an increase in glucagon-secreting alpha-cells was observed. Unfortunately, plasma glucagon levels were not available. In addition, proliferation and dysplasia of exocrine pancreatic cells were observed. It should be noted that this study was conducted in a small number of pancreata from organ donors. These findings are corroborated by 2 studies in rodents.[1,2]

E. Oetjen, MD

References

1. Nachnani JS, Bulchandani DG, Nookala A, et al. Biochemical and histological effects of exendin-4 (exenatide) on the rat pancreas. *Diabetologia*. 2010;53: 153-159.
2. Gier B, Matveyenko AV, Kirakossion D, Dawson D, Dry SM, Butler PC. Chronic GLP-1 receptor activation by exendin-4 induces expansion of pancreatic duct glands in rats and accelerates formation of dysplastic lesions and chronic pancreatitis in the Kras(G12D) mouse model. *Diabetes*. 2012;61:1250-1262.

A small-molecule AdipoR agonist for type 2 diabetes and short life in obesity

Okada-Iwabu M, Yamauchi T, Iwabu M, et al (The Univ of Tokyo, Japan; et al)
Nature 503:493-499, 2013

Adiponectin secreted from adipocytes binds to adiponectin receptors AdipoR1 and AdipoR2, and exerts antidiabetic effects via activation of AMPK and PPAR-α pathways, respectively. Levels of adiponectin in plasma are reduced in obesity, which causes insulin resistance and type 2 diabetes. Thus, orally active small molecules that bind to and activate AdipoR1 and AdipoR2 could ameliorate obesity-related diseases such as type 2 diabetes. Here we report the identification of orally active synthetic small-molecule AdipoR agonists. One of these compounds, AdipoR agonist (AdipoRon), bound to both AdipoR1 and AdipoR2 *in vitro*. AdipoRon showed very similar effects to adiponectin in muscle and liver, such as activation of AMPK and PPAR-α pathways, and ameliorated insulin resistance and glucose intolerance in mice fed a high-fat diet, which was completely obliterated in AdipoR1 and AdipoR2 double-knockout mice. Moreover, AdipoRon ameliorated diabetes of genetically obese rodent model *db/db* mice, and prolonged the shortened lifespan of *db/db* mice on a high-fat diet. Thus, orally active AdipoR agonists such as AdipoRon are a promising therapeutic approach for the treatment of obesity-related diseases such as type 2 diabetes.

▶ Since the detection of adipose tissue as an endocrine-active organ, the function of the cytokines secreted from adipose tissue (ie, adipokines) has received much attention. With the finding that, by attenuating insulin resistance and glucose intolerance in mice, adiponectin exerts antidiabetic effects and that plasma adiponectin levels are reduced in obesity, insulin resistance, and type 2 diabetes, promoting adiponectin action has become a novel goal in the treatment of type 2 diabetes. This study by Okada-Iwabu et al addresses this goal. These authors have already described 2 adiponectin receptors that have slightly different functions and signal via activation of AMPK and peroxisome proliferator–activated receptor-α. They now describe 2 dual agonists for both adiponectin receptors. In an elegant experiment using mice deficient in these receptors, the authors confirm that these small molecules indeed act by binding to the adiponectin receptors. Thus, the panel of a potential novel antidiabetic is expanded by these agonists of the adiponectin receptors.

E. Oetjen, MD

Pathogenesis

Betatrophin: A Hormone that Controls Pancreatic β Cell Proliferation
Yi P, Park J-S, Melton DA (Harvard Univ, Cambridge, MA)
Cell 153:747-758, 2013

Replenishing insulin-producing pancreatic β cell mass will benefit both type I and type II diabetics. In adults, pancreatic β cells are generated primarily by self-duplication. We report on a mouse model of insulin resistance that induces dramatic pancreatic β cell proliferation and β cell mass expansion. Using this model, we identify a hormone, betatrophin, that is primarily expressed in liver and fat. Expression of betatrophin correlates with β cell proliferation in other mouse models of insulin resistance and during gestation. Transient expression of betatrophin in mouse liver significantly and specifically promotes pancreatic β cell proliferation, expands β cell mass, and improves glucose tolerance. Thus, betatrophin treatment could augment or replace insulin injections by increasing the number of endogenous insulin-producing cells in diabetics.

▶ The hepatocyte-derived factor enhancing β-cell proliferation in insulin resistance was identified in this report using a different murine model of insulin resistance. Betatrophin was expressed in the liver and white adipose tissue. The peptide hormone betatrophin might constitute a new class of β-cell mass–enhancing drugs. However, many questions remain open. Why does betatrophin act only on β-cells? What does its receptor look like, and how does it signal? In addition, enhancing β-cell mass will undoubtedly result in a more physiologic pattern of insulin secretion. However, the mechanism of insulin secretion (first and second phase) itself is disturbed in type 2 diabetes. Furthermore, more secreted insulin to overcome insulin resistance will result in more glucose uptake and ultimately more weight gain, thereby perhaps impairing the metabolic condition even more with its low-grade inflammation of the metabolic tissues.

E. Oetjen, MD

Inactivation of specific β cell transcription factors in type 2 diabetes

Guo S, Dai C, Guo M, et al (Vanderbilt Univ Med Ctr, Nashville, TN; Vanderbilt Univ, Nashville, TN; et al)

J Clin Invest 2013 Jul 1 [Epub ahead of print]

Type 2 diabetes (T2DM) commonly arises from islet β cell failure and insulin resistance. Here, we examined the sensitivity of key islet-enriched transcription factors to oxidative stress, a condition associated with β cell dysfunction in both type 1 diabetes (T1DM) and T2DM. Hydrogen peroxide treatment of β cell lines induced cytoplasmic translocation of MAFA and NKX6.1. In parallel, the ability of nuclear PDX1 to bind endogenous target gene promoters was also dramatically reduced, whereas the activity of other key β cell transcriptional regulators was unaffected. MAFA levels were reduced, followed by a reduction in NKX6.1 upon development of hyperglycemia in *db/db* mice, a T2DM model. Transgenic expression of the glutathione peroxidase-1 antioxidant enzyme (GPX1) in *db/db* islet β cells restored nuclear MAFA, nuclear NKX6.1, and β cell function in vivo. Notably, the selective decrease in MAFA, NKX6.1, and PDX1 expression was found in human T2DM islets. MAFB, a MAFA-related transcription factor expressed in human β cells, was also severely compromised. We propose that MAFA, MAFB, NKX6.1, and PDX1 activity provides a gauge of islet β cell function, with loss of MAFA (and/or MAFB) representing an early indicator of β cell inactivity and the subsequent deficit of more impactful NKX6.1 (and/or PDX1) resulting in overt dysfunction associated with T2DM.

▶ Oxidative stress is a common feature in type 1 and type 2 diabetes, and the β-cell is particularly poorly equipped to protect itself against this stress. Oxidative stress arises when too much glucose is metabolized by the mitochondria. Hence, even slightly elevated postprandial glucose levels might lead to oxidative β-cell stress. This study shows that oxidative stress inhibits the function of the β-cell transcription factors MAFA, MAFB, NKX6.1, and PDX, all known to maintain β-cell function. The authors propose a model in which the loss of MAFA and MAFB in rodent or in human islet β-cells represents an early indicator of β-cell inactivity followed by the deficit of NKX6.1 and PDX1. This study is corroborated by the findings of Butler et al,[1] showing a decrease of MAFA in the islets from type 2 diabetic donors. These findings emphasize the importance of MAFA, the long-sought-after glucose-responsive transcription factor.

E. Oetjen, MD

Reference

1. Butler AE, Robertson RP, Hernandez R, Matveyenko AV, Gurlo T, Butler PC. Beta cell nuclear musculoaponeurotic fibrosarcoma oncogen family A (MafA) is deficient in type 2 diabetes. *Diabetologia*. 2012;55:2985-2988.

Prevention and Reversal of Diabetes

Achievement of Goals in U.S. Diabetes Care, 1999–2010

Ali MK, Bullard KM, Saaddine JB, et al (Emory Univ, Atlanta, GA; et al)
N Engl J Med 368:1613-1624, 2013

Background.—Tracking national progress in diabetes care may aid in the evaluation of past efforts and identify residual gaps in care.

Methods.—We analyzed data for adults with self-reported diabetes from the National Health and Nutrition Examination Survey and the Behavioral Risk Factor Surveillance System to examine risk-factor control, preventive practices, and risk scores for coronary heart disease over the 1999–2010 period.

Results.—From 1999 through 2010, the weighted proportion of survey participants who met recommended goals for diabetes care increased, by 7.9 percentage points (95% confidence interval [CI], 0.8 to 15.0) for glycemic control (glycated hemoglobin level <7.0%), 9.4 percentage points (95% CI, 3.0 to 15.8) for individualized glycemic targets, 11.7 percentage points (95% CI, 5.7 to 17.7) for blood pressure (target, <130/80 mm Hg), and 20.8 percentage points (95% CI, 11.6 to 30.0) for lipid levels (target level of low-density lipoprotein [LDL] cholesterol, <100 mg per deciliter [2.6 mmol per liter]). Tobacco use did not change significantly, but the 10-year probability of coronary heart disease decreased by 2.8 to 3.7 percentage points. However, 33.4 to 48.7% of persons with diabetes still did not meet the targets for glycemic control, blood pressure, or LDL cholesterol level. Only 14.3% met the targets for all three of these measures and for tobacco use. Adherence to the recommendations for annual eye and dental examinations was unchanged, but annual lipid-level measurement and foot examination increased by 5.5 percentage points (95% CI, 1.6 to 9.4) and 6.8 percentage points (95% CI, 4.8 to 8.8), respectively. Annual vaccination for influenza and receipt of pneumococcal vaccination for participants 65 years of age or older rose by 4.5 percentage points (95% CI, 0.8 to 8.2) and 6.9 percentage points (95% CI, 3.4 to 10.4), respectively, and daily glucose monitoring increased by 12.7 percentage points (95% CI, 10.3 to 15.1).

Conclusions.—Although there were improvements in risk-factor control and adherence to preventive practices from 1999 to 2010, tobacco use remained high, and almost half of U.S. adults with diabetes did not meet the recommended goals for diabetes care.

▶ Obesity and diabetes are among the diseases showing the greatest increase worldwide and are reaching close to epidemic dimensions. Thus, the search for new antidiabetic therapies and efforts to improve antidiabetic therapy are important areas of research. The question remains of whether the goal of improved diabetes care is being achieved. These authors from the United States investigated this concern in a retrospective study, and the results are not encouraging. Despite a slight reduction in the 10-year probability of coronary heart disease, almost half of the adults with self-reported diabetes do not meet the recommended goals for diabetes care. Particularly, tobacco use remains high, and improvement of glycemic control (measured as HbA1c) is low. This study highlights the importance of diabetes care, putting the individual with diabetes into focus, and argues for improved individual diabetes care, control, and education.

E. Oetjen, MD

2 Lipoproteins and Atherosclerosis

Introduction

The past year has not seen the publication of any major new lipid-modifying drug trials. Much of the new information depended on findings from prospective longitudinal cohorts, post hoc analyses of previously published trials, and registry data. It will be some time before the next wave of prospective randomized clinical trials with new agents is completed. One slated to finish later this year is the IMPROVE-IT trial, which compares simvastatin to simvastatin/ezetimibe therapy in patients who have sustained an acute coronary syndrome. The REDUCE-IT and STRENGTH trials will be evaluating the impact of omega-3 fish oils on cardiovascular events against a statin background. The REVEAL and ACCELERATE trials are testing the impact of cholesteryl ester transfer protein inhibitors on risk for cardiovascular events in patients with coronary artery disease (CAD) already on statin therapy. Two fibrate outcomes trials in patients with CAD and with high triglycerides and low HDL-C will also be getting underway later in 2014. Finally, two large outcomes trials are also randomizing patients now and test the efficacy of PCSK9 monoclonal antibodies in patients with CAD and receiving statin therapy. It is hoped these trials demonstrate reduction in residual risk and open doors to novel pharmacologic interventions in patients with dyslipidemia and cardiovascular disease (CVD).

The American College of Cardiology (ACC) and the American Heart Association (AHA) also published their new guidelines on the management of elevated blood cholesterol. Clearly controversial and out of sync with guidelines from Europe, Canada, and Australia, uptake of these new guidelines will likely be slow. The guidelines have eliminated LDL-C and non-HDL-C targets and thresholds and have moved from an LDL-centric model to a risk-centric model. Intensity of statin therapy depends on risk stratification.

The difficulties and contradictions with high-density lipoproteins continue. In the SMART trial, investigators show that with maximal statin therapy and very low LDL-C, low HDL-C does not portend augmented risk for CVD related events. In contrast, in the COURAGE trial, even in patients with LDL-C < 70 mg/dL, low HDL-C was associated with significant elevations in risk for CVD events. Neither the AIM-HIGH or HPS-2

THRIVE trials were able to demonstrate any efficacy for niacin adjuvant therapy against a statin background in patients with CAD. Moreover, in comprehensive post hoc subgroup analyses, no benefit from niacin could be discerned. Other studies continue to reveal that in patients with established CAD or who have elevated systemic inflammatory tone, HDL particles are dysfunctional and may actually potentiate atherosclerosis. HDL-C is not currently a target of therapy. We still have a very long way to go before HDL therapeutics re-enter the mainstream of medicine.

Consistent with the 4D, AURORA, and SHARP trials, the EVENT registry demonstrates that statin therapy in patients receiving dialysis provides no reduction in risk for CVD events. The study does, however, demonstrate that statin therapy in patients with chronic kidney disease and not on dialysis undergoing stent deployment for CAD is beneficial. A somewhat shocking finding from the ROOBY trial is that among patients who undergo coronary artery bypass grafting and achieve an LDL-C < 70 mg/dL with lipid lowering medication, the risk of saphenous vein graft or internal mammary artery occlusion is not reduced compared to patients who did not take lipid lowering medication. In addition, risk for myocardial infarction and need for revascularization were also not reduced.

Lipoprotein(a) [Lp(a)] is receiving increasing attention. It is exciting that studies with PCSK9 monoclonal antibodies and the CETP inhibitors anacetrapib and evacetrapib all reduce Lp(a) significantly. This offers unique new therapeutic possibilities with which to evaluate what role, if any, Lp(a) reduction has on CAD events. In a post hoc analysis of the JUPITER trial, Ridker and coworkers demonstrate that although statin therapy does not impact Lp(a) levels, Lp(a) contributes significantly to residual risk even when patients are aggressively treated with statin therapy. In an elegant study of German patients with CAD and elevated Lp(a), Leebman and coworkers show that the addition of apheresis therapy to maximal drug therapy reduces risk significantly and quickly for CVD events.

Interesting surprises also arise in relation to triglyceride metabolism and inflammation. Shoajee-Moradie and coworkers show that insulin resistance not only increases hepatic secretion of VLDLs, but jejunal enterocytes also increase chylomicron production and secretion compared to lean controls consuming the identical meal. This finding is not exactly intuitive and changes our view of the impact of insulin resistance on the production and metabolism of triglyceride-rich lipoproteins. Varbo et al show that elevated levels of remnant lipoproteins are independently associated with significant elevations in systemic inflammatory tone even after comprehensive adjustment for covariate risk factors. Makadia and coworkers demonstrate in a Brazilian cohort that atherogenic dyslipidemia correlates with hepatic steatosis even in the absence of obesity and elevations in C-reactive protein (CRP). A new analysis from the Framingham investigators firmly establishes that visceral adiposity, but not subcutaneous adiposity, correlate, with increased risk for both CVD and cancer. Finally, in a post hoc analysis from the SATURN trial, coronary artery atherosclerotic plaque progression and regression correlated highly with CRP levels.

Dyslipidemia remains a widely prevalent and undertreated disorder. Future clinical trials will hopefully fill in some of the blanks and answer some long-standing questions. In the meantime, clinical judgment will have to suffice for a wide range of issues.

Peter P. Toth, MD, PhD

Pharmacologic Therapy

Lipoprotein(a) Concentrations, Rosuvastatin Therapy, and Residual Vascular Risk: An Analysis from the JUPITER Trial

Khera AV, Everett BM, Caulfield MP, et al (Brigham and Women's Hosp, Boston, MA; Quest Diagnostics Nichols Inst, San Juan Capistrano, CA)

Circulation 129:635-642, 2014

Background.—Lipoprotein(a) [Lp(a)] is a low-density lipoprotein-like particle largely independent of known risk factors and predictive of cardiovascular disease. Statins may offset the risk associated with elevated Lp(a), but it is unknown whether Lp(a) is a determinant of residual risk in the setting of low low-density lipoprotein cholesterol after potent statin therapy.

Methods and Results.—Baseline and on-treatment Lp(a) concentrations were assessed in 9612 multiethnic participants in the JUPITER trial (Justification for the Use of Statins in Prevention: An Intervention Trial Evaluating Rosuvastatin) before and after random allocation to rosuvastatin 20 mg/d or placebo, with outcomes reported for whites (n = 7746). Lp(a) concentrations (median [25th-75th percentile], in nmol/L) were highest in blacks (60 [34-100]), then Asians (38 [18-60]), Hispanics (24 [11-46]), and whites (23 [10-50]; $P < 0.001$). Although the median change in Lp(a) with rosuvastatin and placebo was zero, rosuvastatin nonetheless resulted in a small but statistically significant positive shift in the overall Lp(a) distribution ($P < 0.0001$). Baseline Lp(a) concentrations were associated with incident cardiovascular disease (adjusted hazard ratio per 1-SD increment in Ln[Lp(a)], 1.18; 95% confidence interval, 1.03–1.34; $P = 0.02$). Similarly, on-statin Lp(a) concentrations were associated with residual risk of cardiovascular disease (adjusted hazard ratio, 1.27; 95% confidence interval, 1.01-1.59; $P = 0.04$), which was independent of low-density lipoprotein cholesterol and other factors. Rosuvastatin significantly reduced incident cardiovascular disease among participants with baseline Lp(a) ≥ median (hazard ratio, 0.62; 95% confidence interval, 0.43-0.90) and Lp(a) < median (hazard ratio, 0.46; 95% confidence interval, 0.30-0.72), with no evidence of interaction. Similar results were obtained when analyses included nonwhites.

Conclusion.—Among white JUPITER participants treated with potent statin therapy, Lp(a) was a significant determinant of residual risk. The magnitude of relative risk reduction with rosuvastatin was similar among participants with high or low Lp(a).

Clinical Trials Registration Information.—clinicaltrials.gov. Unique identifier: NCT00239681 (Fig 1, Table 3).

▶ In a post hoc analysis of the JUPITER trial, Khera et al evaluate the impact of rosuvastatin therapy on serum lipoprotein(a) (Lp[a]) as well as the size effect of Lp(a) on residual risk for cardiovascular (CV) events. Consistent with other studies, statin therapy did not reduce serum levels of Lp(a). Lp(a) was associated with incident CV events even after comprehensive adjustment for covariates, including age, sex, treatment group (rosuvastatin or placebo), smoking, family history of premature coronary disease, body mass index, systolic blood pressure, fasting glucose, high-density lipoprotein cholesterol, low-density lipoprotein cholesterol, natural logarithm of triglycerides, and natural logarithm of high-sensitivity C-reactive protein (Table 3). Lp(a) was associated with a significant 27% increase in residual risk. There was no discernible difference in magnitude of benefit from rosuvastatin, regardless of whether baseline Lp(a) was higher or lower than the median (Fig 1).

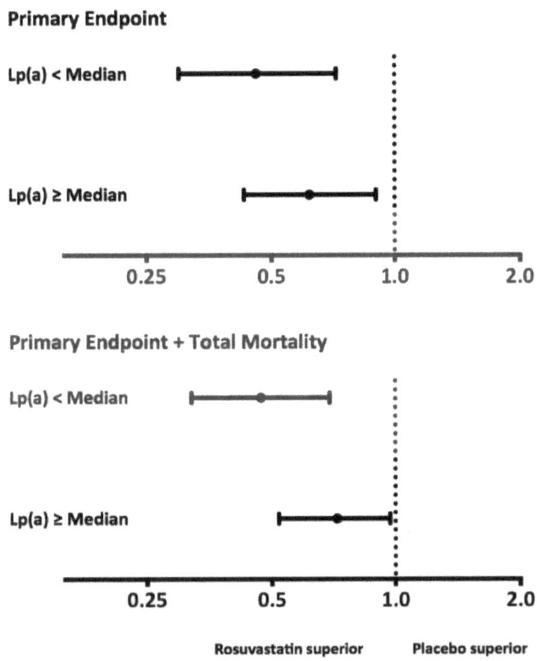

FIGURE 1.—Efficacy of rosuvastatin according to baseline lipoprotein(a) concentration. Hazard ratios and 95% confidence intervals according to intention-to-treat analysis for the primary endpoint (top) and the expanded endpoint (bottom) by baseline lipoprotein(a) concentrations. For the primary endpoint, hazard ratio with rosuvastatin therapy was 0.47 (95%CI 0.30 – 0.72) for participants with baseline Lp(a) concentration below the median and 0.62 (95%CI 0.43 – 0.90) in those above the median (p-interaction = 0.33). Similarly, for the expanded endpoint, hazard ratios were 0.46 (95%CI 0.32 – 0.69) and 0.72 (95%CI 0.52 – 0.97) for those below and above the median, respectively (p-interaction = 0.10). (Reprinted from Khera AV, Everett BM, Caulfield MP, et al. Lipoprotein(a) concentrations, rosuvastatin therapy, and residual vascular risk: an analysis from the JUPITER Trial. *Circulation.* 2014;129:635-642, © 2014, American Heart Association, Inc.)

TABLE 3.—Association Between Baseline Lipoprotein(a) and Incident CVD Among White JUPITER Participants

	Quartile One	Quartile Two	Quartile Three	Quartile Four	*P*-trend	HR/SD increment	*P*-value
Range (nmol/L)	≤10	11–23	24–49	≥50			
Primary Endpoint							
# of events/N	44/1991	50/1884	45/1957	71/1898		210/7730	
Incidence rate, per 100 person years	0.99	1.17	1.02	1.62	0.02	1.20	
Model One	1.00	1.18 (0.79–1.78) $P = 0.44$	1.04 (0.68–1.58) $P = 0.87$	1.70 (1.16–2.47) $P = 0.006$	0.01	1.19 (1.05–1.36)	0.008
Model Two	1.00	1.19 (0.79–1.79) $P = 0.40$	1.02 (0.67–1.56) $P = 0.93$	1.64 (1.12–2.41) $P = 0.01$	0.02	1.18 (1.03–1.35)	0.02
Primary Endpoint Plus Total Mortality							
# of events/N	59/1991	63/1884	67/1957	94/1898		283/7730	
Incidence rate, per 100 person years	1.32	1.47	1.53	2.14	0.004	1.62	
Model One	1.00	1.11 (0.78–1.59) $P = 0.56$	1.15 (0.81–1.63) $P = 0.44$	1.66 (1.20–2.29) $P = 0.002$	0.002	1.22 (1.09–1.37)	0.0005
Model Two	1.00	1.12 (0.78–1.60) $P = 0.54$	1.14 (0.80–1.63) $P = 0.47$	1.61 (1.16–2.25) $P = 0.005$	0.005	1.21 (1.08–1.36)	0.001

Hazard ratios are expressed per 1-SD increment in ln Lp(a), with 1-SD representing an approximately 2.5-fold increment in Lp(a). N = 7,730 reflective of number of white participants with baseline Lp(a) value availables.

Model One: Adjusted for age, gender, and treatment group.

Model Two: Adjusted for age, gender, treatment group, smoking, family history of premature coronary disease, body mass index, systolic blood pressure, fasting glucose, HDL-cholesterol, LDL-cholesterol, ln triglycerides, ln hsCRP.

This analysis emphasizes a number of important points. First, statin therapy benefited patients to an equal degree whether Lp(a) was higher or lower than the median. Second, Lp(a) contributes significantly and independently of other risk factors to residual risk. This confirms the results from prospective longitudinal cohorts and genomewide association studies that Lp(a) is an important and legitimate CV risk factor. The prospective, randomized clinical outcomes trials currently underway with cholesterol ester transfer protein inhibitors (anacetrapib, evacetrapib) and PCSK9 monoclonal antibody inhibitors (alirocumab, evolocumab) will certainly attempt to discern whether Lp(a) reductions with these agents contribute to any decreases seen in primary composite endpoints in patients with established coronary artery disease.

P. P. Toth, MD, PhD

Lipoprotein Apheresis in Patients With Maximally Tolerated Lipid-Lowering Therapy, Lipoprotein(a)-Hyperlipoproteinemia, and Progressive Cardiovascular Disease: Prospective Observational Multicenter Study

Leebmann J, for the Pro(a)LiFe Study Group (General Hosp, Passau, Germany; et al)

Circulation 128:2567-2576, 2013

Background.—Lipoprotein(a) (Lp(a)) hyperlipoproteinemia is a major risk factor for cardiovascular disease, which is not affected by treatment of other cardiovascular risk factors. This study sought to assess the effect of chronic lipoprotein apheresis (LA) on the incidence of cardiovascular events in patients with progressive cardiovascular disease receiving maximally tolerated lipid-lowering treatment.

Methods and Results.—In a prospective observational multicenter study, 170 patients were investigated who commenced LA because of Lp(a)-hyperlipoproteinemia and progressive cardiovascular disease. Patients were characterized regarding plasma lipid status, lipid-lowering drug treatment, and variants at the LPA gene locus. The incidence rates of cardiovascular events 2 years before (y−2 and y−1) and prospectively 2 years during LA treatment (y+1, y+2) were compared. The mean age of patients was 51 years at the first cardiovascular event and 57 years at the first LA. Before LA, mean low-density lipoprotein cholesterol and Lp(a) were $2.56 \pm 1.04\ mmol \cdot L^{-1}$ ($99.0 \pm 40.1\ mg \cdot dL^{-1}$) and Lp(a) $3.74 \pm 1.63\ \mu mol \cdot L^{-1}$ ($104.9 \pm 45.7\ mg \cdot dL^{-1}$), respectively. Mean annual rates for major adverse coronary events declined from 0.41 for 2 years before LA to 0.09 for 2 years during LA ($P < 0.0001$). Event rates including all vascular beds declined from 0.61 to 0.16 ($P < 0.0001$). Analysis of single years revealed increasing major adverse coronary event rates from 0.30 to 0.54 ($P = 0.001$) for y−2 to y−1 before LA, decline to 0.14 from y−1 to y+1 ($P < 0.0001$) and to 0.05 from y+1 to y+2 ($P = 0.014$).

Conclusions.—In patients with Lp(a)-hyperlipoproteinemia, progressive cardiovascular disease, and maximally tolerated lipid-lowering medication, LA effectively lowered the incidence rate of cardiovascular events.

Clinical Trial Registration.—URL: https://drks-neu.uniklinik-freiburg.de. Unique identifier: DRKS00003119 (Fig 3, Table 5).

▶ Apheresis is an established means by which to reduce serum elevated levels of lipoprotein(a) (Lp[a]). Leebmann et al evaluated the impact of apheresis therapy in 170 patients with established coronary artery disease (CAD) and elevated Lp(a) (mean, 104.9 mg/dL). All patients were on maximally tolerated lipid-lowering medication and had a mean baseline low-density lipoprotein cholesterol (LDL-C) level of 99 mg/dL. Incident cardiovascular events and need for revascularization were monitored for 2 years before initiating apheresis and for 2 years after apheresis therapy was started. There was a rapid reduction in all cardiovascular endpoints evaluated within 1 year of initiating apheresis (Fig 3). Major coronary events, myocardial infarction, and revascularization

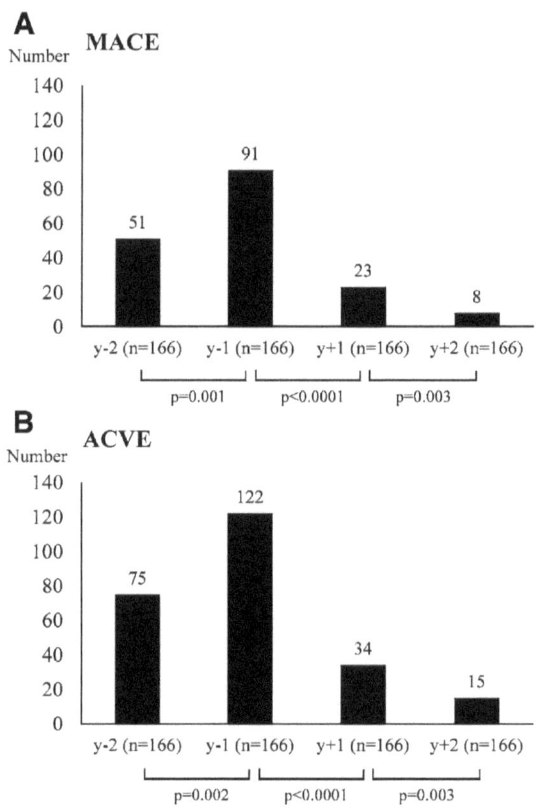

FIGURE 3.—Absolute numbers of MACE (**A**) and ACVE (**B**) for single years before (y−2, y−1) and after (y+1, y+2) commencing chronic LA. Depicted P values are derived from the analysis of corresponding mean annual rates. ACVE indicates Adverse cardiac or vascular events; LA, lipoprotein apheresis; and MACE, major adverse coronary events. (Reprinted from Leebmann J, for the Pro(a)LiFe Study Group. Lipoprotein apheresis in patients with maximally tolerated lipid-lowering therapy, lipoprotein(a)-hyperlipoproteinemia, and progressive cardiovascular disease: prospective observational multicenter study. *Circulation.* 2013;128:2567-2576, with permission from American Heart Association, Inc.)

TABLE 5.—Mean Annual Rates for MACE, ACVE, MI, PCI, and CABG for 2 Years Before (y−2, y−1) and After (y+1, y+2) Commencing Chronic LA and Percentage Changes (Δ) Between Periods Before and During Apheresis

	(y−2 + y−1)	(y+1 + y+2)	Δ, %	*P* Value
MACE	0.41±0.45	0.09±0.22	−78.0	<0.0001
ACVE	0.58±0.53	0.14±0.31	−75.9	<0.0001
MI	0.14±0.24	0.02±0.10	−85.7	<0.0001
PCI	0.22±0.35	0.07±0.19	−68.2	<0.0001
CABG	0.05±0.15	0.01±0.05	−80.0	0.001

ACVE indicates adverse cardiac or vascular events; CABG, coronary artery bypass graft; LA, lipoprotein apheresis; MACE, major adverse coronary events; MI, myocardial infarction; and PCI, percutaneous coronary intervention.

by percutaneous coronary intervention or coronary artery bypass grafting were reduced significantly and dramatically (Table 5). The number of incident events decreased further during the second year of therapy.

This study shows very convincingly that until pharmacologic interventions are available that can significantly reduce circulating levels of Lp(a), apheresis provides a viable treatment that is safe and highly efficacious. The patients in this study had severe elevations in Lp(a) and had established CAD. Apheresis dramatically attenuated risk for acute cardiovascular events and need for coronary revascularization within 1 year of treatment initiation. Benefit was sustained and increased during the second year of therapy. This study provides clear demonstration that Lp(a) reduction decreases risk for coronary heart disease events and attenuates an aggressive course of disease progression in patients with severe elevations in this lipoprotein.

P. P. Toth, MD, PhD

Relationship of Lipoproteins to Cardiovascular Events: The AIM-HIGH Trial (Atherothrombosis Intervention in Metabolic Syndrome With LOW HDL/ High Triglycerides and Impact on Global Health Outcomes)

Guyton JR, Slee AE, Anderson T, et al (Duke Univ Med Ctr, Durham, NC; Axio Res, Seattle, WA; Univ of Calgary, Alberta, Canada; et al)

J Am Coll Cardiol 62:1580-1584, 2013

Objectives.—This study sought to examine the relationship between niacin treatment, lipoproteins, and cardiovascular (CV) outcomes in this secondary analysis of the AIM-HIGH (Atherothrombosis Intervention in Metabolic Syndrome With Low HDL/High Triglycerides and Impact on Global Health Outcomes) trial.

Background.—During a 3-year follow-up in 3,414 patients with established CV disease and low high-density lipoprotein cholesterol (HDL-C) levels, combined niacin + low-density lipoprotein cholesterol (LDL-C)-lowering therapy did not reduce CV events compared with LDL-C-lowering therapy alone.

Methods.—Subjects taking simvastatin and/or ezetimibe were randomized to receive extended-release (ER) niacin 1,500 to 2,000 mg or minimal immediate-release niacin (≤150 mg) as placebo at bedtime. LDL-C levels in both groups were maintained from 40 to 80 mg/dl. Hazard ratios were estimated by using Cox proportional hazards models for relationships between lipoproteins and the composite endpoint of CV death, myocardial infarction, acute coronary syndrome, ischemic stroke, or symptom-driven revascularization.

Results.—CV outcomes were not associated with ER niacin in any baseline lipoprotein tertile. In a subset of patients in both the highest triglyceride (≥198 mg/dl) and lowest HDL-C (<33 mg/dl) tertiles, ER niacin showed a trend toward benefit (hazard ratio: 0.74, $p = 0.073$). In-trial LDL-C levels, non-HDL-C levels, and the total cholesterol/HDL-C ratio were positively associated with CV events in the control group, but these relationships were absent in the ER niacin group.

Conclusions.—Baseline lipoprotein tertiles did not predict differential benefit or harm with ER niacin added to LDL-C-lowering therapy, but a small dyslipidemic subgroup may benefit. ER niacin attenuated expected relationships of lipoprotein risk factors with CV events, raising the possibility that nonlipoprotein actions of niacin could affect risk. (Niacin Plus Statin to Prevent Vascular Events [AIM-HIGH]; NCT00120289) (Fig 1).

▶ Both the AIM-HIGH (Atherothrombosis Intervention in Metabolic Syndrome With Low HDL/High Triglycerides and Impact on Global Health Outcomes)[1] and HPS-2 THRIVE (Heart Protection Study-2 Treatment of HDL to Reduce the Incidence of Vascular Events) (http://www.ctsu.ox.ac.uk/~thrive/) trials tested the efficacy of niacin versus placebo in patients with coronary artery disease and already receiving intensive background therapy. In both studies, patients began with low levels of atherogenic lipoprotein burden. Neither study found differences in their primary endpoints compared with placebo. There is widespread agreement that currently, in patients with well-controlled low-density lipoprotein cholesterol (LDL-C) and non–high-density lipoprotein cholesterol (HDL-C), there is no reason to use adjuvant niacin therapy irrespective of serum HDL-C levels.

In a post hoc analysis of AIM-HIGH, Guyton et al evaluated a variety of tertile subgroups with different lipid and lipoprotein baseline values (Fig 1). None of the groups derived benefit from niacin therapy irrespective of baseline LDL-C, non–HDL-C, HDL-C, triglyceride, total cholesterol to HDL-C ratio, or triglyceride to HDL-C ratio. However, in the group with triglyceride level greater than 198 and HDL-C level less than 33 mg/dL, there was a nonsignificant trend toward a 36% reduction in the primary endpoint. The result is hypothesis generating only.

This was an exhaustive analysis of AIM-HIGH, and no statistically positive finding emerged. It is highly unlikely that another large niacin outcomes trial will be done to either confirm or refute the nonsignificant trend for benefit in patients with high triglycerides and low HDL-C. Although niacin has been found to promote atherosclerotic disease regression in the carotid arteries[2]

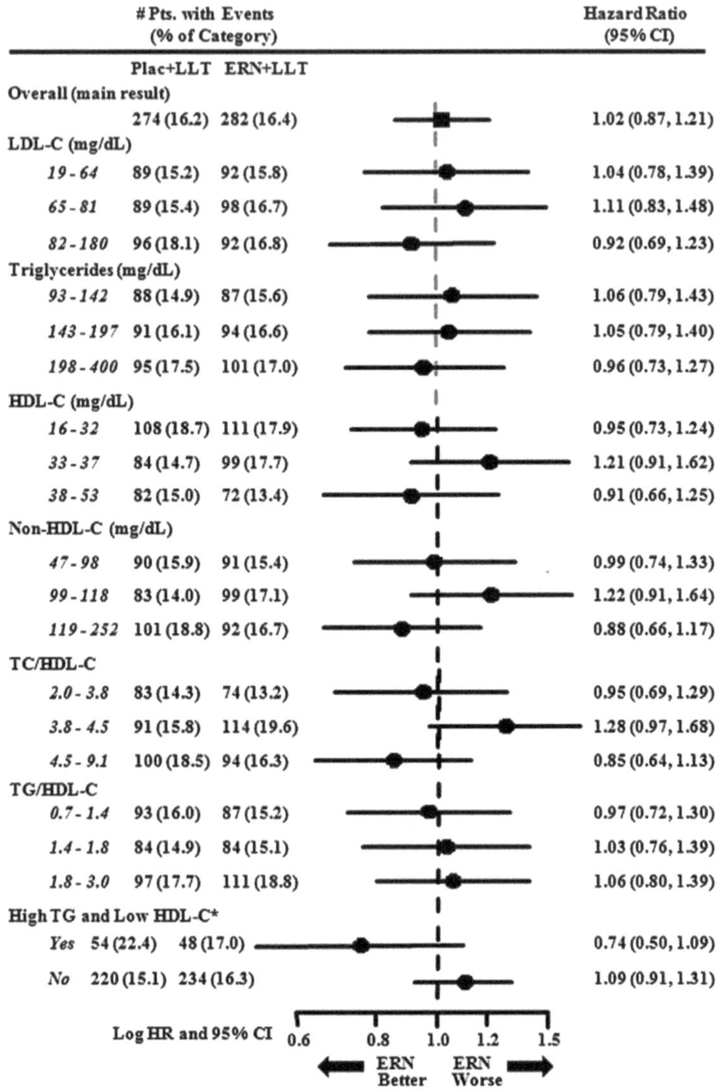

FIGURE 1.—Effect of treatment on CV events by baseline lipoprotein/lipid tertiles. Hazard ratios (HR) for the effect of treatment assignment were calculated by using Cox proportional hazards models, including terms for sex and diabetes. *High triglycerides (TG) and low high-density lipoprotein cholesterol (HDL-C) designates subjects with highest-tertile TG and lowest-tertile HDL-C levels. Placebo (Plac) tablets included 100- to 150-mg immediate-release niacin. CI = confidence interval; CV = cardiovascular; ERN = extended-release niacin; LLT = low-density lipoprotein cholesterol–lowering therapy; Pts = Patients; TC = total cholesterol. (Reprinted from the Journal of the American College of Cardiology. Guyton JR, Slee AE, Anderson T, et al. Relationship of lipoproteins to cardiovascular events: The aim-high trial (atherothrombosis intervention in metabolic syndrome with low HDL/high triglycerides and impact on global health outcomes). *J Am Coll Cardiol.* 2013;62:1580-1584, Copyright 2013, with permission from the American College of Cardiology.)

and has been found to reduce event rates in two small studies,[3,4] its utility in managing cardiovascular disease and dyslipidemia appears to be negligible.

P. P. Toth, MD, PhD

References

1. Boden WE, Probstfield JL, Anderson T, et al. Niacin in patients with low HDL cholesterol levels receiving intensive statin therapy. *N Engl J Med.* 2011;365: 2255-2267.
2. Taylor AJ, Villines TC, Stanek EJ, et al. Extended-release niacin or ezetimibe and carotid intima-media thickness. *N Engl J Med.* 2009;361:2113-2122.
3. Brown BG, Zhao XQ, Chait A, et al. Simvastatin and niacin, antioxidant vitamins, or the combination for the prevention of coronary disease. *N Engl J Med.* 2001; 345:1583-1592.
4. Brown BG, Zambon A, Poulin D, et al. Use of niacin, statins, and resins in patients with combined hyperlipidemia. *Am J Cardiol.* 1998;81:52B-59B.

Statin Therapy in Patients With Chronic Kidney Disease Undergoing Percutaneous Coronary Intervention (from the Evaluation of Drug Eluting Stents and Ischemic Events Registry)

Dasari TW, Cohen DJ, Kleiman NS, et al (Univ of Oklahoma Health Sciences Ctr; St Luke's Mid America Heart Inst, KS; Methodist DeBakey Heart & Vascular Ctr, Houston, TX; et al)

Am J Cardiol 113:621-625, 2014

Secondary prevention trials have demonstrated the efficacy of statins in reducing cardiovascular morbidity and mortality in patients with coronary artery disease and events after percutaneous coronary intervention (PCI). However, there are few data describing the clinical value of statins in patients with coronary artery disease and chronic kidney disease (CKD) undergoing PCI. Of 10,148 patients who entered into Evaluation of Drug Eluting Stents and Ischemic Events, a multicenter registry of unselected patients undergoing PCI from July 2004 to December 2007, we studied 2,306 patients with CKD (estimated glomerular filtration rate ≤60 ml/min based on the Modified Diet in Renal Disease calculation). Patients were stratified into those receiving statins at discharge (n = 1,833, 79%) or not (n = 473, 21%). Patients in the statin group had a greater prevalence of hypertension, recent myocardial infarction (MI), and use of β blockers and angiotensin-converting enzyme inhibitors. Outcomes were assessed from discharge through 1-year follow-up. One-year all-cause mortality was 5.7% in statin group versus 8.7% in the no statin group (adjusted hazard ratio 0.55, 95% confidence interval 0.34 to 0.88). The composite of death, MI, and repeat revascularization was lower in statin group (adjusted hazard ratio 0.71, 95% confidence interval 0.51 to 0.99). In conclusion, among patients with CKD undergoing PCI, the prescription of statins at hospital discharge was associated with a significant improvement in subsequent outcomes including mortality and composite end point of death, MI, and repeat revascularization (Figs 1 and 2, Table 1).

▶ Chronic kidney disease (CKD) is recognized by some specialty organizations as a coronary artery disease (CAD) risk equivalent. CKD is associated with multiple disturbances in lipid lipoprotein metabolism, including elevated triglycerides, low high-density lipoprotein cholesterol (HDL-C), and increased numbers of small, dense low-density lipoprotein (LDL) particles independent of insulin resistance. The Study of Heart and Renal Protection trial found that treatment with a combination of simvastatin and ezetimibe in patients with a mean glomerular filtration rate (GFR) of 27 mL/min reduced risk for cardiovascular events compared with placebo, although mortality was not decreased.[1] In contrast, statin therapy has not been found to be efficacious in patients with end-stage renal disease (ESRD) and receiving dialysis.[2,3] CKD is widely prevalent, and a significant percentage of patients undergoing percutaneous coronary intervention (PCI) have CKD. To date, there has been no investigation to ascertain if statin therapy in patients with CKD undergoing PCI reduces risk for mortality or cardiovascular events.

Dasari and coworkers evaluated this issue with the Evaluation of Drug Eluting Stents and Ischemic Events (EVENT) registry. Data were from 2306 patients with CKD. A total of 1833 patients were given a statin at the time of discharge, whereas 473 were not. The groups were not evenly matched for use of β blockade, angiotensin-converting enzyme inhibition, or nonstatin lipid lowering, but data were adjusted for these differences as well as for age, sex, hypertension, heart failure class, and recent myocardial infarction (MI) using multivariable Cox proportional hazard models (Table 1). Follow-up was for 1 year. At the end of 1 year, all-cause mortality was reduced significantly by 45% and the composite of death, MI, and need for revascularization was reduced significantly by

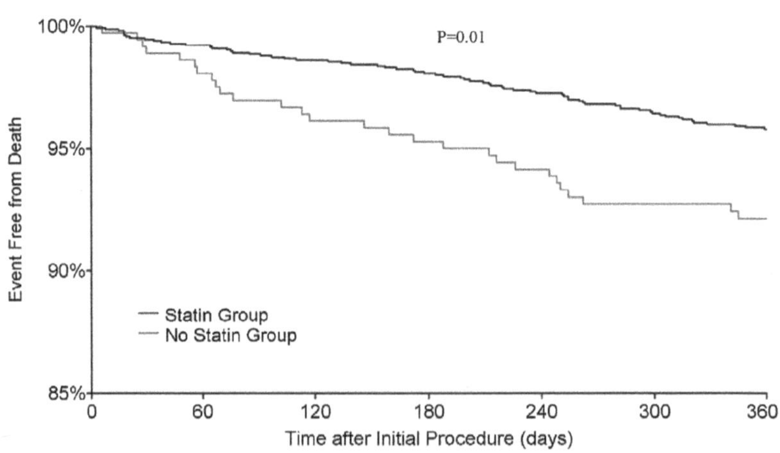

FIGURE 1.—All-cause mortality during follow-up. (Reprinted from the American Journal of Cardiology. Dasari TW, Cohen DJ, Kleiman NS, et al. *Statin* therapy in patients with chronic kidney disease undergoing percutaneous coronary intervention (from the Evaluation of Drug Eluting Stents and Ischemic Events Registry). *Am J Cardiol.* 2014;113:621-625, Copyright 2014, with permission from Elsevier.)

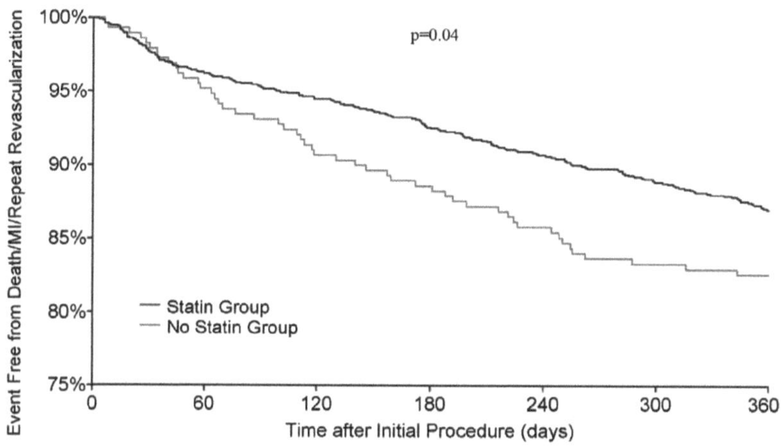

FIGURE 2.—Composite of death, MI, and repeat revascularization during follow-up. (Reprinted from Dasari TW, Cohen DJ, Kleiman NS, et al. *Statin* therapy in patients with chronic kidney disease undergoing percutaneous coronary intervention (from the Evaluation of Drug Eluting Stents and Ischemic Events Registry). *Am J Cardiol.* 2014;113:621-625, with permission from Elsevier.)

TABLE 1.—Baseline Demographic and Clinical Characteristics of the Study Population

Characteristic	Statin Therapy Yes (n = 1,833), %	Statin Therapy No (n = 473), %	*p* Value
Age (yrs), mean ± SD	74 ± 10	75 ± 10	0.16
Men	54	48	0.01
Body mass index (mean ± SD)	27 ± 5	26 ± 5	0.12
Diabetes mellitus	36	37	0.66
Hypertension	87	82	0.004
Current smoker	14	13	0.59
Renal dialysis	7	7	0.58
Previous stroke	14	18	0.07
Heart failure	18	20	0.36
Peripheral arterial disease	17	19	0.45
Previous MI	41	36	0.06
Previous PCI	39	36	0.36
Previous coronary bypass	30	25	0.06
MI within 7 days	16	11	0.002
Number of narrowed coronary arteries			0.26
1	43	46	
2	30	29	
3	27	25	

29% (Figs 1 and 2). Separation of the Kaplan-Meier survival curves for these outcomes was apparent within 30 days. Consistent with previous studies, patients receiving dialysis did not derive benefit from statin therapy.

Although these patients were not randomly selected, the magnitude of between-group differences is striking. This study provides the first evidence supporting the use of statin therapy in patients with CAD and CKD undergoing PCI. It will be of interest to better ascertain long-term outcomes in these patients. It remains poorly understood why statin therapy consistently offers no benefit in patients with ESRD. Until a randomized study is completed (unlikely to be performed), patients with CKD and not on dialysis undergoing PCI for CAD should receive a statin.

P. P. Toth, MD, PhD

References

1. Baigent C, Landray MJ, Reith C, et al. The effects of lowering LDL cholesterol with simvastatin plus ezetimibe in patients with chronic kidney disease (Study of Heart and Renal Protection): a randomised placebo-controlled trial. *Lancet.* 2011;377:2181-2192.
2. Fellström BC, Jardine AG, Schmieder RE, et al. Rosuvastatin and cardiovascular events in patients undergoing hemodialysis. *N Engl J Med.* 2009;360:1395-1407.
3. Wanner C, Krane V, März W, et al. Atorvastatin in patients with type 2 diabetes mellitus undergoing hemodialysis. *N Engl J Med.* 2005;353:238-248.

Impact of Lipid-Lowering Medications and Low-Density Lipoprotein Levels on 1-Year Clinical Outcomes after Coronary Artery Bypass Grafting

Quin JA, Hattler B, Bishawi M, et al (VA Boston Healthcare System, West Roxbury, MA; Eastern Colorado Health Care System, Denver, CO; Northport VA Med Ctr, NY; et al)

J Am Coll Surg 217:452-460, 2013

Background.—Studies investigating lipid-lowering medication (LLM) use and LDL levels in coronary artery bypass grafting patients are limited.

Study Design.—The Veterans Affairs Randomized On/Off Bypass Trial's patient records were analyzed for LLM use and 1-year LDL levels. Mortality, acute MI (AMI), and repeat revascularization rates were compared at 1 year between patients with and without LLM at discharge. In addition, AMI, repeat revascularization, and graft patency were compared between patients that did and did not achieve a 1-year LDL target level of <100 mg/dL.

Results.—The LLM data were available for 86.4% (1,904 of 2,203) of patients. Rates of LLM use were 83.4% (1,316 of 1,577) at discharge and 90.0% (1,713 of 1,904) at 1 year. Patients discharged after coronary artery bypass grafting on LLMs had a significantly lower 1-year mortality rate (1.9% vs 5.4%; $p < 0.01$) than those not discharged on LLM, and 1-year AMI and repeat revascularization rates were not significantly different. Of the patients with 1-year LDL measurements, 69.4% (1,200 of 1,729) achieved an LDL target level of <100 mg/dL. No differences were seen in AMI, revascularization, or graft occlusion rates between patients who achieved target LDL levels and those who did not.

Conclusions.—Rates of LLM use among veterans post–coronary artery bypass grafting are high. Discharge on LLM might be associated with improved intermediate-term survival. Patients who achieved an LDL target of <100 mg/dL at 1-year did not experience improved 1-year clinical outcomes or graft patency. Longer-term follow-up might reveal differences in cardiac outcomes related to achievement of target LDL levels (Tables 1 and 2).

► It is highly established that lipid lowering with statin therapy reduces risk for cardiovascular (CV) events in the secondary prevention setting. In the Post-CABG trial, intensive lipid-lowering therapy targeting low-density lipoprotein cholesterol (LDL-C) levels less than 100 mg/dL coupled with intensive lifestyle modification reduced rates of saphenous vein graft stenosis compared with less-aggressive lipid lowering (LDL-C < 135 mg/dL) in patients who had undergone coronary artery bypass grafting (CABG) surgery.[1] Cardiovascular events rate reductions did not attain significance after 4.5 years of follow-up. However, during a 3-year extended follow-up period (7.5 years total), a composite of

TABLE 1.—Patient Characteristics Based on Lipid-Lowering Medication Use at Discharge after Coronary Artery Bypass Grafting for 1,577 Randomized On/Off Pump Bypass Patients with Discharge Lipid-Lowering Medication Use Data

Patient Characteristics	Discharge LLM Use	No Discharge LLM Use	*p* Value
Age, y, mean (SD); n	62.6 (8.3); 1,316	63.0 (8.2); 261	0.46
Earlier MI, n (%)	360/1,300 (27.7)	77/258 (29.8)	0.48
Elective surgery, n (%)	1,143/1,316 (86.9)	227/261 (87.0)	0.96
Baseline EF, n (%)			
<35%	63/1,285 (4.9)	14/250 (5.6)	0.70
35–44%	149/1,285 (11.6)	25/250 (10.0)	
>45%	1073/1,285 (83.5)	211/250 (84.4)	
Diabetes, n (%)	604/1,316 (45.9)	104/261 (39.8)	0.07
Serum creatinine >1.5 mg/dL, n (%)	106/1,316 (8.1)	22/261 (8.4)	0.84
Preoperative SGPT, U/L, mean (SD); n	31.4 (22.5); 1,278	34.2 (20.2); 254	0.05
Preoperative total bilirubin, mg/dL, mean (SD); n	0.65 (0.31); 1,283	0.64 (0.33); 255	0.79
Preoperative tobacco use, n (%)			
Never	213/1,314 (16.2)	49/261 (18.8)	0.59
Former smoker	662/1,314 (50.4)	129/261 (49.4)	
Current smoker	439/1,314 (33.4)	83/261 (31.8)	
COPD, n (%)	277/1,316 (21.0)	53/261 (20.3)	0.79
CVA, n (%)	101/1,316 (7.7)	15/261 (5.7)	0.28
Peripheral vascular disease, n (%)	190/1,316 (14.4)	44/261 (16.9)	0.31
Hypertension, n (%)	1,152/1,305 (88.3)	222/259 (85.7)	0.25
Aspirin use preoperatively, n (%)	1,103/1,306 (84.5)	220/260 (84.6)	0.95
β-blocker use preoperatively, n (%)	847/1,023 (82.8)	142/181 (78.5)	0.16
Plavix use preoperatively, n (%)	229/1,307 (17.5)	38/260 (14.6)	0.25
Aspirin use at discharge, n (%)	1,211/1,316 (92.0)	226/261 (86.6)	<0.01
β-blocker use at discharge, n (%)	1,237/1,316 (94.0)	226/261 (86.6)	<0.01
Aspirin use at 1 y, n (%)	1,126/1,225 (91.9)	215/233 (92.3)	0.85
β-blocker use at 1 y, n (%)	1,106/1,233 (89.7)	206/235 (87.7)	0.35
Plavix use a 1 y, n (%)	274/1,231 (22.3)	46/235 (19.6)	0.36
LLM use preoperatively, n (%)	916/1,023 (89.5)	116/181 (64.1)	<0.01
LDL level <100 mg/dL at 1 y, n (%)	777/1,088 (71.4)	127/193 (65.8)	0.11
On pump cases, n (%)	657/1,316 (49.9)	127/261(48.7)	0.71
Perioperative stroke, n (%)	9/1,316 (0.7)	5/261 (1.9)	0.05
LIMA use, n (%)	1,250/1,314 (95.1)	246/261 (94.3)	0.55
Postoperative tobacco use, n (%)	179/769 (23.3)	21/114 (18.4)	0.25

CABG, coronary artery bypass grafting; EF, ejection fraction; LIMA, left internal mammary artery; LLM, lipid-lowering medication; SGPT, serum glutamic pyruvate transaminase.

TABLE 2.—One-Year Clinical Outcomes Based on Randomized On/Off Pump Bypass Patients with Lipid-Lowering Medication Use Data at Discharge (n = 1,577)

	Discharge LLM Use (Total n = 1,316)		No Discharge LLM Use (Total n = 261)		
Clinical Outcomes at 1-Year	n	%	n	%	p Value
Post-discharge deaths	25	1.9	14	5.4	<0.01
Post-discharge cardiovascular/vascular deaths	18	1.4	5	1.9	0.50
Acute MI within 1 y	22	1.7	3	1.1	0.54
Revascularization within 1 y	55	4.2	9	3.4	0.58
Composite of the post-discharge deaths and acute MI or revascularization within 1 y	90	6.8	25	9.6	0.12

LLM, lipid-lowering medication.

cardiovascular (CV) events (death or myocardial infarction [MI]) and need for revascularization were both significantly reduced.[2,3] Graft closure in both saphenous veins and internal mammary arteries remains a significant issue in modern cardiovascular medicine. Understanding the dynamics of graft atherosclerotic disease, inflammation, and vessel wall hyperplasia is critical.

The Veterans Affairs Randomized On/Off Bypass (ROOBY) trial evaluated the rates of acute coronary events, need for revascularization, and graft closure in patients who underwent CABG surgery. Outcomes were evaluated retrospectively in 1577 patients after 1 year in patients who did and did not receive lipid-lowering therapy. Target LDL-C on therapy was less than 100 mg/dL. In a multivariable logistic regression model (controlling for age, history of chronic obstructive pulmonary disease, and serum creatinine level greater than 1.5 mg/dL; history of stroke, peripheral arterial disease, diabetes mellitus, or MI; low left ventricular ejection fraction; and non-lipid lowering medication), lipid-lowering medication (statin, fibrate, bile acid binding resin, niacin, or cholesterol absorption inhibition either as monotherapy or used in combination) was associated with reduced risk for all-cause mortality but not CV events (Table 1). Lipid-lowering therapy was also not associated with reductions in MI, need for revascularization, or graft patency in either saphenous veins or internal mammary arteries (Table 2).

These results are somewhat surprising. However, not all patients were receiving statin therapy. Benefit from statin therapy is discernible within months of initiating these medications.[4] In Post-CABG, it required 7.5 years of follow-up to detect reductions in CV events, although benefit on saphenous graft closure was discernible sooner. New trials are indicated to better define optimal approaches to graft closure and CV event rate reduction in patients who undergo bypass surgery.

P. P. Toth, MD, PhD

References

1. Campeau L, Hunninghake DB, Knatterud GL, et al. Aggressive cholesterol lowering delays saphenous vein graft atherosclerosis in women, the elderly, and patients

with associated risk factors. NHLBI post coronary artery bypass graft clinical trial. Post CABG Trial Investigators. *Circulation.* 1999;99:3241-3247.
2. Knatterud GL, Rosenberg Y, Campeau L, et al. Long-term effects on clinical outcomes of aggressive lowering of low-density lipoprotein cholesterol levels and low-dose anticoagulation in the post coronary artery bypass graft trial. Post CABG Investigators. *Circulation.* 2000;102:157-165.
3. Hoogwerf BJ, Hunninghake DB, Knatterud G, Campeau L. A summary of the findings from the Post-CABG trial. *Minerva Cardioangiol.* 2002;50:291-299.
4. Schwartz GG, Olsson AG, Ezekowitz MD, et al. Effects of atorvastatin on early recurrent ischemic events in acute coronary syndromes: the MIRACL study: a randomized controlled trial. *JAMA.* 2001;285:1711-1718.

C-reactive Protein, but not Low-Density Lipoprotein Cholesterol Levels, Associate With Coronary Atheroma Regression and Cardiovascular Events After Maximally Intensive Statin Therapy

Puri R, Nissen SE, Libby P, et al (Cleveland Clinic, OH; Brigham and Women's Hosp, Boston, MA; et al)
Circulation 128:2395-2403, 2013

Background.—Baseline C-reactive protein (CRP) levels predict major adverse cardiovascular events (MACE: death, myocardial infarction, stroke, coronary revascularization, and hospitalization for unstable angina). The association between changes in CRP levels with plaque progression and MACE in the setting of maximally intensive statin therapy is unknown.

Methods and Results.—The Study of Coronary Atheroma by Intravascular Ultrasound: Effect of Rosuvastatin Versus Atorvastatin (SATURN) used serial intravascular ultrasound measures of coronary atheroma volume in patients treated with rosuvastatin 40 mg or atorvastatin 80 mg for 24 months. The treatment groups did not differ significantly in the change from baseline of percent atheroma volume on intravascular ultrasound, CRP-modulating effects, or MACE rates, thus allowing for a (prespecified) post hoc analysis to test associations between the changes in CRP levels with coronary disease progression and MACE. Patients with nonincreasing CRP levels (n = 621) had higher baseline (2.3 [1.1−4.7] versus 1.1 [0.5−1.8] mg/L; $P < 0.001$) and lower follow-up CRP levels (0.8 [0.5−1.7] versus 1.6 [0.7−4.1] mg/L; $P < 0.001$) versus those with increasing CRP levels (n = 364). Multivariable analysis revealed a nonincreasing CRP level to independently associate with greater percent atheroma volume regression ($P = 0.01$). Although the (log) change in CRP did not associate with MACE (hazard ratio, 1.18; 95% confidence interval, 0.93−1.50; $P = 0.17$), the (log) on-treatment CRP associated significantly with MACE (hazard ratio, 1.28; 95% confidence interval, 1.04−1.56; $P = 0.02$). On-treatment low-density lipoprotein cholesterol levels did not correlate with MACE (hazard ratio, 1.09; 95% confidence interval, 0.88−1.35; $P = 0.45$).

Conclusions.—Following 24 months of potent statin therapy, on-treatment CRP levels associated with MACE. Inflammation may be an important driver of residual cardiovascular risk in patients with coronary artery disease despite aggressive statin therapy.

Clinical Trial Registration.—URL: http://clinicaltrials.gov. Unique identifier: NCT000620542 (Figs 1 and 2, Table 3).

► Atherosclerosis is now widely acknowledged as an inflammatory disease. As arterial walls are exposed to cardiovascular disease risk factors, progressive endothelial dysfunction and lipid uptake into the subendothelial space are followed by a plethora of inflammatory responses driven by T lymphocytes and monocytes. The inflammatory response potentiates low-density lipoprotein (LDL) oxidation and macrophage scavenging, giving rise to foam cells and the progenitors to fatty streaks and atherosclerotic lesions.[1,2] Serum C-reactive protein (CRP) levels are highly correlated with risk for cardiovascular events. Post hoc analyses from the JUPITER, PROVE-IT, and A to Z trials all suggest

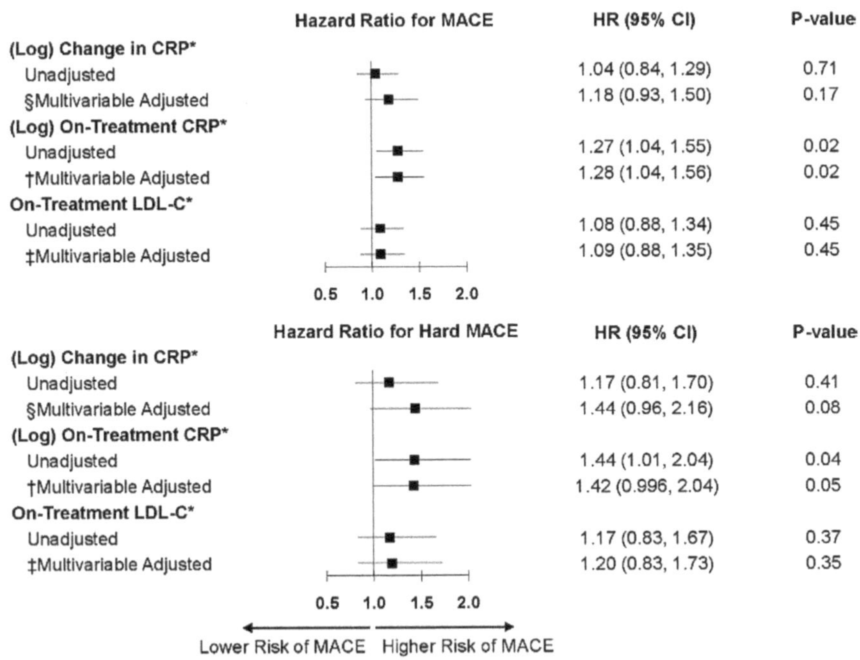

FIGURE 1.—Cox proportional hazard ratios for time to first MACE or hard MACE, according to the change from baseline of CRP levels, on-treatment CRP levels, or on-treatment LDL-C levels. *Values of log-transformed change in CRP, on-treatment CRP, and on-treatment LDL-C were per standard deviation. §Adjusted for history of diabetes mellitus, concomitant ACE inhibitor use, and log-transformed baseline CRP. †Adjusted for history of diabetes mellitus, history of acute coronary syndrome, and concomitant use of ACE inhibitor. ‡Adjusted for history of diabetes mellitus, history of acute coronary syndrome, concomitant ACE inhibitor use, and log-transformed on-treatment CRP. ACE indicates angiotensin-converting enzyme; CI, confidence interval; CRP, C-reactive protein; HR, hazard ratio; LDL-C, low-density lipoprotein cholesterol; and MACE, major adverse cardiovascular events. (Reprinted from Puri R, Nissen SE, Libby P, et al. C-reactive protein, but not low-density lipoprotein cholesterol levels, associate with coronary atheroma regression and cardiovascular events after maximally intensive statin therapy. *Circulation.* 2013;128:2395-2403, Copyright 2013, with permission from American Heart Association, Inc.)

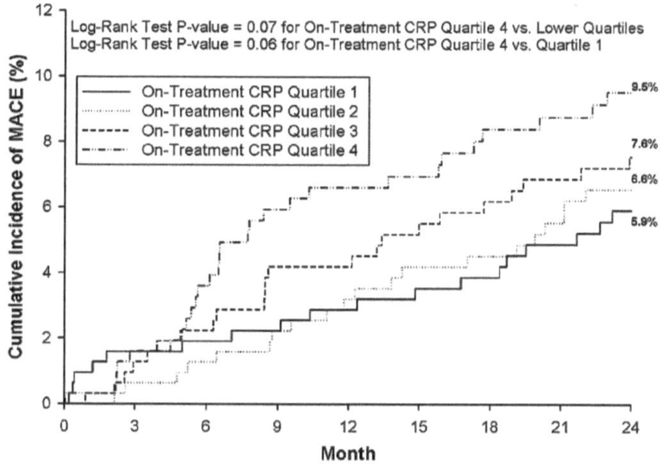

No. Patients At Risk									
On-Treatment CRP Quartile 1	315	308	306	303	299	294	290	284	272
On-Treatment CRP Quartile 2	316	312	309	304	299	293	290	278	270
On-Treatment CRP Quartile 3	316	309	305	295	295	282	277	272	265
On-Treatment CRP Quartile 4	316	303	290	282	277	269	253	245	235

FIGURE 2.—Kaplan–Meier survival curve analysis of quartiles of on-treatment CRP levels and MACE. The cumulative incidence of MACE in patients with the lowest quartile of on-treatment CRP was 5.9% in comparison with 9.5% in those with the highest quartile of baseline coronary PAV ($P = 0.06$). CRP indicates C-reactive protein; MACE, major adverse cardiovascular events; and PAV, percent atheroma volume. (Reprinted from Puri R, Nissen SE, Libby P, et al. C-reactive protein, but not low-density lipoprotein cholesterol levels, associate with coronary atheroma regression and cardiovascular events after maximally intensive statin therapy. *Circulation.* 2013;128:2395-2403, Copyright 2013, with permission from American Heart Association, Inc.)

TABLE 3.—Ultrasonic Measures of Atheroma Volume and Vascular Dimensions

IVUS Parameter	Total (n = 985)	Change From Baseline CRP: No Increase (n = 621)	Change From Baseline CRP: Increase (n = 364)	*P* Value*
Percent atheroma volume, %				
Baseline	36.4 ± 8.2	36.6 ± 8.0	36.0 ± 8.4	0.29
Change from baseline	−1.23 ± 0.09	−1.42 ± 0.11	−0.91 ± 0.15	0.007
P value for change from baseline	<0.001	<0.001	<0.001	
Lumen volume, mm^3				
Baseline	248.0 ± 87.8	248.8 ± 86.8	246.6 ± 89.7	0.54
Change from baseline	1.08 ± 0.93	2.30 ± 1.17	−1.00 ± 1.53	0.09
P value for change from baseline	0.25	0.05	0.52	
EEM volume, mm^3				
Baseline	392.2 ± 134.9	394.8 ± 134.6	387.7 ± 135.3	0.40
Change from baseline	−6.11 ± 1.17	−5.40 ± 1.47	−7.33 ± 1.92	0.43
P value for change from baseline	<0.001	<0.001	<0.001	

Baseline and follow-up values are reported as mean ± SD, and change values are reported as least squares mean ± SE. CRP indicates C-reactive protein; EEM, external elastic membrane; IVUS, intravascular ultrasound; SD, standard deviation; and SE, standard error.

*P value reflects comparisons between groups dichotomized according to change in CRP level.

that the patients who experienced the greatest reductions in risk for cardiovascular events were able to achieve both an LDL cholesterol <70 mg/dL and a CRP <1.0 mg/L.[3-5]

The Study of Coronary Atheroma by Intravascular Ultrasound: Effect of Rosuvastatin versus Atorvastatin (SATURN) compared 2 high-dose regimens of statin therapy (rosuvastatin 40 mg daily and atorvastatin 80 mg daily) in patients with established coronary artery disease and evaluated their impact on rates of target atherosclerotic plaque progression.[6] There was a difference between groups in the primary outcome of change in percent atheroma volume. In this post hoc analysis, the authors evaluate the impact of on-treatment changes in CRP on disease progression. Compared with patients who experienced an increase of CRP during the course of the trial, those with no increase had significantly greater regression of target lesions (Table 1 in the original article). In both unadjusted and multivariable adjusted models, on-treatment CRP correlated with risk for major coronary events whereas LDL cholesterol did not (Fig 1). There was a rising gradient of risk for major coronary events as CRP levels rose (Fig 2).

These results are remarkable and suggest that CRP contributes significantly to likelihood of disease progression or regression. To date CRP is regarded as a risk biomarker. However, it is possible it may evolve into a target of therapy. Multiple trials are underway to test this hypothesis. In the meantime, it is reasonable to intensify lifestyle modification in patients whose CRP is elevated despite intensive background therapy for risk factor burden.

P. P. Toth, MD, PhD

References

1. Ross R. Atherosclerosis—an inflammatory disease. *N Engl J Med.* 1999;340: 115-126.
2. Libby P. Inflammation in atherosclerosis. *Nature.* 2002;420:868-874.
3. Ridker PM, MacFadyen J, Libby P, Glynn RJ. Relation of baseline high-sensitivity C-reactive protein level to cardiovascular outcomes with rosuvastatin in the Justification for Use of statins in Prevention: an Intervention Trial Evaluating Rosuvastatin (JUPITER). *Am J Cardiol.* 2010;106:204-209.
4. Ridker PM, Cannon CP, Morrow D, et al. C-reactive protein levels and outcomes after statin therapy. *N Engl J Med.* 2005;352:20-28.
5. Morrow DA, de Lemos JA, Sabatine MS, et al. Clinical relevance of C-reactive protein during follow-up of patients with acute coronary syndromes in the Aggrastat-to-Zocor Trial. *Circulation.* 2006;114:281-288.
6. Nicholls SJ, Ballantyne CM, Barter PJ, et al. Effect of two intensive statin regimens on progression of coronary disease. *N Engl J Med.* 2011;365:2078-2087.

AMG145, a Monoclonal Antibody Against Proprotein Convertase Subtilisin Kexin Type 9, Significantly Reduces Lipoprotein(a) in Hypercholesterolemic Patients Receiving Statin Therapy: An Analysis From the LDL-C Assessment With Proprotein Convertase Subtilisin Kexin Type 9 Monoclonal Antibody Inhibition Combined With Statin Therapy (LAPLACE)–Thrombolysis in Myocardial Infarction (TIMI) 57 Trial

Desai NR, Kohli P, Giugliano RP, et al (Brigham and Women's Hosp, Boston, MA; et al)

Circulation 128:962-969, 2013

Background.—Lipoprotein(a) [Lp(a)] is an emerging risk factor for cardiovascular disease. Currently, there are few available therapies to lower Lp(a). We sought to evaluate the impact of AMG145, a monoclonal antibody against proprotein convertase subtilisin kexin type 9 (PCSK9), on Lp(a).

Methods and Results.—As part of the LDL-C Assessment With PCSK9 Monoclonal Antibody Inhibition Combined With Statin Therapy (LAPLACE)–Thrombolysis in Myocardial Infarction (TIMI) 57 trial, 631 patients with hypercholesterolemia receiving statin therapy were randomized to receive AMG145 at 1 of 3 different doses every 2 weeks or 1 of 3 different doses every 4 weeks versus placebo. Lp(a) and other lipid parameters were measured at baseline and at week 12. Compared with

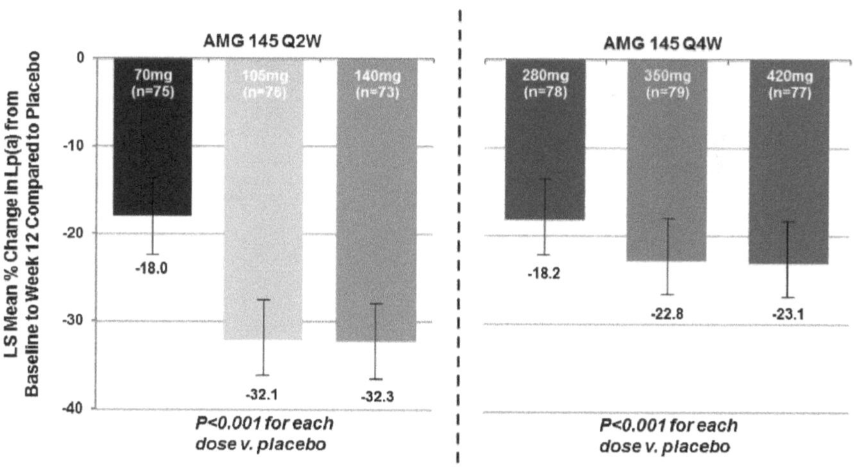

FIGURE 1.—Least squares (LS) mean percent change in lipoprotein(a) [Lp(a)] from baseline to week 12 among subjects with Lp(a) assessed at both of those time points (n = 612). The mean percent change was +3.4% for placebo every 2 weeks (Q2W) and −0.08% for placebo every 4 weeks (Q4W). The bars show the mean percent change by AMG145 treatment arm compared with the corresponding placebo. Error bars depict the standard error. (Reprinted from Desai NR, Kohli P, Giugliano RP, et al. AMG145, a monoclonal antibody against proprotein convertase subtilisin kexin type 9, significantly reduces lipoprotein(a) in hypercholesterolemic patients receiving statin therapy: an analysis from the LDL-C Assessment With Proprotein Convertase Subtilisin Kexin Type 9 Monoclonal Antibody Inhibition Combined With Statin Therapy (LAPLACE)–Thrombolysis in Myocardial Infarction (TIMI) 57 trial. *Circulation.* 2013;128:962-969, with permission from American Heart Association, Inc.)

placebo, AMG145 70 mg, 105 mg, and 140 mg every 2 weeks reduced Lp(a) at 12 weeks by 18%, 32%, and 32%, respectively ($P < 0.001$ for each dose versus placebo). Likewise, AMG145 280 mg, 350 mg, and 420 mg every 4 weeks reduced Lp(a) by 18%, 23%, and 23%, respectively ($P < 0.001$ for each dose versus placebo). The reduction in Lp(a) correlated with the reduction in low-density lipoprotein cholesterol ($\rho = 0.33$, $P < 0.001$). The effect of AMG145 on Lp(a) was consistent regardless of age, sex, race, history of diabetes mellitus, and background statin regimen. Patients with higher levels of Lp(a) at baseline had larger absolute reductions but comparatively smaller percent reductions in Lp(a) with AMG145 compared with those with lower baseline Lp(a) values.

Conclusions.—AMG145 significantly reduces Lp(a), by up to 32%, among subjects with hypercholesterolemia receiving statin therapy, offering an additional, complementary benefit beyond robust low-density

A

Subgroup	AMG 145 140mg Q2W N	AMG 145 140mg Q2W Δ	Placebo Q2W N	Placebo Q2W Δ	P-int
Baseline Lp(a) Level					0.003
Below limit of detection	8	0.0	7	0.1	
Quartile 1	15	-5.0	20	1.8	
Quartile 2	13	-13.7	17	-0.3	
Quartile 3	23	-23.4	12	-0.9	
Quartile 4	14	-49.1	21	-8.5	

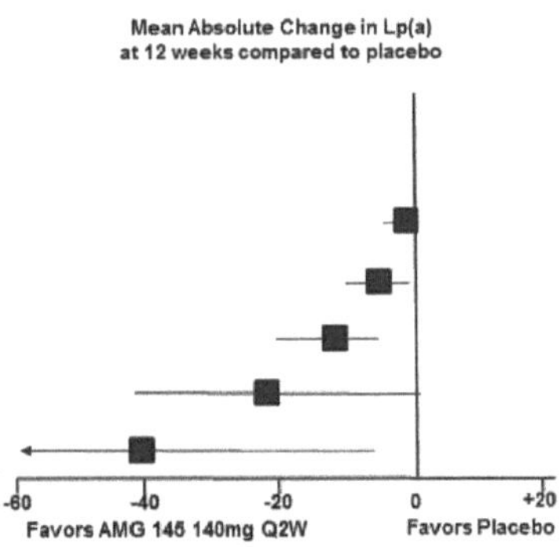

B

Subgroup	AMG 145 420mg Q4W N	AMG 145 420mg Q4W Δ	Placebo Q4W N	Placebo Q4W Δ	P-int
Baseline Lp(a) Level					0.32
Below limit of detection	8	0.2	6	0.2	
Quartile 1	10	-4.4	19	0.9	
Quartile 2	19	-14.3	16	-1.2	
Quartile 3	19	-21.8	25	-3.0	
Quartile 4	21	-54.7	11	-39.7	

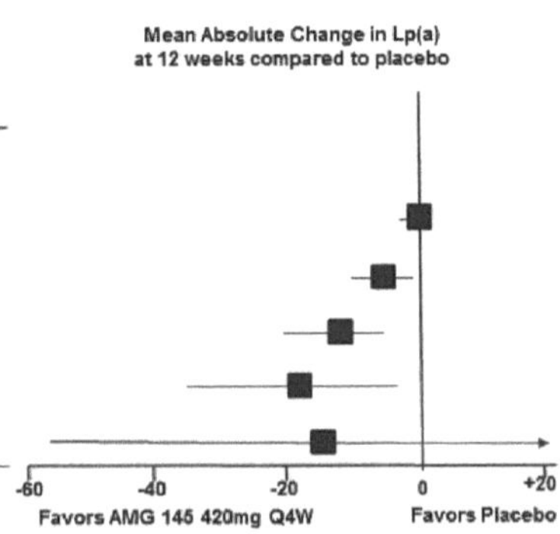

FIGURE 5.—Forest plot of the mean absolute change in lipoprotein(a) [Lp(a)] from baseline to week 12 for AMG145 140 mg every 2 weeks (Q2W; **A**) and AMG145 420 mg every 4 weeks (Q4W; **B**) across quartiles of baseline Lp(a). (Reprinted from Desai NR, Kohli P, Giugliano RP, et al. AMG145, a monoclonal antibody against proprotein convertase subtilisin kexin type 9, significantly reduces lipoprotein(a) in hypercholesterolemic patients receiving statin therapy: an analysis from the LDL-C Assessment With Proprotein Convertase Subtilisin Kexin Type 9 Monoclonal Antibody Inhibition Combined With Statin Therapy (LAPLACE)–Thrombolysis in Myocardial Infarction (TIMI) 57 trial. *Circulation.* 2013;128:962-969, Copyright 2013, with permission from American Heart Association, Inc.)

lipoprotein cholesterol reduction with regard to a patient's atherogenic lipid profile (Figs 1 and 5).

▶ Lipoprotein(a) is widely recognized as a risk factor for atherosclerotic disease.[1,2] Niacin is currently the only approved lipid-modifying agent that can reduce serum levels of Lp(a). However, there is no evidence that lowering Lp(a) with niacin impacts risk for atherosclerotic cardiovascular disease (ASCVD) events. Given the strength of association between Lp(a) levels and risk for ASCVD, new pharmacologic interventions that impact serum levels of this lipoprotein are urgently needed so we can better ascertain through prospective, randomized clinical trials whether reducing this moiety results in reduced risk for acute cardiovascular events.

The monoclonal antibodies against PCSK9 show significant capacity to reduce serum levels of Lp(a). Desai et al show in the LDL-C Assessment With PCSK9 Monoclonal Antibody Inhibition Combined With Statin Therapy (LAPLACE)—Thrombolysis in Myocardial Infarction (TIMI) 57 trial, that AMG 145 given every 2 weeks can reduce Lp(a) by about one-third (Fig 1). The magnitude of Lp(a) reduction is directly related to baseline level of this lipoprotein: higher levels correlate with larger absolute reductions from baseline (Fig 5).

With major outcomes trials underway with PCSK9 monoclonal antibodies, it is possible that benefit from Lp(a) reduction will be discerned. This would be an exciting development and a major advance toward reducing residual risk. It remains to be seen if different isoforms of Lp(a) are reduced to differing degrees by these agents.

P. P. Toth, MD, PhD

References

1. Davidson MH, Ballantyne CM, Jacobson TA, et al. Clinical utility of inflammatory markers and advanced lipoprotein testing: advice from an expert panel of lipid specialists. *J Clin Lipidol.* 2011;5:338-367.
2. Nordestgaard BG, Chapman MJ, Ray K, et al. Lipoprotein(a) as a cardiovascular risk factor: current status. *Eur Heart J.* 2010;31:2844-2853.

Low High-Density Lipoprotein Cholesterol Is Not a Risk Factor for Recurrent Vascular Events in Patients With Vascular Disease on Intensive Lipid-Lowering Medication

van de Woestijne AP, for the SMART Study Group (Univ Med Ctr Utrecht, the Netherlands; et al)

J Am Coll Cardiol 62:1834-1841, 2013

Objectives.—This study sought to evaluate the vascular risk of low high-density lipoprotein-cholesterol (HDL-C) in relation to the use and intensity of lipid-lowering medication in patients with clinically manifest vascular diseases.

Background.—Low levels of HDL-C are associated with an increased risk for vascular diseases and may contribute to residual vascular risk in patients already treated for other risk factors. However, post-hoc analyses from statin trials indicate that the vascular risk associated with low HDL-C may be low or even absent in patients using intensive statin therapy.

Methods.—We performed a prospective cohort study of 6,111 patients with manifest vascular disease. Cox proportional hazards models were used to evaluate the risk of HDL-C on vascular events in patients using no, usual dose, or intensive lipid-lowering therapy.

Results.—New vascular events (myocardial infarction, stroke, or vascular death) occurred in 874 subjects during a median follow-up of 5.4 years (interquartile range: 2.9 to 8.6 years). In patients not using lipid-lowering medication at baseline (n = 2,153), a 0.1 mmol/l increase in HDL-C was associated with a 5% reduced risk for all vascular events (hazard ratio [HR]: 0.95; 95% confidence interval [CI]: 0.92 to 0.99). In patients on usual dose lipid-lowering medication (n = 1,910) there was a 6% reduced risk (HR: 0.94; 95% CI: 0.90 to 0.98). However, in patients using intensive lipid-lowering treatment (n = 2,046), HDL-C was not associated with recurrent vascular events (HR: 1.02; 95% CI: 0.98 to 1.07) irrespective of low-density lipoprotein cholesterol level.

Conclusions.—In patients with clinically manifest vascular disease using no or usual dose lipid-lowering medication, low plasma HDL-C levels are related to increased vascular risk, whereas in patients using intensive lipid-lowering medication, HDL-C levels are not related to vascular risk (Fig 1).

▶ Confusion continues to reign with respect to the role of high-density lipoprotein cholesterol (HDL-C) in the prevention and management of atherosclerotic cardiovascular disease (ASCVD). For decades, prospective epidemiologic cohorts from around the world have consistently shown that HDL-C is among the most important of risk factors for ASCVD. To date, however, no prospective, randomized, controlled clinical trial using HDL-C—raising agents have been able to show a benefit on ASCVD outcomes.[1-3] Do we have it wrong when it comes to HDL-C? Is the relationship between HDL-C and ASCVD simply an epidemiologic epiphenomenon? Is a low HDL-C noncontributory to ASCVD risk once atherogenic lipoprotein burden in serum is reduced significantly by lipid-lowering therapies?

The Second Manifestation of ARTerial (SMART) disease cohort was probed to discern the impact of low HDL-C on risk for ASCVD events. This cohort comprises 6123 patients with established vascular disease (coronary artery disease, peripheral vascular disease, cerebrovascular disease, or aortic aneurysm). The investigators evaluated the impact of low HDL-C on risk for ASCVD events over a median of 5.4 years in patients on no lipid-lowering therapy, usual dose (reduce low-density lipoprotein cholesterol [LDL-C] < 30%), or intensive lipid-lowering therapy (reduce LDL-C > 45%). Among patients on no or usual intensity of lipid-lowering therapy, increasing serum HDL-C correlated with reductions in risk for ASCVD events (Fig 1). However, among patients on intensive lipid-lowering therapy, increased HDL-C had no impact on risk

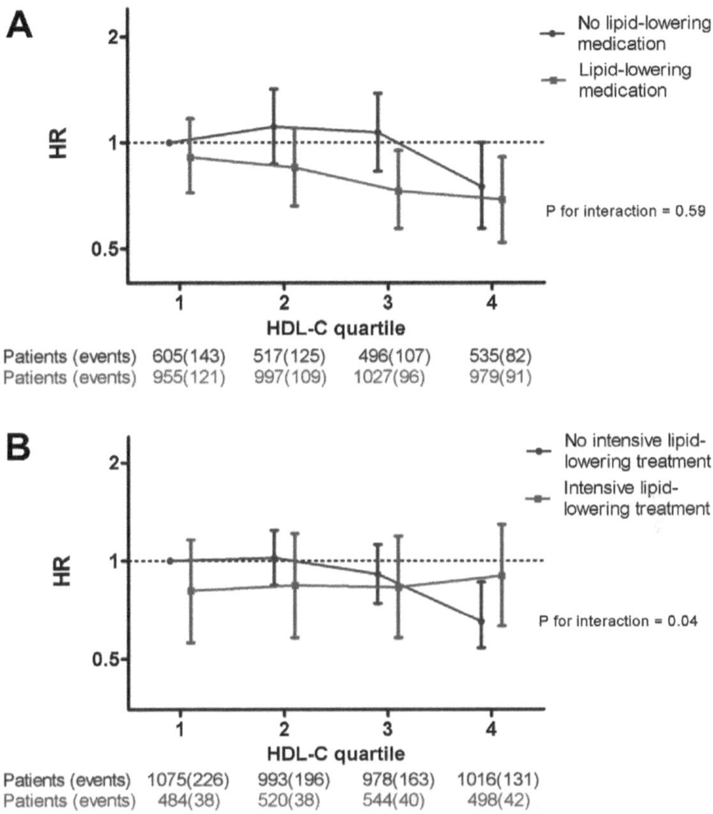

FIGURE 1.—Risk for All Vascular Events Across Quartiles of HDL-C (**A**) Hazard ratio (HR) (95% confidence interval) by increasing quartiles of high-density lipoprotein cholesterol (HDL-C), stratified for yes versus no lipid-lowering therapy, adjusted for age, sex, body mass index, type 2 diabetes mellitus, plasma triglyceride level, alcohol use, and smoking. (**B**) HR (95% confidence interval) by increasing quartiles of HDL-C, stratified for yes versus no intensive lipid-lowering therapy (defined as ≥40% low-density lipoprotein cholesterol reduction), adjusted for age, sex, body mass index, type 2 diabetes mellitus, plasma triglyceride level, alcohol use, and smoking. The reference group includes both patients using no lipid-lowering medication and patients using usual dose lipid-lowering medication. (Reprinted from van de Woestijne AP, for the SMART Study Group. Low high-density lipoprotein cholesterol is not a risk factor for recurrent vascular events in patients with vascular disease on intensive lipid-lowering medication. *J Am Coll Cardiol.* 2013;62:1834-1841, with permission from the American College of Cardiology Foundation.)

for ASCVD events. HDL-C in the latter patients did not correlate with risk for myocardial infarction (MI), ischemic stroke, or vascular death.

These findings are largely consistent with those of the JUPITER[4] and PROVE-IT[5] trials, which no showed relationship between HDL-C and risk in patients treated with intensive statin therapy and aggressive LDL-C reduction. This may help partly explain why such studies as AIM-HIGH[3] and HPS-2 THRIVE (http://www.ctsu.ox.ac.uk/~thrive/), which randomly assigned patients on aggressive lipid-lowering therapy and very low atherogenic lipoprotein burden in serum to placebo versus niacin, were negative. Of note, however, the SMART cohort suggests that a low HDL-C remains a significant risk factor in patients on no lipid-lowering medication and in those receiving low-intensity therapy that reduces LDL-C less than 30%. This important finding will require confirmation in other studies. In the meantime, current guidelines do not specify HDL-C levels as a target for therapeutic intervention.[6,7]

P. P. Toth, MD, PhD

References

1. Schwartz GG, Olsson AG, Ballantyne CM, et al. Rationale and design of the dal-OUTCOMES trial: efficacy and safety of dalcetrapib in patients with recent acute coronary syndrome. *Am Heart J.* 2009;158:896-901.e3.
2. Barter PJ, Caulfield M, Eriksson M, et al. Effects of torcetrapib in patients at high risk for coronary events. *N Engl J Med.* 2007;357:2109-2122.
3. Boden WE, Probstfield JL, Anderson T, et al. Niacin in patients with low HDL cholesterol levels receiving intensive statin therapy. *N Engl J Med.* 2011;365: 2255-2267.
4. Ridker PM, Genest J, Boekholdt SM, et al. HDL cholesterol and residual risk of first cardiovascular events after treatment with potent statin therapy: an analysis from the JUPITER trial. *Lancet.* 2010;376:333-339.
5. Ray KK, Cannon CP, Cairns R, Morrow DA, Ridker PM, Braunwald E. Prognostic utility of apoB/AI, total cholesterol/HDL, non-HDL cholesterol, or hs-CRP as predictors of clinical risk in patients receiving statin therapy after acute coronary syndromes: results from PROVE IT-TIMI 22. *Arterioscler Thromb Vasc Biol.* 2009; 29:424-430.
6. Stone NJ, Robinson J, Lichtenstein AH, et al. 2013 ACC/AHA Guideline on the Treatment of Blood Cholesterol to Reduce Atherosclerotic Cardiovascular Risk in Adults: A Report of the American College of Cardiology/American Heart Association Task Force on Practice Guidelines. *Circulation.* 2013.
7. Toth PP, Barter PJ, Rosenson RS, et al. High-density lipoproteins: a consensus statement from the National Lipid Association. *J Clin Lipidol.* 2013;7:484-525.

Effect of the Proprotein Convertase Subtilisin/Kexin 9 Monoclonal Antibody, AMG 145, in Homozygous Familial Hypercholesterolemia

Stein EA, Honarpour N, Wasserman SM, et al (Metabolic and Atherosclerosis Research Ctr, Cincinnati, OH; Amgen Inc, Thousand Oaks, CA; et al)
Circulation 128:2113-2120, 2013

Background.—Homozygous familial hypercholesterolemia is a rare, serious disorder with a substantial reduction in low-density lipoprotein (LDL) receptor function, severely elevated LDL cholesterol, cardiovascular disease, and often death in childhood. Response to conventional drug therapies is modest. Monoclonal antibodies to proprotein convertase subtilisin/kexin 9 (PCSK9) reduce LDL cholesterol in heterozygous familial hypercholesterolemia. The effect in homozygous familial hypercholesterolemia is unknown and uncertain. We evaluated the efficacy and safety of AMG 145 in an open-label, single-arm, multicenter, dose-scheduling pilot study in patients with homozygous familial hypercholesterolemia.

Methods and Results.—Eight patients with LDL receptor–negative or –defective homozygous familial hypercholesterolemia on stable drug therapy were treated with subcutaneous 420 mg AMG 145 every 4 weeks for ≥12 weeks, followed by 420 mg AMG 145 every 2 weeks for an additional 12 weeks. All patients completed both treatment periods. Mean change from baseline in LDL cholesterol at week 12 was −16.5% (range, 5.2% to −43.6%; $P = 0.0781$) and −13.9% (range, 39.9% to −43.3%; $P = 0.1484$) with 4- and 2-week dosing, respectively. No reduction was seen in the 2 receptor—negative patients. Over the treatment periods, mean ± SD LDL cholesterol reductions in the 6 LDL receptor-defective patients were 19.3 ± 16% and 26.3 ± 20% with 4- and 2-week dosing, respectively ($P = 0.0313$ for both values), ranging from 4% to 48% with 2-week dosing. No serious side effects were reported.

Conclusion.—This study demonstrates significant and dose-related LDL cholesterol lowering with a PCSK9 monoclonal antibody in homozygous familial hypercholesterolemia patients with defective LDL receptor activity but no reduction in those who were receptor negative (Tables 1 and 3).

► Lomitapide (a microsomal triglyceride transfer protein inhibitor) and mipomersen (an oligonucleotide antisense inhibitor of apoprotein B100 mRNA translation) are both indicated for the treatment of homozygous familial hypercholesterolemia (HoFH). HoFH is highly associated with premature-onset multivessel coronary artery disease (CAD).[1] The disease is caused by the complete loss or near complete loss of low-density lipoprotein (LDL) receptor expression and activity. HoFH can be secondary to homozygous loss of LDL receptor functionality or to compound heterozygosity.[2] Negative receptor function and defective receptor function are defined as LDL receptor activity of less than 2% and 2% to 25%, respectively. A new drug class in phase 3 development comprises monoclonal antibodies directed against proprotein convertase/subtilisin/kexin 9 (PCSK9), an enzyme that functions as a chaperone molecule to guide LDL receptors into the lysosomal compartment for proteolytic degradation.[3] Loss of function mutations in the gene for PCSK9 are associated with reduced lifetime serum levels of LDL cholesterol (LDL-C) and decreased

TABLE 1.—Patient Genotypes

Patient	Mutation Allele 1 (Estimated LDLR Function)	Mutation Allele 2 (Estimated LDLR Function)	Overall LDLR Function
1	Asp266Glu (15%–30%)	Asp266Glu (15%–30%)	Receptor defective
2	1187-10 G>A* (not determined)	Asp266Glu (15%–30%)	Receptor defective
3	Asp224Asn (<2%)	Cys296Tyr (not determined)	Negative†
4	Deletion exons 4–18 (not determined)	Cys197Gly (not determined)	Negative†
5	Asp221Gly (<2%)	Asp227Glu (5%–15%)	Receptor defective
6‡§	Asp227Glu (5%–15%)	Asp227Glu (5%–15%)	Receptor defective
7‡§	Asp227Glu (5%–15%)	Asp227Glu (5%–15%)	Receptor defective
8	Asp175Asn (not determined)	Asp227Glu (5%–15%)	Receptor defective

LDLR indicates low-density lipoprotein receptor.
*Mutation at splice acceptor site 10 nucleotides upstream of the first nucleotide of exon 9, 1187.
†Confirmed by fibroblast culture.
‡True homozygous patient.
§Patients share the same genotype.

TABLE 3.—Efficacy Outcomes Based on Mutation Status

Mutation Status	Percentage Change From Baseline, Mean (SD), %					
	Week 12, Every-4-Week Dosing			Week 12, Every-2-Week Dosing		
	UC LDL-C	Apolipoprotein B	Lipoprotein(a)*	UC LDL-C	Apolipoprotein B	Lipoprotein(a)
Defective LDL receptor (n = 6)	−22.9 (17.5)	−18.3 (14.9)	−10.0 (11.5)	−23.6 (18.5)	−17.9 (18.0)	−18.7 (14.1)
Negative LDL receptor (n = 2)	2.6 (3.7)	−4.5 (3.5)	−16.8 (8.0)	15.3 (34.7)	3.4 (14.0)	−18.5 (5.3)
	Average of Week 4, 8, and 12, Every-4-Week Dosing			Average of Week 4, 8, and 12, Every-2-Week Dosing		
Defective LDL receptor (n = 6)	−19.3 (15.5) $P = 0.0313$[†]	−18.0 (13.1)	−10.0 (11.5)	−26.3 (20.4) ($P = 0.0313$)[†]	−22.1 (18.7)	−20.0 (12.1)
Negative LDL receptor (n = 2)	4.4 (10.3)	1.4 (5.6)	−16.8 (8.0)	11.0 (23.6)	2.1 (7.9)	−22.7 (11.2)

LDL indicates low-density lipoprotein; LDL-C, low-density lipoprotein cholesterol; and UC, ultracentrifugation.
*Lipoprotein(a) was collected only at week 12 for every-4-week dosing.
[†]Signed-rank test.

risk for atherosclerotic cardiovascular disease—related events.[4] When a monoclonal antibody binds to PCSK9, it induces steric hindrance and abolishes its ability to bind to LDL receptors. This results in a substantial elevation in LDL receptor expression and augmented LDL-C clearance from the systemic circulation with significant reduction in serum LDL-C.

In a proof-of-concept study, patients with HoFH were treated with PCSK9 monoclonal antibody AMG 145. Eight patients who were confirmed by genotyping to have receptor-negative or receptor-defective mutations were included (Table 1). As expected, the 2 receptor-negative patients did not experience a reduction in LDL-C (Table 2 in the original article). Receptor-defective patients experienced a significant reduction in LDL-C with both dosing regimens of AMG 145. Of interest, all patients experienced an approximately 20% reduction in serum levels of lipoprotein(a) (Lp[a]), a finding that is not yet explained, especially because it was also observed in the patients who were receptor negative.

It would be intuitively apparent that a monoclonal antibody directed against PCSK9 would not lower serum LDL-C in patients homozygous for LDL receptor—negative polymorphisms. Compound heterozygotes or patients homozygous for receptor-defective mutations do experience a significant reduction in LDL-C. Consequently, genotyping in these patients will likely turn out to be of some value. It is also intriguing that these patients all experienced a similar reduction in Lp(a), an effect likely mediated via a mechanism that is independent of the LDL receptor and yet to be identified. The PCSK9 monoclonal antibodies may provide benefit because of their capacity to lower Lp(a). This is certainly a possibility that warrants intensive investigation given the consistency between epidemiology, genomewide association studies, and mechanistic studies evaluating the relationship between Lp(a) and atherosclerosis.

P. P. Toth, MD, PhD

References

1. Goldberg AC, Hopkins PN, Toth PP, et al. Familial hypercholesterolemia: screening, diagnosis and management of pediatric and adult patients: clinical guidance from the National Lipid Association Expert Panel on Familial Hypercholesterolemia. *J Clin Lipidol.* 2011;5:S1-S8.
2. Watts GF, Gidding S, Wierzbicki AS, et al. Integrated guidance on the care of familial hypercholesterolaemia from the International FH Foundation. *Int J Cardiol.* 2014;171:309-325.
3. Abifadel M, Varret M, Rabes JP, et al. Mutations in PCSK9 cause autosomal dominant hypercholesterolemia. *Nat Genet.* 2003;34:154-156.
4. Cohen JC, Boerwinkle E, Mosley TH Jr, Hobbs HH. Sequence variations in PCSK9, low LDL, and protection against coronary heart disease. *N Engl J Med.* 2006;354:1264-1272.

Prevention of Atherosclerosis

High-Density Lipoprotein Mediated Cellular Cholesterol Efflux in Acute Coronary Syndromes

Hafiane A, Jabor B, Ruel I, et al (McGill Univ Faculty of Medicine, Montreal, Quebec, Canada)

Am J Cardiol 113:249-255, 2014

Systemic inflammation at the development of an acute coronary syndrome (ACS) might alter the high-density lipoprotein (HDL) components and function. One of the major functions of HDL particles is their ability to remove cellular cholesterol from macrophages. The aim of the present study was to characterize the HDL efflux capacity in patients with ACS. We analyzed the cholesterol efflux in those ACS (within 72 hours of symptoms [ACS1]) and, again, 3 months later (ACS2). As controls, we used normal subjects without coronary artery disease (CAD) and patients with chronic, stable CAD. The 4 groups were matched for age and HDL cholesterol levels. We used a cell-based efflux system in ^{3}[H]-cholesterol–labeled J774 macrophages to measure cholesterol efflux from apolipoprotein B–depleted plasma. The present study included 20 patients with ACS. Their mean age was 58 ± 9 years, and the mean HDL cholesterol level was 1.06 ± 0.22 mmol/L (41 ± 9 mg/dl). The ACS1 group showed a marked increase in high-sensitivity C-reactive protein and serum amyloid A, reflecting systemic inflammation. The HDL cholesterol efflux capacity was reduced in ACS1 subjects and remained reduced 12 weeks later and in those with stable CAD. These results suggest that the acute presence of serum amyloid A does not account for the impairment of HDL-mediated cholesterol efflux capacity in the ACS1 group. Little correlation was found between HDL cholesterol and HDL efflux capacity ($r = 0.233$; $p = 0.049$), suggesting that HDL cholesterol is a poor marker of HDL function in inflammatory states and CAD. In conclusion, our data support the concept that atherogenic HDL dysfunction and impaired efflux occur in ACS, independent of changes in plasma HDL cholesterol and apolipoprotein A-I levels (Fig 1, Table 1).

► Among the most important functions attributed to high-density lipoprotein (HDL) particles is the ability to engage in reverse cholesterol transport (RCT), a series of reactions by which cholesterol is removed from macrophage foam cells in the subendothelial space and returned to the liver for disposal. If RCT is impaired, then vascular wall lipid homeostasis becomes disrupted, and net accumulation of lipid potentiates atherosclerosis.[1] The capacity of HDL particles to promote lipid externalization from macrophages correlates with risk for coronary artery disease (CAD).[2] Studies that define HDL as dysfunctional most frequently attribute this to impaired capacity to antagonize oxidative and proinflammatory reactions. It is also important to establish if the dysfunction induced by CAD is also associated with reduced capacity to stimulate cholesterol and lipid efflux from macrophages.

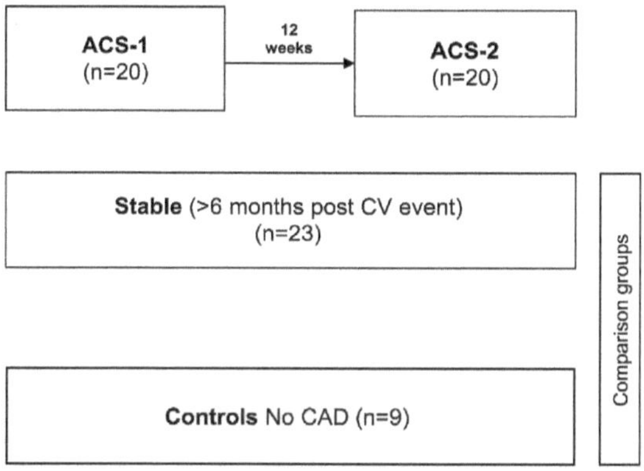

FIGURE 1.—Schematic diagram of study protocol. (Reprinted from the American Journal of Cardiology. Hafiane A, Jabor B, Ruel I, et al. High-Density lipoprotein mediated cellular cholesterol efflux in acute coronary syndromes. *Am J Cardiol.* 2014;113:249-255, Copyright 2014, with permission from Elsevier.)

TABLE 1.—Patient Characteristics

Variable	ACS1 (n = 20)	ACS2 (n = 20)	CAD (n = 23)	Controls (n = 9)
Age (yrs)	58.1 ± 8.9	58.3 ± 8.8	61.6 ± 9.5	56.2 ± 17.5
Male gender	16 (80)	16 (80)	21 (91)	8 (89)
Hypertension	5	5	10	5
ACS NSTEMI/STEMI	4/16	4/16	6/15	0/0
Smoking	7 (35)	7 (35)	2 (9)	0
Diabetes	5 (25)	5 (25)	2 (7)	0
BMI (kg/m^2)	27.3 ± 4.2	27.5 ± 4.3	27.8 ± 3.6	34.0 ± 6.4*
Total cholesterol (mmol/L; mg/dl)	4.24 ± 0.87 (164.0 ± 33.6)	3.12 ± 0.63 (120.5 ± 24.4)†	3.86 ± 0.61 (149.4 ± 23.7)	5.10 ± 0.80 (197.2 ± 31.1)‡
TG (mmol/L; mg/dl)	1.56 ± 0.89 (138.4 ± 79.0)	1.12 ± 0.44 (99.4 ± 39.2)‡	1.52 ± 0.97 (134.7 ± 85.7)	2.16 ± 0.77 (191.1 ± 68.1)
HDL cholesterol (mmol/L; mg/dl)	1.06 ± 0.22 (41.1 ± 8.7)	1.04 ± 0.28 (40.4 ± 11.0)	1.10 ± 0.30 (42.5 ± 11.5)	1.11 ± 0.20 (43.0 ± 7.8)
LDL cholesterol (mmol/L; mg/dl)	2.47 ± 0.70 (95.5 ± 27.1)	1.56 ± 0.39 (60.4 ± 15.2)†	2.08 ± 0.43 (80.2 ± 16.8)‡	3.01 ± 0.58 (116.2 ± 22.5)
apoA-I (g/L)	1.23 ± 0.25	1.28 ± 0.25	1.38 ± 0.26	1.44 ± 0.13‡
apoB (g/L)	0.91 ± 0.30	0.62 ± 0.11†	0.76 ± 0.14‡	0.98 ± 0.20
hs-CRP (mg/L)	37.95 ± 62.62	1.85 ± 1.35‡	1.50 ± 1.32‡	6.70 ± 11.04
SAA (ng/ml)	303.3 ± 123.7	100.8 ± 85.6†	61.6 ± 45.8†	116.8 ± 46.2†
Statin	6 (30)	6 (30)	23 (100)	0
Cholesterol efflux	16.9 ± 2.8	17.0 ± 3.2	15.4 ± 7.0	25.9 ± 6.1†

Data are presented as mean ± SD or n (%).
For cholesterol conversion to mg/dl, multiply by 38.67, and for triglycerides, multiply by 88.57.
The level of significance is indicated for pairwise comparisons between ACS1 and other groups: *$p < 0.01$; †$p < 0.001$; ‡$p < 0.05$.
apoA-I = apolipoprotein A-I; apoB = apolipoprotein B; BMI = body mass index; hs-CRP = high sensitivity C-reactive protein; LDL = low-density lipoprotein; NSTEMI = non–ST-segment elevation myocardial infarction; STEMI = ST-segment elevation myocardial infarction; TG = triglycerides.

Hafiane et al investigated whether HDL-induced lipid efflux is impaired in patients who sustained an acute coronary syndrome (ACS). Twenty patients with ACS were included. Efflux capacity was measured at baseline and after

12 weeks of therapy. ACS patients were compared with patients with stable ischemic heart disease (SIHD) and healthy controls without CAD. Not unexpectedly, efflux capacity correlated weakly with HDL cholesterol (HDL-C) levels. Despite having similar baseline levels of HDL-C (Table 1), the efflux capacity of the HDL extracted from patients with ACS, both at baseline and after 12 weeks, and the patients with SIHD were reduced to nearly identical levels compared with healthy controls (Fig 1). Of great interest, despite therapeutic intervention, the efflux capacity of the patients with ACS remained impaired. After ACS, HDL particles became significantly enriched with serum amyloid A, consistent with enrichment of the particle with acute-phase reactants and displacement of components of the HDL proteome.

This study suggests that SIHD and ACS reduce HDL efflux capacity to a nearly identical degree. It is also fascinating that efflux capacity remained depressed even 12 weeks after an ACS despite therapeutic interventions. There is urgent need to quantify more precisely how much HDL dysfunction, either through loss of efflux capacity/rates of RCT or secondary to reduced capacity to antagonize oxidation, inflammation, and endothelial dysfunction, contributes to residual risk. This is especially true of patients who sustain an ACS or who have unstable disease despite maximally intensive therapy and yet continue to experience recurrent ACS or require frequent percutaneous revascularization.

P. P. Toth, MD, PhD

References

1. Toth PP. Reverse cholesterol transport: high-density lipoprotein's magnificent mile. *Curr Atheroscler Rep*. 2003;5:386-393.
2. Khera AV, Cuchel M, de la Llera-Moya M, et al. Cholesterol efflux capacity, high-density lipoprotein function, and atherosclerosis. *N Engl J Med*. 2011;364:127-135.

Lack of protective role of HDL-C in patients with coronary artery disease undergoing elective coronary artery bypass grafting

Angeloni E, Paneni F, Landmesser U, et al (Univ of Rome 'Sapienza', Italy; IRCCS Neuromed, Pozzilli, Italy; Univ Hosp Zürich, Switzerland)
Eur Heart J 34:3557-3562, 2013

Aims.—Primary prevention studies have confirmed that high-density lipoprotein cholesterol (HDL-C) levels are strongly associated with reduced cardiovascular events. However, recent evidence suggests that HDL-C functionality may be impaired under certain conditions. In the present study, we hypothesize that HDL-C may lose their protective role in the secondary prevention of coronary artery disease (CAD).

Methods and Results.—A consecutive series of 1548 patients undergoing isolated first-time elective CABG at one institution between 2004 and 2009 was studied. According to the ATPIII criteria, pre-operative HDL-C values were used to identify patients with high (Group A) vs.

low HDL-C (Group B). To eliminate biased estimates, a propensity score model was built and two cohorts of 1:1 optimally matched patients were obtained. Cumulative survival and major adverse cardiovascular events (MACE) were analysed by means of Kaplan–Meier method. Cox proportional-hazards regression models were used to identify independent predictors of MACE and death. Propensity matching identified two cohorts of 502 patients each. At a median follow-up time of 32 months, there were 44 out of 502 (8.8%) deaths in Group A and 36 out of 502 deaths in Group B (7.2%, HR 1.19; $P = 0.42$). MACE occurred in 165 out of 502 (32.9%) in Group A and 120 out of 502 (23.9%) in Group B ($P = 0.04$). Regression analysis showed that pre-operative HDL-C levels were not associated with reduced but rather increased MACE occurrence during follow-up (HR 1.43, $P = 0.11$).

Conclusion.—Higher HDL-C levels are not associated with reduced risk of vascular events in CAD patients undergoing CABG. Our findings may support efforts to improve HDL-C functionality instead of increasing their levels.

▶ The high-density lipoproteins (HDLs) carry several components as part of their proteome and lipidome. The HDLs also transport microRNAs. It is believed that the specific molecular cargo they are endowed with at any given time modulates their capacity to engage in such anti-atherogenic activities as reverse cholesterol transport, reverse endothelial cell dysfunction, reduce oxidative and inflammatory tone, decrease platelet activation, and even regulate islet cell insulin secretion.[1,2] The functionality of HDLs has been found to be impaired in several pathophysiologic states, including coronary artery disease (CAD),[3] chronic kidney disease,[4] and rheumatologic disease.[5] Given these findings, there is emerging consensus that HDL cholesterol (HDL-C) is not likely to emerge as a meaningful therapeutic target. Focus is turning toward therapeutic modulation of HDL particle functionality.

Adding to this burgeoning literature is a study by Angeloni et al who evaluated the functionality of HDL particles in patients with CAD undergoing coronary artery bypass grafting (CABG). These investigators evaluated the impact of high and low levels of HDL-C (< 40 mg/dL in men and < 50 mg/dL in women) on outcomes in 1548 patients. High HDL-C was associated with trends for a 33% increase in mortality (Fig 1 in the original article) and a 41% increase in risk for major acute coronary events (Fig 2 in the original article), although these did not achieve statistical significance.

This study confirms the findings of others that in patients with CAD, HDL-C loses at least some of its capacity to protect against atherosclerotic cardiovascular disease events. The heightened systemic inflammation associated with CAD is known to induce the substitution of key anti-oxidative and anti-inflammatory components with acute phase reactants. The authors correctly point out that until this issue is understood in greater detail, it is perhaps harmful to engage in therapeutic effort to increase HDL if the particles are dysfunctional and possibly incurring vascular injury. The statins have been found to convert dysfunctional HDL from a proinflammatory phenotype to an anti-inflammatory one.[6]

P. P. Toth, MD, PhD

References

1. Toth PP, Barter PJ, Rosenson RS, et al. High-density lipoproteins: a consensus statement from the National Lipid Association. *J Clin Lipidol.* 2013;7:484-525.
2. Bays HE, Toth PP, Kris-Etherton PM, et al. Obesity, adiposity, and dyslipidemia: a consensus statement from the National Lipid Association. *J Clin Lipidol.* 2013;7: 304-383.
3. Ansell BJ. Targeting the anti-inflammatory effects of high-density lipoprotein. *Am J Cardiol.* 2007;100:3-9.
4. Yamamoto S, Yancey PG, Ikizler TA, et al. Dysfunctional high-density lipoprotein in patients on chronic hemodialysis. *J Am Coll Cardiol.* 2012;60:2372-2379.
5. Dessein PH, Stanwix AE, Joffe BI. Cardiovascular risk in rheumatoid arthritis versus osteoarthritis: acute phase response related decreased insulin sensitivity and high-density lipoprotein cholesterol as well as clustering of metabolic syndrome features in rheumatoid arthritis. *Arthritis Res.* 2002;4:R5.
6. Navab M, Anantharamaiah GM, Reddy ST, Van Lenten BJ, Ansell BJ, Fogelman AM. Mechanisms of disease: proatherogenic HDL—an evolving field. *Nat Clin Pract Endocrinol Metab.* 2006;2:504-511.

Statin Safety

Lipid-Modifying Therapies and Risk of Pancreatitis: A Meta-analysis

Preiss D, Tikkanen MJ, Welsh P, et al (Univ of Glasgow, UK; Helsinki Univ Hosp, Finland; et al)
JAMA 308:804-811, 2012

Context.—Statin therapy has been associated with pancreatitis in observational studies. Although lipid guidelines recommend fibrate therapy to reduce pancreatitis risk in persons with hypertriglyceridemia, fibrates may lead to the development of gallstones, a risk factor for pancreatitis.

Objective.—To investigate associations between statin or fibrate therapy and incident pancreatitis in large randomized trials.

Data Sources.—Relevant trials were identified in literature searches of MEDLINE, EMBASE, and Web of Science (January 1, 1994, for statin trials and January 1, 1972, for fibrate trials, through June 9, 2012). Published pancreatitis data were tabulated where available (6 trials). Unpublished data were obtained from investigators (22 trials).

Study Selection.—We included randomized controlled cardiovascular end-point trials investigating effects of statin therapy or fibrate therapy. Studies with more than 1000 participants followed up for more than 1 year were included.

Data Extraction.—Trial-specific data described numbers of participants developing pancreatitis and change in triglyceride levels at 1 year. Trial-specific risk ratios (RRs) were calculated and combined using random-effects model meta-analysis. Between-study heterogeneity was assessed using the I^2 statistic.

Results.—In 16 placebo- and standard care–controlled statin trials with 113 800 participants conducted over a weighted mean follow-up of 4.1 (SD, 1.5) years, 309 participants developed pancreatitis (134 assigned to statin, 175 assigned to control) (RR, 0.77 [95% CI, 0.62-0.97; $P = .03$; $I^2 = 0\%$]). In 5 dose-comparison statin trials with 39 614 participants conducted over 4.8 (SD, 1.7) years, 156 participants developed pancreatitis (70 assigned to intensive dose, 86 assigned to moderate dose) (RR, 0.82 [95% CI, 0.59-1.12; $P = .21$; $I^2 = 0\%$]). Combined results for all 21 statin trials provided RR 0.79 (95% CI, 0.65-0.95; $P = .01$; $I^2 = 0\%$). In 7 fibrate trials with 40 162 participants conducted over 5.3 (SD, 0.5) years, 144 participants developed pancreatitis (84 assigned to fibrate therapy, 60 assigned to placebo) (RR, 1.39 [95% CI, 1.00-1.95; $P = .053$; $I^2 = 0\%$]).

Conclusion.—In a pooled analysis of randomized trial data, use of statin therapy was associated with a lower risk of pancreatitis in patients with normal or mildly elevated triglyceride levels.

▶ Pancreatitis is a serious and potentially life-threatening complication of severe hypertriglyceridemia (SHTG). In patients with SHTG, it is generally recommended that risk for pancreatitis be reduced by treating patients with fibrates, high-dose fish oil, a low-fat diet, and intensive lifestyle modification so as to relieve any insulin resistance that might be exacerbating the SHTG. To date, none of these interventions had randomized data to support their application, although it makes intuitive sense to reduce exposure to triglycerides as much as possible.

In an intriguing meta-analysis by Preiss et al, the impact of statin and fibrate therapy on risk for pancreatitis was explored. These investigators pooled from 21 prospective randomized statin trials (16 statin vs placebo and 5 dose-comparison trials) and found a significant 21% ($P = .01$) reduction in risk for acute pancreatitis (Fig 1 in the original article). They also pooled data from 7 prospective randomized fibrate trials (including 2 with gemfibrozil, 2 with clofibrate, 1 with bezafibrate, and 2 with fenofibrate) and showed a trend for a 39% increased risk for pancreatitis ($P = .053$; number needed to harm over 5 years, 935; Fig 2 in the original article). In addition, meta-regression analysis found no relationship across the trials between risk of pancreatitis and triglyceride reduction with fibrate therapy after 1 year of therapy.

These data are intriguing. Although hypothesis generating only and requiring confirmation in a prospective randomized study, it possible that statin therapy is more efficacious for reducing risk of pancreatitis than the fibrates, despite a lower capacity to reduce serum triglycerides. One explanation for these findings may relate to the ability of statins to reduce the cholesterol content of bile, thereby reducing risk for gallstone pancreatitis. The impact of fish oils on risk for pancreatitis in patients with hypertriglyceridemia is being evaluated as a prespecified secondary endpoint in the REDUCE-IT trial using eicosapentaenoic acid monotherapy.

P. P. Toth, MD, PhD

Epidemiology and Diagnosis

Body Fat Distribution, Incident Cardiovascular Disease, Cancer, and All-Cause Mortality

Britton KA, Massaro JM, Murabito JM, et al (Brigham and Women's Hosp, Boston, MA; Boston Univ, MA; Framingham Heart Study, MA; et al)
J Am Coll Cardiol 62:921-925, 2013

Objectives.—The aim of this study was to determine whether ectopic fat depots are prospectively associated with cardiovascular disease, cancer, and all-cause mortality.

Background.—The morbidity associated with excess body weight varies among individuals of similar body mass index. Ectopic fat depots may underlie this risk differential. However, prospective studies of directly measured fat are limited.

Methods.—Participants from the Framingham Heart Study (n = 3,086; 49% women; mean age of 50.2 years) underwent assessment of fat depots (visceral adipose tissue, pericardial adipose tissue, and periaortic adipose tissue) using multidetector computed tomography and were followed up longitudinally for a median of 5.0 years. Cox proportional hazards regression models were used to examine the association of each fat depot (per 1 SD increment) with the risk of incident cardiovascular disease, cancer, and all-cause mortality after adjustment for standard risk factors, including body mass index.

Results.—Overall, there were 90 cardiovascular events, 141 cancer events, and 71 deaths. After multivariable adjustment, visceral adipose tissue was associated with cardiovascular disease (hazard ratio: 1.44; 95% confidence interval: 1.08 to 1.92; $p = 0.01$) and cancer (hazard ratio: 1.43; 95% confidence interval: 1.12 to 1.84; $p = 0.005$). Addition of visceral adipose tissue to a multivariable model that included body mass index modestly improved cardiovascular risk prediction (net reclassification improvement of 16.3%). None of the fat depots were associated with all-cause mortality.

Conclusions.—Visceral adiposity is associated with incident cardiovascular disease and cancer after adjustment for clinical risk factors and generalized adiposity. These findings support the growing appreciation of a pathogenic role of ectopic fat (Fig 2, Table 2).

▶ There is a global obesity epidemic. Obesity is widely credited with increasing the prevalence of metabolic syndrome, diabetes mellitus, and cardiovascular disease. The obesity paradox, however, casts lingering doubt about whether obesity is truly associated with increased morbidity and mortality, as in patients afflicted with coronary artery disease or congestive heart failure, obesity is associated with reduced mortality.[1,2] It is highly established that excess visceral fat serves multiple toxic functions, which include nonspecific free fatty acid release and increased inflammatory mediator and resistin expression, among others.[3]

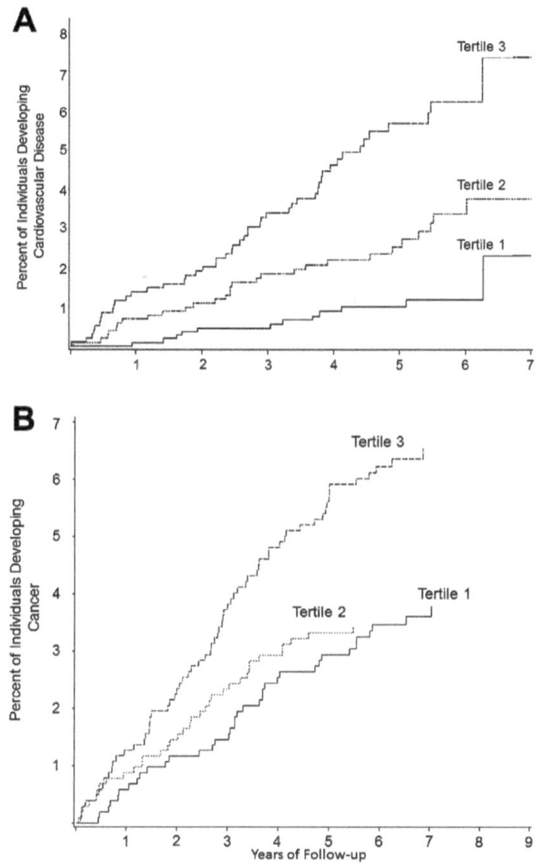

FIGURE 2.—Kaplan-Meier curve of time to cardiovascular disease and cancer by tertile of VAT Vertical axes show the percentage of subjects developing (**A**) cardiovascular disease and (**B**) cancer during follow-up; horizontal axes reflect years of follow-up. Tertile cutpoints for VAT are 1,242.2 and 2,168.4 cm^3. Abbreviation as in Figure 1. (Reprinted from the Journal of the American College of Cardiology. Britton KA, Massaro JM, Murabito JM, et al. Body fat distribution, incident cardiovascular disease, cancer, and all-cause mortality. *J Am Coll Cardiol.* 2013;62:921-925, Copyright 2013, with permission from the American College of Cardiology.)

The toxic effects of ectopic fat deposition is an important issue and is being investigated intensely worldwide.

In an analysis from the Framingham Offspring Study, 3086 men and women underwent imaging to evaluate the volume of visceral, pericardial, and periaortic adipose tissue. After multivariable adjustments (age, gender, systolic blood pressure, hypertension treatment, diabetes mellitus, smoking, total cholesterol and HDL-C, and body mass index), only visceral adipose tissue volume correlated with risk for cardiovascular events and cancer (Table 2). There was a clear gradient of increasing risk for developing cardiovascular disease and cancer as tertile of visceral adipose tissue volume increased (Fig 2). There was no correlation between subcutaneous adipose tissue and risk for either CV disease or cancer.

TABLE 2.—The Association of Ectopic Fat Depots With Incident CVD (n = 90), Cancer (n = 141), and All-Cause Mortality (n = 71)

	Age- and Sex-Adjusted Model, HR (95% CI)	*p* Value	Multivariable* Model, HR (95% CI)	*p* Value
CVD				
VAT	1.48 (1.21–1.81)	<0.001	1.44 (1.08–1.92)†	0.014
Periaortic fat	1.41 (1.16–1.71)	<0.001	1.31 (1.03–1.67)	0.03
Pericardial fat	1.24 (1.05–1.46)	0.01	1.11 (0.91–1.35)	0.3
SAT	1.23 (0.99–1.53)	0.06	0.99 (0.66–1.49)	1.0
Cancer				
VAT	1.22 (1.03–1.46)	0.03	1.43 (1.12–1.84)	0.005
Periaortic fat	1.21 (1.02–1.44)	0.03	1.22 (0.99–1.50)	0.06
Pericardial fat	1.20 (1.05–1.39)	0.02	1.17 (0.98–1.38)	0.08
SAT	0.98 (0.82–1.18)	0.9	0.90 (0.65–1.26)	0.5
All-cause mortality				
VAT	1.26 (1.01–1.57)	0.04	1.05 (0.77–1.43)	0.7
Periaortic fat	1.28 (1.05–1.55)	0.01	1.08 (0.85–1.38)	0.5
Pericardial fat	1.31 (1.10–1.55)	0.002	1.17 (0.95–1.44)	0.1
SAT	1.07 (0.81–1.40)	0.7	0.72 (0.45–1.15)	0.2

A p value of <0.017 was considered statistically significant.

CI = confidence interval; CVD = cardiovascular disease; HR = hazard ratio. Abbreviations as in Table 1.

*Adjusted for age, sex, systolic blood pressure, diabetes, total cholesterol, high-density lipoprotein cholesterol, current smoking, hypertension treatment, and body mass index.

†For the CVD outcome, the integrated discrimination index was 0.082 (95% CI: −0.003 to 0.176) after the addition of VAT to the multivariable model. The chi-square statistic (p value) for model calibration was 12.9 ($p = 0.2$), suggesting good calibration.

Visceral adipose tissue clearly regulates substantial pathophysiology. The Framingham Offspring Study shows that increased visceral adipose tissue, but not subcutaneous adipose tissue, correlates with increased risk for cardiovascular disease even after comprehensive adjustment for established risk factor covariates. It is anticipated that as more studies are better controlled and data from other cohorts are appropriately adjusted, this will be a consistent finding and will render the obesity paradox obsolete.

P. P. Toth, MD, PhD

References

1. Uretsky S, Messerli FH, Bangalore S, et al. Obesity paradox in patients with hypertension and coronary artery disease. *Am J Med.* 2007;120:863-870.
2. Curtis JP, Selter JG, Wang Y, et al. The obesity paradox: body mass index and outcomes in patients with heart failure. *Arch Intern Med.* 2005;165:55-61.
3. Bays HE, Toth PP, Kris-Etherton PM, et al. Obesity, adiposity, and dyslipidemia: a consensus statement from the National Lipid Association. *J Clin Lipidol.* 2013;7: 304-383.

Low Levels of High-Density Lipoprotein Cholesterol and Increased Risk of Cardiovascular Events in Stable Ischemic Heart Disease Patients: A Post-Hoc Analysis From the COURAGE Trial (Clinical Outcomes Utilizing Revascularization and Aggressive Drug Evaluation)

Acharjee S, Boden WE, Hartigan PM, et al (Einstein Med Ctr Philadelphia, PA; Samuel S. Stratton VA Med Ctr and Albany Med College; Cooperative Studies Program Coordinating Ctr and VA Connecticut Health Care System, West Haven, CT; et al)

J Am Coll Cardiol 62:1826-1833, 2013

Objectives.—This study sought to assess the independent effect of high-density lipoprotein-cholesterol (HDL-C) level on cardiovascular risk in patients with stable ischemic heart disease (SIHD) who were receiving optimal medical therapy (OMT).

Background.—Although low HDL-C level is a powerful and independent predictor of cardiovascular risk, recent data suggest that this may not apply when low-density lipoprotein-cholesterol (LDL-C) is reduced to optimal levels using intensive statin therapy.

Methods.—We performed a post-hoc analysis in 2,193 men and women with SIHD from the COURAGE trial. The primary outcome measure was the composite of death from any cause or nonfatal myocardial infarction (MI). The independent association between HDL-C levels measured after 6 months on OMT and the rate of cardiovascular events after 4 years was assessed. Similar analyses were performed separately in subjects with LDL-C levels below 70 mg/dl (1.8 mmol/l).

Results.—In the overall population, the rate of death/MI was 33% lower in the highest HDL-C quartile as compared with the lowest quartile, with quartile of HDL-C being a significant, independent predictor of death/MI ($p = 0.05$), but with no interaction for LDL-C category ($p = 0.40$). Among subjects with LDL-C levels <70 mg/dl, those in the highest quintile of HDL-C had a 65% relative risk reduction in death or MI as compared with the lowest quintile, with HDL-C quintile demonstrating a significant, inverse predictive effect ($p = 0.02$).

Conclusions.—In this post-hoc analysis, patients with SIHD continued to experience incremental cardiovascular risk associated with low HDL-C levels despite OMT during long-term follow-up. This relationship persisted and appeared more prominent even when LDL-C was reduced to optimal levels with intensive dyslipidemic therapy (Figs 1 and 2).

▶ The Treating to New Targets (TNT) study found that even among patients with stable coronary artery disease receiving statin therapy, as high-density lipoprotein cholesterol (HDL-C) progressively decreased, risk for arteriosclerotic cardiovascular disease (ASCVD)-related events increased continuously.[1] These findings are in agreement with a meta-analysis by Jafri and coworkers[2] who showed that although statin therapy decreased risk for ASCVD events, it did not alter the inverse relationship between HDL-C and risk for cardiovascular events. This is in clear contradistinction to the results of the JUPITER[3] and

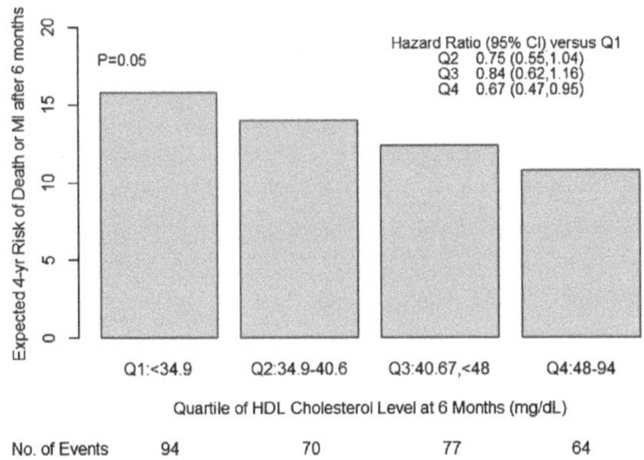

FIGURE 1.—Multivariate analysis of the relationship between death or MI and quartiles of HDL cholesterol. Hazard ratios are adjusted for age, sex, body mass index, hypertension, diabetes, current smoking, and triglycerides, and use lowest quartile (Q1) as referent. CI = confidence interval; HDL = high-density lipoprotein; MI = myocardial infarction. (Reprinted from the Journal of the American College of Cardiology. Acharjee S, Boden WE, Hartigan PM, et al. Low levels of high-density lipoprotein cholesterol and increased risk of cardiovascular events in stable ischemic heart disease patients: a post-hoc analysis from the COURAGE trial (clinical outcomes utilizing revascularization and aggressive drug evaluation). *J Am Coll Cardiol.* 2013;62:1826-1833, Copyright 2013, with permission from the American College of Cardiology.)

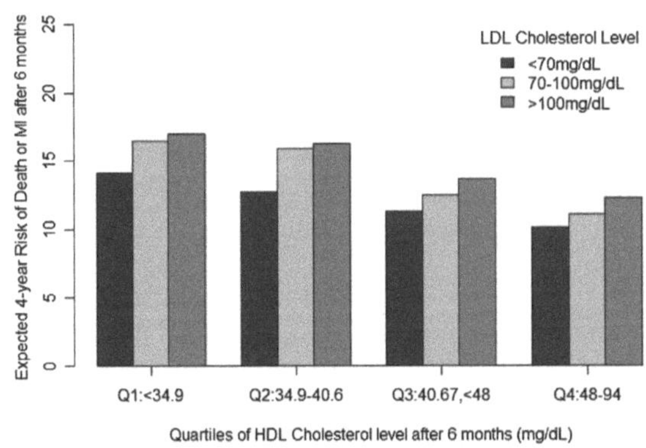

FIGURE 2.—Relationship between HDL-C quartiles and death or MI across categories of LDL-C The effect of HDL-C quartile on death or MI was independent, with no apparent interaction with LDL-C category ($p = 0.40$). LDL = Low-density lipoprotein; other abbreviations as in Fig 1. (Reprinted from the Journal of the American College of Cardiology. Low levels of high-density lipoprotein cholesterol and increased risk of cardiovascular events in stable ischemic heart disease patients: a post-hoc analysis from the COURAGE trial (clinical outcomes utilizing revascularization and aggressive drug evaluation). *J Am Coll Cardiol.* 2013;62:1826-1833, Copyright 2013, with permission from the American College of Cardiology.)

PROVE-IT[4] trials, which found that high-intensity statin therapy and aggressive reductions in low-density lipoprotein cholesterol (LDL-C) obviated any contribution of low HDL-C to ASCVD risk.

The inconsistency of these results is further heightened by another post hoc analysis. In the Clinical Outcomes Utilizing Revascularization and Aggressive Drug Evaluation (COURAGE) study, optimal medical therapy with or without percutaneous coronary intervention was evaluated in 2287 patients with stable ischemic heart disease (SIHD). This trial showed that prophylactic stenting offered no outcome advantage for patients with SIHD and whose risk factor burden was tightly controlled with lifestyle modification and intensive background pharmacologic therapy. In this analysis, the impact of HDL-C levels on ASCVD risk was investigated. Even after rigorous multivariate adjustment (age, gender, triglycerides, hypertension, diabetes, smoking, body mass index), risk for the primary endpoint (myocardial infarction [MI] or death) was reduced by 33% ($P = .02$) when comparing the highest with the lowest quartile of HDL-C after 4 years of follow-up (Fig 1). The secondary endpoints of death, MI, or stroke and death or acute coronary syndrome were both reduced by 28%. At any level of LDL-C, as HDL-C increased, risk for events decreased (Fig 2). Among patients with LDL-C level less than 70 mg/dL, when comparing the highest with lowest quintile of HDL-C, risk was 65% lower even after multivariate adjustment ($P = .006$).

In the COURAGE trial, low HDL-C clearly contributed to residual risk for ASCVD events, even in patients whose LDL-C on therapy was less than 70 mg/dL. It is not clear why different studies have disparate results. These data are consistent with those of TNT as well as the corpus of epidemiologic investigation showing a strong, continuous inverse relationship between HDL-C and risk for ASCVD. Clearly, simply reducing atherogenic lipoprotein burden to low levels is not always adequate to render a low HDL-C noncontributory to residual risk. This is an issue that clearly requires further definition.

P. P. Toth, MD, PhD

References

1. Barter P, Gotto AM, LaRosa JC, et al. HDL cholesterol, very low levels of LDL cholesterol, and cardiovascular events. *N Engl J Med.* 2007;357:1301-1310.
2. Jafri H, Alsheikh-Ali AA, Karas RH. Meta-analysis: statin therapy does not alter the association between low levels of high-density lipoprotein cholesterol and increased cardiovascular risk. *Ann Intern Med.* 2010;153:800-808.
3. Ridker PM, Genest J, Boekholdt SM, et al. HDL cholesterol and residual risk of first cardiovascular events after treatment with potent statin therapy: an analysis from the JUPITER trial. *Lancet.* 2010;376:333-339.
4. Ray KK, Cannon CP, Cairns R, Morrow DA, Ridker PM, Braunwald E. Prognostic utility of apoB/AI, total cholesterol/HDL, non-HDL cholesterol, or hs-CRP as predictors of clinical risk in patients receiving statin therapy after acute coronary syndromes: results from PROVE IT-TIMI 22. *Arterioscler Thromb Vasc Biol.* 2009; 29:424-430.

Elevated Remnant Cholesterol Causes Both Low-Grade Inflammation and Ischemic Heart Disease, Whereas Elevated Low-Density Lipoprotein Cholesterol Causes Ischemic Heart Disease Without Inflammation

Varbo A, Benn M, Tybjærg-Hansen A, et al (Copenhagen Univ Hosp, Denmark)
Circulation 128:1298-1309, 2013

Background.—Elevated nonfasting remnant cholesterol and low-density lipoprotein (LDL) cholesterol are causally associated with ischemic heart disease (IHD), but whether elevated nonfasting remnant cholesterol and LDL cholesterol both cause low-grade inflammation is currently unknown.

Methods and Results.—We studied 60 608 individuals from the Copenhagen General Population Study, the Copenhagen City Heart Study, and the Copenhagen Ischemic Heart Disease study, of whom 10 668 had IHD diagnosed between 1977 and 2011. We genotyped for variants affecting levels of nonfasting remnant cholesterol, LDL cholesterol, C-reactive protein by *CRP* alleles, and C-reactive protein by *IL6R* alleles. Using a multidirectional mendelian randomization design, we investigated possible causal associations between the lipoproteins and C-reactive protein and between the lipoproteins and IHD. A 1-mmol/L(39 mg/dL) higher level of nonfasting remnant cholesterol was associated observationally with a 37% (95% confidence interval, 35–39) higher C-reactive protein level and causally with a 28% (95% confidence interval, 10–48) higher level. For LDL cholesterol, a 1-mmol/L (39-mg/dL) higher level was associated observationally with a 7% (95% confidence interval, 6–7) higher C-reactive protein level, but we found no causal association. Likewise, higher levels of C-reactive protein did not associate causally with elevated nonfasting remnant cholesterol or LDL cholesterol. Finally, the causal risk ratio for IHD for a 1-mmol/L (39-mg/dL) higher level was 3.3 (95% confidence interval, 2.1–5.2) for nonfasting remnant cholesterol and 1.8 (95% confidence interval, 1.5–2.2) for LDL cholesterol. The causal associations for remnant cholesterol were present even in those without diabetes mellitus and obesity.

Conclusions.—Elevated nonfasting remnant cholesterol is causally associated with low-grade inflammation and with IHD, whereas elevated LDL cholesterol is associated causally with IHD without inflammation.

► The suggestion that remnant lipoproteins (RLPs) contribute to atherogenesis was first made by Zilversmit in 1979.[1] The RLPs include chylomicron remnants, very low-density lipoprotein (LDL) remnants, and intermediate-density lipoproteins. The RLPs are enriched with triglycerides and are the basis for the association between hypertriglyceridemia and increased risk for coronary artery disease (CAD). In the Framingham Offspring Study, serum levels of RLPs correlate with risk for cardiovascular (CV) events in women with established CAD.[2] Similarly, in the Honolulu Heart Study, serum levels of RLPs were significantly associated with risk for CV events among men of Asian descent.[3] In the ACCORD trial, RLPs correlated with CV events among diabetic women in a postprandial substudy.[4] Remnant levels correlate with risk for acute CV events in Japanese patients with established CAD,[5] carotid intima media thickness,[6] carotid plaque macrophage density,[7] ischemic stroke,[8] and endothelial dysfunction[9] and can be extracted from atherosclerotic plaque.[10] Among patients with Fredrickson type III dyslipoproteinemia (familial dysbetalipoproteinemia; due to defective apolipoprotein E), serum remnants are increased leading to the development of xanthomas and elevated risk for CV events.[11]

Danish investigators with the Copenhagen Heart Study, Copenhagen General Population Study, and the Copenhagen Ischemic Heart Disease Study have taken RLP remnants research to an entirely different level. By applying a multidirectional Mendelian randomization design (genotyping for polymorphisms impacting serum levels of nonfasting RLP LDL cholesterol [LDL-C] and C-reactive protein [CRP]), they were able to ascertain that for every 39-mg/dL increase in nonfasting levels of RLPs, both CRP and risk for ischemic heart disease (IHD) increased significantly by 28% and 37%, respectively. CRP levels increase linearly as a function of serum RLP concentration (Fig 1 in the original article). Serum levels of LDL-C correlated with risk for IHD but not serum levels of CRP. There was no causal association between serum CRP and levels of RLPs or LDL-C. These relationships held across all models for covariate adjustment. It also held in both men and women, in women who were either pre- or postmenopausal, in patients with or without diabetes, and irrespective of obesity (Fig 2 in the original article).

These are remarkable, novel findings. Patients are essentially postprandial almost all of the time. Postprandial states are characterized by elevated RLPs. Remnants are a component of non–high-density lipoprotein cholesterol (HDL-C). The new guidelines have removed any emphasis from non–HDL-C[12] despite the observation that they are more highly predictive of risk for atherosclerotic CVD (ASCVD) and that even when LDL-C is less than 100 mg/dL in high-risk patients, a non–HDL-C level greater than 130 mg/dL still leaves patients with substantial residual risk.[13] Remnants require considerable further study. Investigators from Copenhagen make clear that RLPs heighten risk for ASCVD not just because they increase exposure of the vasculature to elevated cholesterol and triglyceride for substantial periods of the day but also because they are independently associated with increased systemic inflammatory tone.

P. P. Toth, MD, PhD

References

1. Zilversmit DB. Atherogenesis: a postprandial phenomenon. *Circulation.* 1979; 60:473-485.
2. McNamara JR, Shah PK, Nakajima K, et al. Remnant-like particle (RLP) cholesterol is an independent cardiovascular disease risk factor in women: results from the Framingham Heart Study. *Atherosclerosis.* 2001;154:229-236.
3. Imke C, Rodriguez BL, Grove JS, et al. Are remnant-like particles independent predictors of coronary heart disease incidence? The Honolulu Heart study. *Arterioscler Thromb Vasc Biol.* 2005;25:1718-1722.
4. Ginsberg HN, Elam MB, Lovato LC, et al. Effects of combination lipid therapy in type 2 diabetes mellitus. *N Engl J Med.* 2010;362:1563-1574.
5. Kugiyama K, Doi H, Takazoe K, et al. Remnant lipoprotein levels in fasting serum predict coronary events in patients with coronary artery disease. *Circulation.* 1999;99:2858-2860.
6. Karpe F, Boquist S, Tang R, Bond GM, de Faire U, Hamsten A. Remnant lipoproteins are related to intima-media thickness of the carotid artery independently of LDL cholesterol and plasma triglycerides. *J Lipid Res.* 2001;42:17-21.
7. Zambon A, Puato M, Faggin E, Grego F, Rattazzi M, Pauletto P. Lipoprotein remnants and dense LDL are associated with features of unstable carotid plaque: a flag for non-HDL-C. *Atherosclerosis.* 2013;230:106-109.
8. Kim JY, Park JH, Jeong SW, et al. High levels of remnant lipoprotein cholesterol is a risk factor for large artery atherosclerotic stroke. *J Clin Neurol.* 2011;7: 203-209.

9. Maggi FM, Raselli S, Grigore L, Redaelli L, Fantappiè S, Catapano AL. Lipoprotein remnants and endothelial dysfunction in the postprandial phase. *J Clin Endocrinol Metab.* 2004;89:2946-2950.
10. Rapp JH, Lespine A, Hamilton RL, et al. Triglyceride-rich lipoproteins isolated by selected-affinity anti-apolipoprotein B immunosorption from human atherosclerotic plaque. *Arterioscler Thromb.* 1994;14:1767-1774.
11. Vermeer BJ, Frants RR, Havekes LM. Familial dysbetalipoproteinemia: a genetically heterogenous disease caused by mutations of the ligand apolipoprotein E. *J Invest Dermatol.* 1992;98:57S-60S.
12. Stone NJ, Robinson J, Lichtenstein AH, et al. 2013 ACC/AHA Guideline on the Treatment of Blood Cholesterol to Reduce Atherosclerotic Cardiovascular Risk in Adults: A Report of the American College of Cardiology/American Heart Association Task Force on Practice Guidelines. *Circulation.* 2013 Nov 12 [Epub ahead of print].
13. Boekholdt SM, Arsenault BJ, Mora S, et al. Association of LDL cholesterol, non-HDL cholesterol, and apolipoprotein B levels with risk of cardiovascular events among patients treated with statins: a meta-analysis. *JAMA.* 2012;307: 1302-1309.

Metabolic Syndrome

Relation of Hepatic Steatosis to Atherogenic Dyslipidemia

Makadia SS, Blaha M, Keenan T, et al (Johns Hopkins Med Insts, Baltimore, MD; Johns Hopkins Ciccarone Preventative Cardiology Ctr, Baltimore, MD; et al)
Am J Cardiol 112:1599-1604, 2013

Hepatic steatosis is closely associated with the metabolic syndrome. We assessed for an independent association between hepatic steatosis and atherogenic dyslipidemia after adjustment for obesity, physical activity, hyperglycemia, and systemic inflammation. We studied 6,333 asymptomatic subjects without clinical cardiovascular disease undergoing a health screen in Brazil from November 2008 to July 2010. Hepatic steatosis was diagnosed by ultrasound. Atherogenic dyslipidemia was defined using 2 definitions: criteria for (1) metabolic syndrome or (2) insulin resistance (triglyceride/high-density–lipoprotein cholesterol ratio of ≥2.5 in women and ≥3.5 in men). In hierarchical multivariate regression models, we evaluated for an independent association of hepatic steatosis with atherogenic dyslipidemia. Hepatic steatosis was detected in 36% of participants (average age 43.5 years, 79% men, average body mass index 26.3 kg/m^2). Subjects with hepatic steatosis had similar levels of low-density–lipoprotein cholesterol, with significantly lower level of high-density-lipoprotein cholesterol and higher level of triglyceride compared with those without steatosis. Hepatic steatosis remained significantly independently associated with atherogenic dyslipidemia of both definitions (metabolic syndrome [odds ratio 2.47, 95% confidence interval 2.03 to 3.02] and insulin resistance [odds ratio 2.50, 95% confidence interval 2.13 to 2.91]) after multivariate adjustment. Stratified analyses showed a persistent independent association in nonobese subjects, those without metabolic syndrome, those with normal high-sensitivity C-reactive protein, nonalcohol abusers, and those with normal liver enzymes. Hepatic steatosis was significantly associated with atherogenic dyslipidemia independent of obesity, physical activity, hyperglycemia, and systemic inflammation after multivariate adjustment. In conclusion, this adds to the growing body of evidence that hepatic steatosis may play a direct metabolic role in conferring increased cardiovascular risk (Fig 2, Tables 2 and 3).

▶ Hepatic steatosis is widely regarded as a reliable marker of insulin resistance (IR) and is frequently observed in the setting of metabolic syndrome (MS). Hepatic steatosis also correlates with increased risk of ectopic fat deposition in other tissues, such as the pancreas, epicardium, skeletal muscle, and myocardium.[1] Hepatic steatosis results from the excess influx of free fatty acid and inadequate capacity to dispose of this excess lipid via mitochondrial oxidation, increased gluconeogenesis, or augmented secretion within very-low-density lipoprotein particles. MS and IR are well known to be associated with several disturbances in lipid and lipoprotein metabolism.[2] In an elegant study by Makadia et al, the quantitative relationship between atherogenic dyslipidemia and hepatic steatosis was investigated using a cohort of 6333 patients in Sao Paolo, Brazil. Atherogenic dyslipidemia was defined according to (1) the National Cholesterol Education Program's criteria for MS (triglyceride ≥150 mg/dL, high-density lipoprotein cholesterol [HDL-C] less than 40 mg/dL in men and less than 50 mg/dL in women) and (2) established lipid-dependent definition for IR (triglyceride/HDL-C ratio ≥2.5 in women and ≥3.5 in men). Liver ultrasonography was used to establish or negate the presence of steatosis. For multivariable regression analyses, a hierarchical model was applied: model 1 is unadjusted; adjustments were first made for age, gender, alcohol use, and physical activity

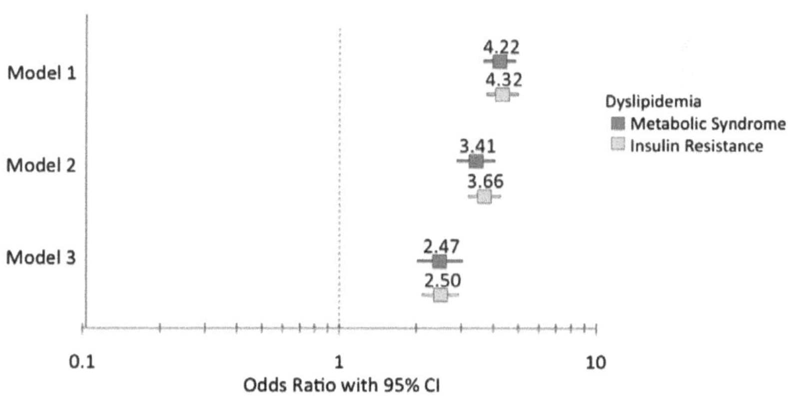

FIGURE 2.—ORs for atherogenic dyslipidemia in subjects with hepatic steatosis by sequential hierarchal regression. Model 1: unadjusted. Model 2: adjusted for age, gender, alcohol use, and physical activity. Model 3: adjusted for model 2 plus BMI, waist circumference, hypertension or antihypertensive medications, diabetes or use of diabetes medications, hyperglycemia, log hs-CRP, smoking, and use of lipid-lowering medications. Dyslipidemia (metabolic syndrome): levels of TG ≥150 mg/dl and HDL-C <40 mg/dl in men or <50 mg/dl in women or the use of lipidlowering medications. Dyslipidemia (insulin resistance): TG/HDL-C ratio of ≥2.5 in women and ≥3.5 in men. (Reprinted from the American Journal of Cardiology. Makadia SS, Blaha M, Keenan T, et al. Relation of hepatic steatosis to atherogenic dyslipidemia. *Am J Cardiol.* 2013;112:1599-1604, Copyright 2013, with permission from Elsevier.)

TABLE 2.—Difference Between Lipid Values in Patients with Hepatic Steatosis and those Without it in Multivariate Linear Regression

	Model 1	Model 2	Model 3
Lipid Parameter	β Coefficient (95% CI)	β Coefficient (95% CI)	β Coefficient (95% CI)
TC (mg/dl)	9.43 (7.50 to 11.37)	6.33 (4.15 to 8.51)	4.49 (1.87 to 7.12)
LDL-C (mg/dl)	7.39 (5.67 to 9.10)	3.28 (1.35 to 5.22)	0.73 (−1.58 to 3.03)
HDL-C (mg/dl)	−8.74 (−9.33 to −8.16)	−5.55 (−6.16 to −4.95)	−2.96 (−3.69 to −2.23)
TGs (mg/dl)*	0.40 (0.37 to 0.42)	0.31 (0.28 to 0.33)	0.23 (0.20 to 0.26)
Non-HDL-C (mg/dl)	18.2 (16.2 to 20.1)	11.9 (9.70 to 14.08)	7.47 (4.83 to 10.11)
TG/HDL ratio*	0.57 (0.54 to 0.61)	0.43 (0.39 to 0.46)	0.29 (0.25 to 0.34)
TC/HDL ratio*	0.22 (0.21 to 0.24)	0.15 (0.13 to 0.16)	0.09 (0.07 to 0.10)

Model 1: unadjusted; n = 6,333.
Model 2: adjusted for age, gender, alcohol use, and physical activity; n = 5,697.
Model 3: adjusted for model 2 plus BMI, waist circumference, hypertension or antihypertensive medications, diabetes or diabetes medications, hyperglycemia, log hs-CRP, smoking, and use of lipid-lowering medications; n = 4,825.
*Log transformed.

TABLE 3.—Stratified ORs of Hepatic Steatosis with Dyslipidemia in Multivariate Logistic Regression

	Dyslipidemia	
	Metabolic Syndrome	Insulin Resistance
Stratifications	OR (95% CI)	OR (95% CI)
Obesity*		
Yes, n = 1,122	2.51 (1.73 to 3.64)	2.20 (1.64 to 2.95)
No, n = 3,703	2.97 (2.39 to 3.68)	3.25 (2.73 to 3.87)
Systemic Inflammation*		
Yes, n = 930	2.74 (1.74 to 4.31)	3.20 (2.25 to 4.56)
No, n = 3,895	2.42 (1.94 to 3.01)	2.39 (2.01 to 2.85)
Metabolic Syndrome†		
Yes, n = 1,108	1.51 (1.12 to 2.03)	1.64 (1.18 to 2.28)
No, n = 4,310	2.26 (1.71 to 2.99)	2.25 (1.87 to 2.70)

Dyslipidemia (metabolic syndrome) is defined as HDL levels of <40 mg/dl in men and <50 mg/dl in women and TG level of ≥150 mg/dl.
Dyslipidemia (insulin resistance) is defined as a TG/HDL ratio of ≥2.5 in women and ≥3.5 in men.
Obesity is defined as a BMI of ≥30 kg/m^2 or waist circumference of >88 cm in women or >102 cm in men if BMI is ≥25 kg/m^2.
Systemic inflammation is defined as an hs-CRP level of ≥3.
*Adjusted for BMI (not in no obesity or obesity), waist circumference (not in no obesity or obesity), hypertension, hypertension medications, diabetes, diabetes medications, log hs-CRP (not in hs-CRP level < or ≥3), smoking, and lipid-lowering medications.
†Regression analysis for no metabolic syndrome or metabolic syndrome subgroups excluded those who met the Harmonizing Definition for metabolic syndrome.

(model 2); in model 3, additional adjustments for obesity, components of the metabolic syndrome, systemic inflammation, body mass index, waist circumference, hypertension, antihypertensive medications, diabetes, diabetes medications, hyperglycemia, log hs–C-reactive protein (hs-CRP), smoking status, and lipid-lowering medications. The associations between hepatic steatosis and dyslipidemia were stratified by alcohol consumption, obesity, log hs-CRP, metabolic syndrome, and liver function studies. Hepatic steatosis correlated significantly with triglycerides, HDL-C, non—HDL-C, triglyceride/HDL-C, and total cholesterol/HDL-C across hierarchical adjustment (Table 2). Even after comprehensive adjustment for covariates (model 3), dyslipidemia correlated highly with hepatic steatosis (metabolic syndrome definition: odds ratio [OR], 2.47; 95% confidence interval [CI], 2.03 to 3.02 and insulin resistance definition: OR, 2.50; 95% CI, 2.13 to 2.91; Fig 2). In addition, in a subgroup analysis using model 3, there were statistically significant associations between hepatic steatosis and dyslipidemia for both MS and IR in subjects with and without obesity, with and without elevated hs-CRP levels, and with and without metabolic syndrome (Table 2). The results were significant even after adjusting for liver function studies.

This study establishes that dyslipidemia is independently associated with hepatic steatosis. Atherogenic dyslipidemia correlated highly with steatosis even after comprehensive multivariable adjustment. It also shows that hepatic steatosis can occur in the absence of obesity, evidence of systemic inflammation, and meeting criteria for MS. Increased serum levels of hepatic enzymes correlated poorly with steatosis.

P. P. Toth, MD, PhD

References

1. Toth PP. Epicardial steatosis, insulin resistance, and coronary artery disease. *Heart Fail Clin.* 2012;8:671-678.
2. Toth PP. Insulin resistance, small LDL particles, and risk for atherosclerotic disease. *Curr Vasc Pharmacol.* 2013 Apr 25 [Epub ahead of print].

Prandial Hypertriglyceridemia in Metabolic Syndrome Is Due to an Overproduction of Both Chylomicron and VLDL Triacylglycerol

Shojaee-Moradie F, Ma Y, Lou S, et al (Univ of Surrey, Guildford, UK; et al)
Diabetes 62:4063-4069, 2013

The aim was to determine whether fed VLDL and chylomicron (CM) triacylglycerol (TAG) production rates are elevated in metabolic syndrome (MetS). Eight men with MetS (BMI 29.7 ± 1.1) and eight lean age-matched healthy men (BMI 23.1 ± 0.4) were studied using a frequent feeding protocol. After 4 h of feeding, an intravenous bolus of $^2H_5$-glycerol was administered to label VLDL1, VLDL2, and TAG. ^{13}C-glycerol tripalmitin was administered orally as an independent measure of CM TAG metabolism. Hepatic and intestinal lipoproteins were separated by an immunoaffinity method. In MetS, fed TAG and the increment in TAG from fasting to feeding were higher ($P = 0.03$ and $P = 0.04$, respectively) than in lean men. Fed CM, VLDL1, and VLDL2 TAG pool sizes were higher ($P = 0.006$, $P = 0.03$, and $P < 0.02$, respectively), and CM, VLDL1, and VLDL2 TAG production rates were higher ($P < 0.002$, $P < 0.05$, and $P = 0.06$, respectively) than in lean men. VLDL1, VLDL2, and CM TAG clearance rates were not different between groups. In conclusion, prandial hypertriglyceridemia in men with MetS was due to an increased production rate of both VLDL and CM TAG. Since both groups received identical meals, this suggests that in MetS the intestine is synthesizing more TAG de novo for export in CMs.

▶ Hypertriglyceridemia and elevated serum levels of very-low-density lipoproteins (VLDLs) and their remnants are hallmarks of insulin resistance (IR). In the setting of IR, insulin is no longer effectively inhibiting the activity of hormone-sensitive lipase and visceral adipose tissue hydrolyzes triglycerides and releases free fatty acids (FFAs) into serum. The FFAs can be oxidized by systemic tissues or can be taken up by hepatocytes. The hepatocytes can, in turn, either oxidize the FFAs within mitochondria or esterify them to glycerol to reassimilate triglycerides. The triglycerides can be packaged into VLDL particles and secreted. In patients with IR, hepatic VLDL secretion is increased. The lipolysis of VLDL and its remnants is impaired because the activity of lipoprotein lipase is decreased secondary to reduced expression of this enzyme and increased expression of its endogenous inhibitor, lipoprotein lipase.[1]

An important question in current endocrinology is whether IR is also associated with increased jejunal secretion of chylomicrons. Shojaee-Moradie et al investigated this issue in men with and without metabolic syndrome in the postprandial state using standard meals. As expected, among the men with metabolic syndrome, fasting glucose, insulin, homeostasis model assessment-estimated insulin resistance, and triglycerides were higher and high-density lipoprotein cholesterol (HDL-C) was lower compared with men without metabolic syndrome. Of considerable interest is the observation that in men with IR, the production rates and pool sizes of chylomicrons and VLDLs were higher than in men without IR (Fig 1 in the original article). Clearance rates as measured by fractional catabolic rate were not significantly different.

This study shows, in humans with IR, that the postprandial increase in serum triglycerides is a product of both increased jejunal and hepatic production of triglyceride-rich lipoproteins. The capacity to clear these lipoproteins through the usual hepatic mechanisms was not impaired. The authors postulate that the jejunum produces higher levels of chylomicrons in the postprandial phase in patients with IR secondary to increased de novo biosynthesis of triglycerides, increased conversion of dietary sources of glucose to FFA, or increased uptake of FFA from the circulation. This study does not differentiate these possibilities. The study establishes that the jejunum participates very intimately in the etiology of the hypertriglyceridemia that associates with IR due to heightened production and secretion of chylomicrons.

P. P. Toth, MD, PhD

Reference

1. Toth PP, Dayspring TD, Pokrywka GS. Drug therapy for hypertriglyceridemia: fibrates and omega-3 fatty acids. *Curr Atheroscler Rep*. 2009;11:71-79.

3 Obesity

New Developments in Obesity

KSR2 Mutations Are Associated with Obesity, Insulin Resistance, and Impaired Cellular Fuel Oxidation

Pearce LR, Atanassova N, Banton MC, et al (Addenbrooke's Hosp, Cambridge, UK; et al)

Cell 155:765-777, 2013

Kinase suppressor of Ras 2 (KSR2) is an intracellular scaffolding protein involved in multiple signaling pathways. Targeted deletion of *Ksr2* leads to obesity in mice, suggesting a role in energy homeostasis. We explored the role of *KSR2* in humans by sequencing 2,101 individuals with severe early-onset obesity and 1,536 controls. We identified multiple rare variants in *KSR2* that disrupt signaling through the Raf-MEKERK pathway and impair cellular fatty acid oxidation and glucose oxidation in transfected cells; effects that can be ameliorated by the commonly prescribed antidiabetic drug, metformin. Mutation carriers exhibit hyperphagia in childhood, low heart rate, reduced basal metabolic rate and severe insulin resistance. These data establish KSR2 as an important regulator of energy intake, energy expenditure, and substrate utilization in humans. Modulation of KSR2-mediated effects may represent a novel therapeutic strategy for obesity and type 2 diabetes.

▶ Obesity is caused by a complex interaction of the environment, genetic predisposition, and human lifestyle. Although environmental factors are major contributors to the obesity epidemic, genetic predisposition does play a major role in the development of obesity. Human genes influence how our bodies capture, store, and release energy from food. Genetic factors are estimated to account for greater than 40% of the population variation in body mass index (BMI).[1,2] Despite a relatively high heritability, the search for obesity susceptibility genes has been a difficult process. Progress until recently has been slow, and success is limited. For instance, although several BMI and obesity genes have been identified via genome-wide association studies (GWAS),[1,2] the proportion of the variability explained by these loci overall remains very low. Next-generation sequencing seeks to complement GWAS findings (which are typically common variants with minor allele frequencies more than 5%) through the intensive interrogation of both common and rare variants contributing to a trait.

Kinase suppressor of Ras 2 (KSR2) is an intracellular scaffolding protein that involves multiple signaling pathways. KSR2 is an important regulator of AMP kinase, energy expenditure, and insulin sensitivity.[3] Disruption of KSR2 in vivo impairs AMP-activated protein kinase—regulated pathways affecting fatty acid oxidation and thermogenesis that leads to obesity. In this study, the researchers examined the role of KSR2 in humans by sequencing 2101 individuals with severe early-onset obesity (mean BMI standard deviation score of 3.5; onset $<$ 10 years old) and 1536 controls. About 2% of obese subjects versus 1% of controls had a rare frameshift, nonsense, or missense variant in KSR2. Twenty-three variants identified were found only in severely obese subjects, 5 variants were found in both obese subjects and controls, and 3 variants were found only in the controls, all of whom were overweight or obese. The family study did not show a classical Mendelian inheritance pattern, suggesting that KSR2 variants predispose to obesity against a background of other genetic or environmental factors. Further physiologic studies showed that KSR2 mutations disrupted signaling through the Ras-Raf-MEK-ERK pathway. Mutations of KSR2 in humans impaired cellular glucose oxidation and fatty acid oxidation in transfected cells; these effects can be rescued by the addition of metformin. Furthermore, the basal metabolic rate (BMR) measured by indirect calorimetry in adults with KSR2 mutations was significantly lower than the predicted BMR based on age, gender, and body composition. In children with mutations, the measured BMR was also less than the predicted value, although this was not statistically significant. Sleeping heart rate was also lower in KSR2 mutation carriers despite normal 24-hour urine catecholamines and serum thyroid-stimulating hormone. Hyperphagia was reported in the children with mutation. These data show that KSR2 is an important regulator of basal metabolic rate, fatty acid oxidation, glucose oxidation, and food intake. Developing medications targeting KSR2 activity may give us a new therapeutic option for obesity and type 2 diabetes. It should be noted that only small numbers of obese subjects have mutations of the KSR2 gene. Not all people who carry obese-susceptible genes will become obese; healthy lifestyle may counteract some of the genetically related obesity risk.

L. Khaodhiar, MD

References

1. Hjelmborg J, Fagnani C, Silventoinen K, et al. Genetic influences on growth traits of BMI: a longitudinal study of adult twins. *Obesity (Silver Spring)*. 2008;16: 847-852.
2. Walley AJ, Asher JE, Froguel P. The genetic contribution to non-syndromic human obesity. *Nat Rev Genet*. 2009;10:431-442.
3. Costanzo-Garvey DL, Pfluger PT, Dougherty MK, et al. KSR2 is an essential regulator of AMP kinase, energy expenditure, and insulin sensitivity. *Cell Metab*. 2009;10:366-378.

Myths, Presumptions, and Facts about Obesity

Casazza K, Fontaine KR, Astrup A, et al (Univ of Alabama at Birmingham; Univ of Copenhagen, Denmark; et al)

N Engl J Med 368:446-454, 2013

Background.—Many beliefs about obesity persist in the absence of supporting scientific evidence (presumptions); some persist despite contradicting evidence (myths). The promulgation of unsupported beliefs may yield poorly informed policy decisions, inaccurate clinical and public health recommendations, and an unproductive allocation of research resources and may divert attention away from useful, evidence-based information.

Methods.—Using Internet searches of popular media and scientific literature, we identified, reviewed, and classified obesity-related myths and presumptions. We also examined facts that are well supported by evidence, with an emphasis on those that have practical implications for public health, policy, or clinical recommendations.

Results.—We identified seven obesity-related myths concerning the effects of small sustained increases in energy intake or expenditure, establishment of realistic goals for weight loss, rapid weight loss, weight-loss readiness, physical-education classes, breast-feeding, and energy expended during sexual activity. We also identified six presumptions about the purported effects of regularly eating breakfast, early childhood experiences, eating fruits and vegetables, weight cycling, snacking, and the built (i.e., human-made) environment. Finally, we identified nine evidence-supported facts that are relevant for the formulation of sound public health, policy, or clinical recommendations.

Conclusions.—False and scientifically unsupported beliefs about obesity are pervasive in both scientific literature and the popular press. (Funded by the National Institutes of Health.) (Tables 1-3).

► In this article, the authors reviewed scientific data on obesity and described 7 obesity-related myths, 6 presumptions, and 9 facts. The myths were defined as beliefs held true despite substantial evidence proving them false, the presumptions were those without enough evidence to prove or disprove them, and the facts were those with sufficient evidence to support them (Tables 1-3). Although I agree with the facts and presumptions, I don't agree with some of the myths. Some of the myths should be classified as presumptions because we do not have evidence one way or the other (as I discuss later). In reality, we cannot perform randomized controlled trials to answer every question we have, whether from practical, ethical, or logical standpoints. We also have to depend on epidemiological studies, and sometimes we cannot prove them right or wrong if there are conflicting results. The first of the "myths" that should be a presumption is that the authors dismissed setting realistic weight loss goals as an important part of obesity treatment. The second myth was the belief that large and rapid weight loss was associated with better long-term outcomes compared with slow, gradual weight loss. We clearly don't have enough long-term data on either of these topics. From a practical standpoint, some

TABLE 1.—Seven Myths about Obesity*

Myth	Basis of Conjecture
Small sustained changes in energy intake or expenditure will produce large, long-term weight changes	National health guidelines and reputable websites advertise that large changes in weight accumulate indefinitely after small sustained daily lifestyle modifications (e.g., walking for 20 minutes or eating two additional potato chips)
Setting realistic goals in obesity treatment is important because otherwise patients will become frustrated and lose less weight	According to goal-setting theory, unattainable goals impair performance and discourage goal-attaining behavior; in obesity treatment, incongruence between desired and actual weight loss is thought to undermine the patient's perceived ability to attain goals, which may lead to the discontinuation of behaviors necessary for weight loss
Large, rapid weight loss is associated with poorer long-term weight outcomes than is slow, gradual weight loss	This notion probably emerged in reaction to the adverse effects of nutritionally insufficient very-low-calorie diets (<800 kcal per day) in the 1960s; the belief has persisted, has been repeated in textbooks and recommendations from health authorities, and has been offered as a rule by dietitians
Assessing the stage of change or diet readiness is important in helping patients who seek weight-loss treatment	Many believe that patients who feel ready to lose weight are more likely to make the required lifestyle changes
Physical-education classes in their current format play an important role in preventing or reducing childhood obesity	The health benefits of physical activity of sufficient duration, frequency, and intensity are well established and include reductions in adiposity
Breast-feeding is protective against obesity	The belief that breast-fed children are less likely to become obese has persisted for more than a century and is passionately defended
A bout of sexual activity burns 100 to 300 kcal for each person involved	Many sources state that substantial energy is expended in typical sexual activity between two adults

*We define myths as beliefs held true despite substantial evidence refuting them. A list of articles in which these myths are espoused is provided in the Supplementary Appendix.

people do better with an aggressive weight loss goal and/or more rapid weight loss whereas others are more content with a smaller weight loss goal and/or slower weight loss. The third "myth" that may be relevant is that the authors disregarded the assessment of the stage of change or diet readiness to help patients who seek weight loss treatment. In this particular topic, the authors reviewed 5 trials that looked at stages of change in people entering weight loss programs and found that it did not predict weight loss outcomes. The authors themselves did point out that, by definition, people voluntarily choosing to enter weight loss programs are at least minimally ready to engage in behavioral changes. From a clinician's standpoint, stage of change assessment is also important for other reasons if not for the treatment success. These assessments can lead to interventions tailored to the individual's readiness. Stage of change can also positively affect the doctor-patient relationship, with patients less likely to create resistance or impede change.[1] The final "myth" that may be true, as stated by the authors, is that breastfeeding is protective against obesity in offspring. The article they cited concluded that

TABLE 2.—Presumptions about Obesity*

Presumption	Basis for Conjecture
Regularly eating (vs. skipping) breakfast is protective against obesity	Skipping breakfast purportedly leads to overeating later in the day
Early childhood is the period during which we learn exercise and eating habits that influence our weight throughout life	Weight-for-height indexes, eating behaviors, and preferences that are present in early childhood are correlated with those later in life
Eating more fruits and vegetables will result in weight loss or less weight gain, regardless of whether one intentionally makes any other behavioral or environmental changes	By eating more fruits and vegetables, a person presumably spontaneously eats less of other foods, and the resulting reduction in calories is greater than the increase in calories from the fruit and vegetables
Weight cycling (i.e., yo-yo dieting) is associated with increased mortality	In observational studies, mortality rates have been lower among persons with stable weight than among those with unstable weight
Snacking contributes to weight gain and obesity	Snack foods are presumed to be incompletely compensated for at subsequent meals, leading to weight gain
The built environment, in terms of sidewalk and park availability, influences obesity	Neighborhood-environment features may promote or inhibit physical activity, thereby affecting obesity

*We define presumptions as unproved yet commonly espoused propositions. A list of articles in which these presumptions are implied is provided in the Supplementary Appendix.

breastfeeding (initiation, longer duration, or exclusivity) no longer appears to be a major determinant on childhood and adolescent obesity but may well exert a modest protective effect (not no effect).[2] Because breastfeeding has other potential benefits and may have some modest protective effect against obesity, it should be encouraged.

In terms of the facts outlined by the authors about obesity, there are sufficient data that meal replacement products, pharmacotherapy, and weight loss surgery can be useful in the treatment of obesity.[3-5] Although this may be true, this article received overwhelming attention in press. People have questioned the purposes of this article and whether it was aimed to promote drugs, meal replacement, and bariatric surgery because many of the authors have deep financial ties to food, beverage, and weight loss product makers. From a clinician's point of view, I do agree that meal replacement products or structured meals can be useful and safe. Weight loss medications provide more weight loss than diet and exercise alone, but they are not suitable for everybody, and there are certain risks and side effects. Patients should be followed appropriately when using weight loss medications. Once medications are discontinued, patients are likely to regain lost weight. Physical activity or exercise has been shown to promote long-term weight maintenance. Weight loss surgery should be considered in patients who meet National Institutes of Health criteria for surgery and have failed medical treatment. Risks of surgery depend on the type of surgery. Gastric bypass is more effective than gastric banding but has a higher rate of complications.

L. Khaodhiar, MD

TABLE 3.—Facts about Obesity*

Fact	Implication
Although genetic factors play a large role, heritability is not destiny; calculations show that moderate environmental changes can promote as much weight loss as the most efficacious pharmaceutical agents available[26]	If we can identify key environmental factors and successfully influence them, we can achieve clinically significant reductions in obesity
Diets (i.e., reduced energy intake) very effectively reduce weight, but trying to go on a diet or recommending that someone go on a diet generally does not work well in the long-term[27]	This seemingly obvious distinction is often missed, leading to erroneous conceptions regarding possible treatments for obesity; recognizing this distinction helps our understanding that energy reduction is the ultimate dietary intervention required and approaches such as eating more vegetables or eating breakfast daily are likely to help only if they are accompanied by an overall reduction in energy intake
Regardless of body weight or weight loss, an increased level of exercise increases health[28]	Exercise offers a way to mitigate the health-damaging effects of obesity, even without weight loss
Physical activity or exercise in a sufficient dose aids in long-term weight maintenance[28,29]	Physical-activity programs are important, especially for children, but for physical activity to affect weight, there must be a substantial quantity of movement, not mere participation
Continuation of conditions that promote weight loss promotes maintenance of lower weight[30]	Obesity is best conceptualized as a chronic condition, requiring ongoing management to maintain long-term weight loss
For overweight children, programs that involve the parents and the home setting promote greater weight loss or maintenance[31]	Programs provided only in schools or other out-of-home structured settings may be convenient or politically expedient, but programs including interventions that involve the parents and are provided at home are likely to yield better outcomes
Provision of meals and use of meal-replacement products promote greater weight loss[32]	More structure regarding meals is associated with greater weight loss, as compared with seemingly holistic programs that are based on concepts of balance, variety, and moderation
Some pharmaceutical agents can help patients achieve clinically meaningful weight loss and maintain the reduction as long as the agents continue to be used[33]	While we learn how to alter the environment and individual behaviors to prevent obesity, we can offer moderately effective treatment to obese persons
In appropriate patients, bariatric surgery results in long-term weight loss and reductions in the rate of incident diabetes and mortality[34]	For severely obese persons, bariatric surgery can offer a life-changing, and in some cases lifesaving, treatment

Editor's Note: Please refer to original journal article for full references.
*We classify the listed propositions as facts because there is sufficient evidence to consider them empirically proved.

References

1. Zimmerman GL, Olsen CG, Bosworth MF. A 'stages of change' approach to helping patients change behavior. *Am Fam Physician.* 2000;61:1409-1416.
2. Gillman MW. Breastfeeding and obesity—the 2011 scorecard. *Int J Epidemiol.* 2011;40:681-684.
3. Wing RR, Jeffery RW. Food provision as a strategy to promote weight loss. *Obes Res.* 2001;9:271S-275S.
4. Wright SM, Aronne LJ. Obesity in 2010: the future of obesity medicine: where do we go from here? *Nat Rev Endocrinol.* 2011;7:69-70.
5. Sjöström L, Lindroos AK, Peltonen M, et al. Lifestyle, diabetes, and cardiovascular risk factors 10 years after bariatric surgery. *N Engl J Med.* 2004;351:2683-2693.

Epidemiology and Complications of Obesity

Are Metabolically Healthy Overweight and Obesity Benign Conditions?: A Systematic Review and Meta-Analysis

Kramer CK, Zinman B, Retnakaran R (Mount Sinai Hosp, Toronto, Ontario, Canada; Univ of Toronto, Ontario, Canada)

Ann Intern Med 159:758-769, 2013

Background.—Recent interest has focused on a unique subgroup of overweight and obese individuals who have normal metabolic features despite increased adiposity. Normal-weight individuals with adverse metabolic status have also been described. However, it remains unclear whether metabolic phenotype modifies the morbidity and mortality associated with higher body mass index (BMI).

Purpose.—To determine the effect of metabolic status on all-cause mortality and cardiovascular events in normal-weight, overweight, and obese persons.

Data Sources.—Studies were identified from electronic databases.

Study Selection.—Included studies evaluated all-cause mortality or cardiovascular events (or both) and clinical characteristics of 6 patient groups defined by BMI category (normal weight/overweight/obesity) and metabolic status (healthy/unhealthy), as defined by the presence or absence of components of the metabolic syndrome by Adult Treatment Panel III or International Diabetes Federation criteria.

Data Extraction.—Two independent reviewers extracted the data. Metabolically healthy people of normal weight made up the reference group.

Data Synthesis.—Eight studies ($n = 61\,386$; 3988 events) evaluated participants for all-cause mortality and/or cardiovascular events. Metabolically healthy obese individuals (relative risk [RR], 1.24; 95% CI, 1.02 to 1.55) had increased risk for events compared with metabolically healthy normal-weight individuals when only studies with 10 or more years of follow-up were considered. All metabolically unhealthy groups had a similarly elevated risk: normal weight (RR, 3.14; CI, 2.36 to 3.93), overweight (RR, 2.70; CI, 2.08 to 3.30), and obese (RR, 2.65; CI, 2.18 to 3.12).

Limitation.—Duration of exposure to the metabolic-BMI phenotypes was not described in the studies and could partially affect the estimates.

Conclusion.—Compared with metabolically healthy normal-weight individuals, obese persons are at increased risk for adverse long-term outcomes even in the absence of metabolic abnormalities, suggesting that there is no healthy pattern of increased weight.

▶ It is well recognized that individuals in the same body mass index (BMI) category can have substantial heterogeneity of metabolic features, including glucose tolerance, lipid profiles, blood pressure, and waist circumference. Up to 30% of obese individuals are considered "metabolically healthy" and some have suggested that this subgroup of healthy obese patients are protected against metabolic and cardiovascular comorbidities and may not need treatment.[1] In this systematic review and meta-analysis, the authors identified 12 prospective or cross-sectional studies that evaluated all-cause mortality or cardiovascular events and clinical characteristics of 6 patient groups defined by BMI category (normal weight/overweight/obesity) and metabolic status (healthy/unhealthy) as defined by the presence or absence of components of the metabolic syndrome by Adult Treatment Panel III or International Diabetes Federation criteria. The most important finding was that the metabolically healthy obese group had 24% increased mortality rate and cardiovascular risk compared with the metabolically healthy normal-weight subjects when studies with 10 or more years of follow-up were considered. The metabolically healthy overweight group, however, had similar risk to the healthy, normal-weight individuals. All metabolically unhealthy groups regardless of BMI category had a 2- to 3-fold increased cardiovascular risk. When they compared persons with the same metabolic status (healthy or unhealthy), those with higher BMI had increased levels of systolic blood pressure, diastolic blood pressure, waist circumference, and Homeostasis Model Assessment of Insulin Resistance. A similar inverse association was observed for high-density lipoprotein cholesterol.

This meta-analysis has limitations. The studies did not account for other factors possibly associated with mortality, such as smoking or physical activity, and they did not have data on weight gain, age, or ethnicity of subjects. Higher BMI has been reported to provide lower relative mortality risk in elderly persons than in young and middle-aged populations; thus, results of this meta-analysis may not be generalizable to older people. Similarly, people of certain ethnic backgrounds are at higher risk of metabolic syndrome despite being normal weight.

It should be noted that complications of obesity are not limited to metabolic syndrome. Obese people are at risk for other medical conditions such as sleep apnea, osteoarthritis, gallbladder disease, infertility, and certain types of cancer.[2] Obese people may experience social stigma, discrimination, and overall reduced quality of life.[3] Even though preventing cardiovascular disease and death is very important, it should not be the only reason obese people should be encouraged to lose weight.

L. Khaodhiar, MD

References

1. Blüher M. The distinction of metabolically 'healthy' from 'unhealthy' obese individuals. *Curr Opin Lipidol.* 2010;21:38-43.
2. Bray GA. Risks of obesity. *Endocrinol Metab Clin North Am.* 2003;32:787-804.
3. Puhl RM, Heuer CA. Weight bias: a review and update. *Obesity (Silver Spring).* 2009;17:941-964.

Diet and Obesity

Cardiovascular Effects of Intensive Lifestyle Intervention in Type 2 Diabetes

The Look AHEAD Research Group (Warren Alpert Med School of Brown Univ, Providence, RI; Natl Insts of Health, Bethesda, MD; Johns Hopkins School of Medicine, Baltimore, MD; et al)

N Engl J Med 369:145-154, 2013

Background.—Weight loss is recommended for overweight or obese patients with type 2 diabetes on the basis of short-term studies, but long-term effects on cardiovascular disease remain unknown. We examined whether an intensive lifestyle intervention for weight loss would decrease cardiovascular morbidity and mortality among such patients.

Methods.—In 16 study centers in the United States, we randomly assigned 5145 overweight or obese patients with type 2 diabetes to participate in an intensive lifestyle intervention that promoted weight loss through decreased caloric intake and increased physical activity (intervention group) or to receive diabetes support and education (control group). The primary outcome was a composite of death from cardiovascular causes, nonfatal myocardial infarction, nonfatal stroke, or hospitalization for angina during a maximum follow-up of 13.5 years.

Results.—The trial was stopped early on the basis of a futility analysis when the median follow-up was 9.6 years. Weight loss was greater in the intervention group than in the control group throughout the study (8.6% vs. 0.7% at 1 year; 6.0% vs. 3.5% at study end). The intensive lifestyle intervention also produced greater reductions in glycated hemoglobin and greater initial improvements in fitness and all cardiovascular risk factors, except for low-density-lipoprotein cholesterol levels. The primary outcome occurred in 403 patients in the intervention group and in 418 in the control group (1.83 and 1.92 events per 100 person-years, respectively; hazard ratio in the intervention group, 0.95; 95% confidence interval, 0.83 to 1.09; $P = 0.51$).

Conclusions.—An intensive lifestyle intervention focusing on weight loss did not reduce the rate of cardiovascular events in overweight or obese adults with type 2 diabetes. (Funded by the National Institutes of Health and others; Look AHEAD ClinicalTrials.gov number, NCT00017953.)

► Overweight and obesity are associated with increased morbidity and mortality. Several short-term studies have demonstrated beneficial effects of moderate weight loss, defined as 5% to 10% weight loss, on many cardiovascular risk factors. The Swedish Obese Subjects (SOS) study showed a long-term reduction in macrovascular disease in participants with type 2 diabetes after bariatric surgery.[1] For all SOS subjects, surgery was associated with 30% reduction in mortality after 16 years of follow-up. The mean weight changes in the study were −23%, −17%, −16%, and −18% at 2, 10, 15, and 20 years, respectively.

The Look AHEAD (Action for HEAlth in Diabetes) was a multicenter randomized study that examined whether an intensive lifestyle intervention designed to achieve weight loss through caloric restriction and increased physical activity would decrease cardiovascular morbidity and mortality among overweight and obese adults with type 2 diabetes. The study was stopped early for futility after a median follow-up of 9.6 years when investigators failed to show that weight loss by intensive lifestyle intervention (one that recommended 1200–1800 calories per day and 175 minutes of moderate-intensity physical activity per week) reduced the risk of cardiovascular events among such patients. Weight loss was significantly greater in the intervention group than the control group throughout the study. At 1 year, patients in the intervention group lost 8.6% of their body weight compared with 0.7% in the control group. As time went on, the intervention group has regained some weight back, whereas the control group gradually lost weight. At the end of the study, the mean weight loss was 6% in the treatment group versus 3.5% in the control group. The intensive lifestyle intervention group had greater improvements than the control group in glycated hemoglobin levels and greater initial improvements in fitness and all other measured cardiovascular risk factors, except low-density lipoprotein cholesterol levels. The difference in the cardiovascular risk factors between the 2 groups also decreased over time, with glycated hemoglobin and systolic blood pressure showing the most sustained differences. The primary end point, which was the first occurrence of cardiovascular outcomes including death from cardiovascular causes, nonfatal myocardial infarction, nonfatal stroke, or hospitalization for angina was similar in both groups (1.83 and 1.92 events per 100 person-years).

The Look AHEAD investigators have considered several possible explanations for the negative results of the study. They noted that the differential weight loss between the intervention and control arms averaged 4.0% over the course of the study but only 2.5% at the end. It is possible that larger weight loss, such as that noted in the SOS study, may be needed to have an effect on cardiovascular events. It should be noted that weight loss in the intervention group represented the excellent weight loss that can be achieved with current lifestyle treatment. The control group did receive diabetes support and education and was able to lose some weight. Other factors such as the intensification of medical management of cardiovascular risk factors in routine medical care in the both study groups and the increased use of statins in the control group may have made the relative benefit of the intensive lifestyle intervention more difficult to demonstrate. So why should clinicians continue to recommend that patients with type 2 diabetes lose weight with diet and exercise even though it does not decrease the risk of heart attack or stroke? Because patients can lose weight safely and improve their glycemic control and their physical fitness. They are more likely to require less insulin, antihypertensive medications, and statins. Some patients may even have a partial remission of diabetes.[2] Other benefits include reductions in urinary incontinence,[3] sleep apnea,[4] and depression[5] and improvements in quality of life,[6] physical functioning,[7] and mobility.

L. Khaodhiar, MD

References

1. Sjöström L. Review of the key results from the Swedish Obese Subjects (SOS) trial—a prospective controlled intervention study of bariatric surgery. *J Intern Med.* 2013; 273:219-234.
2. Gregg EW, Chen H, Wagenknecht LE, et al. Association of an intensive lifestyle intervention with remission of type 2 diabetes. *JAMA.* 2012;308:2489-2496.
3. Phelan S, Kanaya AM, Subak LL, et al. Weight loss prevents urinary incontinence in women with type 2 diabetes: results from the Look AHEAD trial. *J Urol.* 2012; 187:939-944.
4. Foster GD, Borradaile KE, Sanders MH, et al. A randomized study on the effect of weight loss on obstructive sleep apnea among obese patients with type 2 diabetes: the Sleep AHEAF study. *Arch Intern Med.* 2009;169:1619-1626.
5. Faulconbridge LF, Wadden TA, Rubin RR, et al. One-year changes in symptoms of depression and weight in overweight/obese individuals with type 2 diabetes in the Look AHEAD study. *Obesity (Silver Spring).* 2012;20:783-793.
6. Williamson DA, Rejeski J, Lang W, Van Dorsten B, Fabricatore AN, Toledo K. Impact of a weight management program on health-related quality of life in overweight adults with type 2 diabetes. *Arch Intern Med.* 2009;169:163-171.
7. Foy CG, Lewis CE, Hairston KG, et al. Intensive lifestyle intervention improves physical function among obese adults with knee pain: findings from the look AHEAD trial. *Obesity (Silver Spring).* 2011;19:83-93.

Surgical Treatment of Obesity

Review of the key results from the Swedish Obese Subjects (SOS) trial – a prospective controlled intervention study of bariatric surgery

Sjöström L (The Univ of Gothenburg, Sweden)

J Intern Med 273:219-234, 2013

Obesity is a risk factor for diabetes, cardiovascular disease events, cancer and overall mortality. Weight loss may protect against these conditions, but robust evidence for this has been lacking. The Swedish Obese Subjects (SOS) study is the first long-term, prospective, controlled trial to provide information on the effects of bariatric surgery on the incidence of these objective endpoints. The SOS study involved 2010 obese subjects who underwent bariatric surgery [gastric bypass (13%), banding (19%) and vertical banded gastroplasty (68%)] and 2037 contemporaneously matched obese control subjects receiving usual care. The age of participants was 37–60 years and body mass index (BMI) was $\geq$34 kg m^{-2} in men and $\geq$38 kg m^{-2} in women. Here, we review the key SOS study results published between 2004 and 2012. Follow-up periods varied from 10 to 20 years in different reports. The mean changes in body weight after 2, 10, 15 and 20 years were 23%, −17%, −16% and −18% in the surgery group and 0%, 1%, −1% and −1% in the control group respectively. Compared with usual care, bariatric surgery was associated with a long-term reduction in overall mortality (primary endpoint) [adjusted hazard ratio (HR) = 0.71, 95% confidence interval (CI) 0.54– 0.92; $P = 0.01$] and decreased incidences of diabetes (adjusted HR = 0.17; $P < 0.001$), myocardial infarction (adjusted HR = 0.71; $P = 0.02$), stroke (adjusted

HR = 0.66; $P = 0.008$) and cancer (women: adjusted HR = 0.58; $P = 0.0008$; men: n.s.]. The diabetes remission rate was increased severalfold at 2 years [adjusted odds ratio (OR) = 8.42; $P < 0.001$] and 10 years (adjusted OR = 3.45; $P < 0.001$). Whereas high insulin and/or high glucose at baseline predicted favourable treatment effects, high baseline BMI did not, indicating that current selection criteria for bariatric surgery need to be revised.

▶ Overweight and obesity are associated with increased morbidity and mortality. Several short-term studies have demonstrated beneficial effects of moderate weight loss, defined as 5% to 10% weight loss, on many cardiovascular risk factors. The review and meta-analysis of prospective cohort studies showed that intentional weight loss achieved by diet and lifestyle changes had a neutral effect on all-cause mortality.[1] The Look AHEAD (Action for HEAlth in Diabetes) trial, a large randomized controlled study, was stopped early on the basis of futility after 9.6 years when the investigators found no effect of an intensive lifestyle intervention on cardiovascular events in overweight or obese adults with type 2 diabetes.[2] In contrast, the results of retrospective cohort studies in obese subjects have shown that long-term mortality is markedly reduced after gastric bypass surgery in patients both with and without diabetes.[3,4] The Swedish Obese Subjects (SOS) trial is a prospective, nonrandomized controlled intervention study of bariatric surgery. The study involved more than 2000 obese patients who had surgery, compared with more than 2000 obese patients who received usual care. Majority of the patients underwent vertical banded gastroplasty (68%), whereas the remainder underwent either gastric banding (19%) or gastric bypass (13%).

The author has reviewed the results of SOS study published between 2004 to 2012 when the follow-up periods varied from 10 to 20 years. The mean weight losses were 23%, 17%, 16%, and 18% at 2, 10, 15, and 20 years after surgery. Compared with usual care, patients who underwent bariatric surgery had an almost 30% reduction in overall mortality and significantly decreased risks of diabetes, myocardial infarction, stroke, and cancer. The most common cause of death in this cohort was cancer, and fatal myocardial infarction was the second.

Patients with diabetes and/or insulin resistance seem to have multiple benefits from weight loss surgery. Data from the SOS study showed that 72% of patients who had type 2 diabetes at baseline went into remission after 2 years, although about half of these patients had relapsed after 10 years. More importantly, the reduction in cardiovascular death after bariatric surgery was intensified in patients who had higher fasting serum insulin levels. The incidence of myocardial infarction also decreased after surgery in patients with diabetes. In subjects without diabetes, the risk of development of type 2 diabetes diminished by 96%, 84%, and 78% after 2, 10, and 15 years. The reduction in diabetes risk was more pronounced in people with impaired fasting glucose at baseline than people with normal fasting glucose. These numbers are striking considering the risk reduction reported in several intensive lifestyle intervention studies has been on the order of 40% to 60% over 2 to 6 years.[5,6] Serum insulin was a main predictor for the treatment effect after surgery with regard to mortality, cardiovascular events, and incidence of diabetes, whereas body mass index (BMI) did not predict the effect of surgery on any of these end points. The author has suggested current guidelines for bariatric surgery should be modified, giving more importance to metabolic parameters than the BMI value. Similarly, a recent study of the UK General Practice Research Database reported that factors such as type 2 diabetes status and age may be better predictors of 10-year mortality and eligibility for bariatric surgery in obese patients.[7] They concluded that type 2 diabetes mellitus is the most important mortality predictor and suggested prioritizing it over BMI or other comorbidities.

L. Khaodhiar, MD

References

1. Harrington M, Gibson S, Cottrell RC. A review and meta-analysis of the effect of weight loss on all-cause mortality risk. *Nutr Res Rev.* 2009;22:93-108.
2. Look AHEAD Research Group, Wing RR, Bolin P, Brancati FL, et al. Cardiovascular effects of intensive lifestyle intervention in type 2 diabetes. *N Engl J Med.* 2013;369:145-154.
3. Macdonald KG Jr, Long SD, Swanson MS, et al. The gastric bypass operation reduces the progression and mortality of non-insulin-dependent diabetes mellitus. *J Gastrointest Surg.* 1997;1:213-220.
4. Adams TD, Gress RE, Smith SC, et al. Long-term mortality after gastric bypass surgery. *N Engl J Med.* 2007;357:753-761.
5. Knowler WC, Barrett-Connor E, Fowler SE, et al. Diabetes Prevention Program Research Group. Reduction in the incidence of type 2 diabetes with lifestyle intervention or metformin. *N Engl J Med.* 2002;346:393-403.
6. Yamaoka K, Tango T. Efficacy of lifestyle education to prevent type 2 diabetes: a meta-analysis of randomized controlled trials. *Diabetes Care.* 2005;28:2780-2786.
7. Padwal RS, Klarenbach SW, Wang X, et al. A simple prediction rule for all-cause mortality in a cohort eligible for bariatric surgery. *JAMA Surg.* 2013;148:1109-1115.

4 Thyroid

Introduction

A number of recent studies in this section are likely to have an important bearing on the practice of endocrinology. This year, I considered the study by Bath et al, which was published in *The Lancet*, as one of the best in 2013.[1] The aim of this study was to investigate whether women with low iodine status in early pregnancy would have children with poorer cognitive outcomes than those of higher status. A previous Avon Longitudinal Study of Parents and Children (ALSPAC) showed a positive association between maternal seafood consumption and child intelligence quotient (IQ), which the authors suggest could at least partly have been driven by the high iodine content of seafood. Even though this study has several limitations, such as the use of just one spot-urine sample for iodine measurement, the study observed a significant difference in the verbal and the total IQ in children of iodine-deficient mothers compared to children of mothers with normal iodine intake. This study is in line with former studies showing a lower IQ in children of mothers with (subclinical) hypothyroidism during pregnancy compared to children of euthyroid mothers. This, however, is also a matter of discussion. Nonetheless, there is a clear recommendation of the WHO to supplement iodine in iodine-deficient areas and especially in pregnant woman. The present study supports this concept.

Another study by Shields et al investigated the natural history of mild thyroid hormone deficiency during pregnancy and post-delivery.[2] The authors performed the first systematic follow-up study of subclinical hypothyroidism in pregnancy. They found that the majority of women identified as having subclinical hypothyroidism in pregnancy had normal TSH levels after pregnancy; only a few women with maternal hypothyroxinemia had high TSH levels outside pregnancy. The biggest risk factor for raised TSH levels after pregnancy was the presence of TPO antibodies. Irrespective of the limitations of the study, these results highlight the need for reassessment of the thyroid status of pregnant women after pregnancy.

These are just two examples of excellent studies published in 2013. I hope you enjoy reading these and other commentaries.

Matthias Schott, MD, PhD

References

1. Bath SC, Steer CD, Golding J, Emmett P, Rayman MP. Effect of inadequate iodine status in UK pregnant women on cognitive outcomes in their children: results from the Avon Longitudinal Study of Parents and Children (ALSPAC). *Lancet.* 2013; 382:331-337.
2. Shields BM, Knight BA, Hill AV, Hattersley AT, Vaidya B. Five-year follow-up for women with subclinical hypothyroidism in pregnancy. *J Clin Endocrinol Metab.* 2013;98:E1941-E1945.

Autoimmunity

Reduced Effectiveness of $CD4^{+}Foxp3^{+}$Regulatory T Cells in CD28-Deficient NOD.H-2h4 Mice Leads to Increased Severity of Spontaneous Autoimmune Thyroiditis

Ellis JS, Hong S-H, Zaghouani H, et al (Univ of Missouri, School of Medicine, Columbia)

J Immunol 191:4940-4949, 2013

NOD.H-2h4 mice given NaI in their drinking water develop iodine-accelerated spontaneous autoimmune thyroiditis (ISAT) with chronic inflammation of the thyroid by T and B cells and production of anti-mouse thyroglobulin (MTg) autoantibody. $CD28^{-/-}$ NOD.H-2h4 mice, which have reduced numbers of $CD4^{+}Foxp3^{+}$regulatory T cells (Tregs), were developed to examine the role of Tregs in ISAT development. $CD28^{-/-}$ NOD.H2-h4 mice develop more severe ISAT than do wild-type (WT) mice, with collagen deposition (fibrosis) and low serum T4. $CD28^{-/-}$mice have increased expression of proinflammatory cytokines IFN-γ and IL-6, consistent with increased mononuclear cell infiltration and tissue destruction in thyroids. Importantly, transferring purified $CD4^{+}Foxp3^{+}$Tregs from WT mice reduces ISAT severity in $CD28^{-/-}$ mice without increasing the total number of Tregs, suggesting that endogenous Tregs in $CD28^{-/-}$ mice are functionally ineffective. Endogenous $CD28^{-/-}$ Tregs have reduced surface expression of CD27, TNFR2 p75, and glucocorticoid-induced TNFR-related protein compared with transferred $CD28^{+/+}$ Tregs. Although anti-MTg autoantibody levels generally correlate with ISAT severity scores in WT mice, $CD28^{-/-}$ mice have lower anti-MTg autoantibody responses than do WT mice. The percentages of follicular B cells are decreased and those of marginal zone B cells are increased in spleens of $CD28^{-/-}$ mice, and they have fewer thyroid-infiltrating B cells than do WT mice. This suggests that CD28 deficiency has direct and indirect effects on the B cell compartment. B cell-deficient ($B^{-/-}$) NOD.H-2h4 mice are resistant to ISAT, but $CD28^{-/-}B^{-/-}$ mice develop ISAT comparable to WT mice and have reduced numbers of Tregs compared with WT $B^{-/-}$ mice.

► NOD.H-2h4 mice given sodium iodide in their drinking water develop iodine-accelerated spontaneous autoimmune thyroiditis (ISAT). ISAT is characterized by infiltration of the thyroid by T and B cells, with destruction of thyroid follicles and production of Abs to mouse thyroglobulin. In the present study, the authors hypothesized that an early permanent deficiency in regulatory T cells (Tregs), as in NOD mice, would lead to increased activation of autoreactive effector CD4+ T cells and increased ISAT severity in wild-type and B2/2CD28$^{-/-}$ NOD.H-2h4 mice. CD28$^{-/-}$ NOD.H-2h4 mice were developed to test this hypothesis. The results presented in this article suggest that, in addition to having reduced Tregs compared with wild-type NOD.H-2h4 mice, CD28-deficient mice have Tregs that are less effective at suppressing autoimmune thyroiditis. This is shown, for instance, in Fig 4 of the original article. Also of note, B-cell function and/or the effectiveness of T-cell help were affected by the lack of CD28 (Fig 5 of the original article). This is an important study because it shows that thyroiditis in these mice is mediated not only by the lower number of Tregs but also by the lesser effectiveness of T cells in these mice.

M. Schott, MD, PhD

Changes in Serum Adhesion Molecules, Chemokines, Cytokines, and Tissue Remodeling Factors in Euthyroid Women Without Thyroid Antibodies Who Are at Risk for Autoimmune Thyroid Disease: A Hypothesis on the Early Phases of the Endocrine Autoimmune Reaction

Beumer W, Effraimidis G, Drexhage RC, et al (Erasmus Univ, Rotterdam, The Netherlands; Univ of Amsterdam, The Netherlands)

J Clin Endocrinol Metab 98:2460-2468, 2013

Background.—The target glands in spontaneous animal models of endocrine autoimmune disease show, prior to the autoimmune reaction, growth and connective tissue abnormalities, whereas the autoimmune reaction is initiated by an early accumulation of macrophages and dendritic cells in the target glands.

Aim.—The aim of the study was to test the hypothesis that serum factors related to these growth and connective tissue abnormalities and the early accumulation of immune cells, ie, tissue growth/remodeling factors, adhesion molecules, chemokines, and pro- and anti-inflammatory cytokines, are related to thyroid peroxidase autoantibodies (TPO-Abs) seroconversion in subjects at risk to develop autoimmune thyroid disease (AITD).

Design.—A controlled study on 64 TPO-Ab-negative euthyroid female relatives with at least 1 first- or second-degree relative with documented autoimmune hyper- or hypothyroidism, 32 of whom did and 32 who did not seroconvert to TPO-Ab positivity in 5-year follow-up. The relatives were compared with 32 healthy controls. In all subjects we measured serum levels of chemokine (C-C motif) ligand (CCL)-2, CCL3, CCL4, soluble vascular cell adhesion molecule, soluble intercellular adhesion molecule-1, thrombospondin-1, vascular endothelial growth factor-A, angiopoietin 1 receptor-2, metalloproteinase-13, platelet-derived growth factor-BB, fibronectin, IL-1β, IL-6, TNF-α, IL-10, and growth differentiation factor-15 by multiplex (cytometric bead array) or a single commercial ELISA.

Results.—Both seroconverting and nonseroconverting family members showed an up-regulation of fibronectin and a down-regulation of platelet-derived growth factor-BB and the adhesion and migration factors CCL2, CCL4, soluble vascular cell adhesion molecule-1, angiopoietin 1 receptor-2, and metalloproteinase-13. The seroconverters differed from the nonseroconverters by an up-regulation of the proinflammatory compounds Il-1β, IL-6, and CCL3.

Conclusion.—This study shows that euthyroid females within AITD families show a characteristic pattern of abnormalities in serum levels of tissue remodeling factors, growth factors, chemokines, (vascular) adhesion molecules, and cytokines prior to the occurrence of TPO-Abs in serum. The results provide proof of principle that preseroconversion stages and seroconversion to AITD might be predicted using serum analytes related to growth/connective tissue abnormalities and migration/accumulation abnormalities of macrophages and dendritic cells.

▶ There is a generally accepted view that subjects with a family history of autoimmune thyroid disease (AITD) are at increased risk to also get this autoimmune disorder.[1] This observation can be attributed to genetics and also to environmental factors. Presence of thyroid peroxidase autoantibodies (TPO-Abs) is a marker to predict disease progression in an advanced state. Markers to predict the risk for AITD in a very early state are limited and comprise the known genetic predispositions.[2] Because AITD represents an immunologic disorder with macrophages and dendritic cells accumulating in the thyroid gland just before thyroid autoimmunization, the authors hypothesized that immunologic early prediction marker (eg, chemokines, vascular factors, adhesion molecules, matrix remodeling factors, cytokines) might be found in healthy euthyroid individuals known to be at risk for AITD. Comparing euthyroid seroconverting, nonseroconverting, and healthy women, changes in serum adhesion molecules, chemokines, cytokines, and tissue remodeling factors are detected by Beumer and colleagues. Euthyroid seroconverting and nonseroconverting women differed by the level of the proinflammatory compounds interkeukin-1β (IL-1β), IL-6, and chemokine (CC motif) ligand (CCL)-3 as sown in Fig 2 of the original article. Women at risk for AITD showed a higher level of fibronectin (Fig 4 in the original article) and a lower level of platelet-derived growth factor-BB, CCL2, CCL4, soluble vascular cell adhesion molecule-1, angiopoietin 1 receptor-2, and metalloproteinase-13 (Figs 2-4 in the original article). Despite some technical limitations (insufficient sensitivity for some cytokines) and statistical restriction (subject number) Beumer gives the proof of principle that very early stages of AITD (still no TPO-Abs in serum) are detectable in individuals at risk by testing peripheral blood for these immunologic compounds.

M. Ehlers, PhD
M. Schott, MD, PhD

References

1. Strieder TG, Tijssen JG, Wenzel BE, Endert E, Wiersinga WM. Prediction of progression to overt hypothyroidism or hyperthyroidism in female relatives of patients with autoimmune thyroid disease using the Thyroid Events Amsterdam (THEA) score. *Arch Intern Med.* 2008;15:1657-1663.
2. Eschler DC, Hasham A, Tomer Y. Cutting edge: the etiology of autoimmune thyroid diseases. *Clin Rev Allergy Immunol.* 2011;2:190-197.

Thyroid Cancer

Differentiated Thyroid Cancer Is Associated With Less Aggressive Disease and Better Outcome in Patients With Coexisting Hashimotos Thyroiditis

Dvorkin S, Robenshtok E, Hirsch D, et al (Rabin Med Ctr, Petah Tikva, Israel)
J Clin Endocrinol Metab 98:2409-2414, 2013

Background.—Evaluation of surgical specimens suggests that patients with Hashimoto thyroiditis (HT) have a higher prevalence of differentiated thyroid cancer. Although patients with HT are reported to present with earlier stage disease, there is controversy as to whether these patients have better prognosis when adjusted for histology and stage at presentation.

Objectives.—To investigate differences between patients with differentiated thyroid cancer patients and without HT for aggressiveness of disease and clinical outcome, and the decline rate of antithyroglobulin antibodies titers over time.

Methods.—A retrospective study using the Rabin Medical Center Thyroid Cancer Registry. Seven hundred fifty-three patients were included and divided into 2 groups of patients with and without HT at diagnosis. Disease severity at presentation was evaluated using the entire cohort, whereas a control group matched for age, gender, histology, and stage was used to evaluate disease course and outcome.

Results.—HT was present in 14.2% (n = 107) of included patients and was associated with smaller primary tumor (17.9 vs 21.2 mm, $P = .01$) and less lymph node involvement (23% vs 34%, $P = .02$) at presentation. When matched groups were compared, patients with HT received less additional radioactive iodine (RAI) treatments (1.24 vs 1.45, $P = .03$) and showed lower rates of persistence at 1 year (13% vs 26%, $P = .04$) and higher rates of disease remission at the end of follow-up (90% vs 79%, $P = .05$). On multivariate analysis HT was predictive of a lower rate of lymph nodes involvement (odds ratio 0.34, 95% confidence interval 0.17–0.66) and persistent disease at the end of follow-up (odds ratio 0.48, 95% confidence interval 0.24–0.93). Antithyroglobulin antibodies slowly disappeared in most patients with no evidence of disease.

Conclusion.—Our study demonstrates that HT is associated with a less aggressive form of differentiated thyroid cancer and a better long-term outcome (Table 2).

▶ An association of Hashimoto thyroiditis (HT) and papillary thyroid cancer has been suggested for decades as thyroid specimens of HT patients often show

TABLE 2.—Clinical Characteristics and Outcome of PTC Matched Patients With and Without HT

	Hashimoto (n = 98)	Controls (n = 98)	*P* Value
Female, %	93	92	ns
Age, y, mean ± SD	50.5 ± 15	50.5 ± 15	ns
Size, mm, mean ± SD	17.8 ± 12	19.5 ± 13	ns
Multifocal tumor, %	54	55	ns
Extrathyroidal extension, %	19	15	ns
Stage, %			
I	58	56	ns
II	9	11	ns
III	22	23	ns
IV	8	9	ns
RAI ablation dose, mCi, mean ± SD	110 ± 46	101 ± 51	ns
Number of RAI treatments, mean ± SD	1.24 ± 0.5	1.45 ± 0.8	.03
Cumulative RAI dose, mCi, mean ± SD	145 ± 82	177 ± 145	.06
External radiotherapy, %	3	3	ns
Additional surgery, %	4.1	11.2	.12
Persistent disease at 1 y, %	13	26	.04
NED at last follow-up, %	90	79	.05

Abbreviations: NED, no evidence of disease; ns, not significant; RAI, radioactive iodine.

coexisting carcinoma.[1] But in contrast to surgical and pathological series, large population-based clinical studies failed to show any significant increase of the incidence of thyroid cancer in cohorts of patients with HT followed up for more than 10 years.[2] This observation led Dvorkin and his colleagues to the question as to whether differentiated thyroid cancer (DTC), when present, is less aggressive in HT patients. Using the Rabin Medical Center thyroid cancer registry, the impact of HT on the long-term outcome of DTC was investigated. The study included 753 patients with DTC; 107 had coexisting HT (14.2%). When compared with the control group, patients with HT had both significantly smaller primary tumor and less lymph node involvement. Furthermore, HT patients needed fewer additional radioactive iodine treatments, showed lower rates of persistence at 1 year, and were often found with no evidence of disease at the end of follow-up (Table 2). Antithyroglobulin antibodies (Tg-Abs) disappeared in most patients (84%) with no evidence of disease. This study has a few limitations, as it is possible that HT patients have a better prognosis because they are subjected to more intensive surveillance, resulting in earlier diagnosis. Furthermore, the higher prevalence of HT among women should be kept in mind, as women are known to have more thyroid cancers but fewer recurrences and better survival. An interesting result is the detection of Tg-Abs in 16% of patients that have no evidence of persistent disease several years after initial treatment. Whether the persistency of Tg-Abs during follow-up represents persistent disease or immune memory is not clarified.

The study by Dvorkin and colleagues shows that DTC follows a less-aggressive course in HT patients.

M. Ehlers, PhD
M. Schott, MD, PhD

References

1. Hirabayashi RN, Lindsay S. The relation of thyroid carcinoma and chronic thyroiditis. *Surg Gynecol Obstet.* 1965;121:243-252.
2. Rago T, Di Coscio G, Ugolini C, et al. Clinical features of thyroid autoimmunity are associated with thyroiditis on histology and are not predictive of malignancy in 570 patients with indeterminate nodules on cytology who had a thyroidectomy. *Clin Endocrinol (Oxf).* 2007;67:363-369.

Does *BRAF* V600E Mutation Predict Aggressive Features in Papillary Thyroid Cancer? Results From Four Endocrine Surgery Centers

Li C, Aragon Han P, Lee KC, et al (The Johns Hopkins Univ School of Medicine, Baltimore, MD; et al)

J Clin Endocrinol Metab 98:3702-3712, 2013

Background.—Existing evidence is controversial regarding the association between *BRAF* mutation status and aggressive features of papillary thyroid cancer (PTC). Specifically, no study has incorporated multiple surgical practices performing routine central lymph node dissection (CLND) and thus has patients who are truly evaluable for the presence or absence of central lymph node metastases (CLNMs).

Methods.—Consecutive patients who underwent total thyroidectomy and routine CLND at 4 tertiary endocrine surgery centers were retrospectively reviewed. Descriptive and bivariable analyses examined demographic, patient, and tumor-related factors. Multivariable analyses examined the odds of CLNM associated with positive *BRAF* status.

Results.—In patients with classical variant PTC, bivariate analysis found no significant associations between *BRAF* mutation and aggressive clinicopathologic features; multivariate analysis demonstrated that *BRAF* status was not an independent predictor of CLNM. When all patients with PTC were analyzed, including those with aggressive or follicular subtypes, bivariate analysis showed *BRAF* mutation to be associated with LNM, advanced American Joint Committee on Cancer (AJCC) stage, and histologic subtype. Multivariable analyses showed *BRAF*, age, size, and extrathyroidal extension to be associated with CLNM.

Conclusion.—Although *BRAF* mutation was found to be an independent predictor of central LNM in the overall cohort of patients with PTC, this relationship lost significance when only classical variant PTC was included in the analysis. The usefulness of *BRAF* in predicting the presence of LNM remains questionable. Prospective studies are needed before *BRAF* mutation can be considered a reliable factor to guide the treatment of patients with PTC, specifically whether to perform prophylactic CLND (Table 14).

▶ A high proportion of papillary thyroid carcinomas (PTC) are characterized by somatic aberrations in the *BRAF* kinase gene. The most frequent mutation is

TABLE 14.—Multivariate Analysis of Predictors Available Preoperatively of Central LNM in All Patients With PTC

Preoperative Features	Odds Ratio	95% Confidence Interval	*P*
BRAF mutation	2.20	1.34–3.61	.002[a]
Gender (female)	1.47	0.87–2.48	.150
Age (≥45 y)	0.43	0.28–0.67	<.001[b]
Tumor size (>2 cm)	1.82	1.16–2.85	.010[a]

[a]Denotes significant positive association.
[b]Denotes significant negative association.

caused by an amino acid change (T1799A/p.V600E) and associated with gain of function. This study aims to address the important controversy regarding the prognostic value of *BRAF* mutation status, with particular emphasis on lymph node metastases, by incorporating patients from 4 tertiary endocrine surgery centers whose surgeons perform routine central lymph node dissection for all patients with PTC. The authors investigated 315 patients with classical variant PTC (CVPTC). In the subgroup of patients with CVPTC only, the bivariate analysis found no significant associations between *BRAF* mutation and aggressive clinicopathologic features, including the presence of lymph node metastases (LNM). Multivariable analysis in our CVPTC subgroup found that only increased tumor size and extrathyroidal extension (ETE) were independent predictors of central LNM (Table 14). When similar analyses were applied to patients with follicular variant PTC, significant bivariate associations between *BRAF* mutation and older age as well as advanced American Joint Committee on Cancer stage were seen. *BRAF* mutation and ETE were also found to be independent predictors of central LNM in this subgroup.

As stated by the authors, the results of this study emphasize that the existing evidence behind the use of *BRAF* V600E mutation as a prognostic indicator, specifically to guide whether to perform a central lymph node dissection in patients with PTC, is insufficient. Although *BRAF* mutation was found to be an independent predictor of central LNM in the overall cohort of patients with PTC, this relationship lost significance when follicular and aggressive variants were excluded from the analysis, and only patients with CVPTC, the most common subtype, were examined. Based on these results, the usefulness of *BRAF* mutation in the management algorithm of patients of PTC remains questionable. Prospective, multi-institutional studies should be carried out before *BRAF* mutation can be considered a reliable factor to guide the treatment of patients with PTC.

M. Schott, MD, PhD

Aberrant Overexpression of Pyruvate Kinase M2 Is Associated With Aggressive Tumor Features and the *BRAF* Mutation in Papillary Thyroid Cancer

Feng C, Gao Y, Wang C, et al (The First Hosp of China Med Univ, Liaoning, People's Republic of China; Feng Tian Hosp, Liaoning, People's Republic of China)

J Clin Endocrinol Metab 98:E1524-E1533, 2013

Context.—Many tumor cells predominantly generate energy through high rates of glycolysis. Pyruvate kinase M2 (PKM2) has been identified as being necessary for aerobic glycolysis.

Objective.—The aim of this study was to investigate the expression pattern of PKM2 in papillary thyroid cancer (PTC) and the possible role of PKM2 in PTC.

Design.—The expression of PKM2 in human thyroid tissues was examined using immunocytochemistry. PKM2 expression in PTC correlated with clinicopathological features and the *BRAF* mutation. PTC cells were transfected with small interfering RNA against *PKM2*. PKM2 expression in cells was analyzed by Western blotting and real-time RT-PCR. Cell growth was evaluated both in vitro and in vivo. Lactate and ATP production and glucose consumption by cells were determined using commercial assay kits.

Results.—PKM2 was aberrantly overexpressed in PTC. This overexpression was associated with poor clinicopathological features including advanced tumor stages and lymph node metastasis. More intensive immunostaining of PKM2 was detected in PTCs harboring the *BRAF* mutation. Specific small interfering RNA against *PKM2* in PTC cell lines retarded cell growth both in vitro and in xenograft mouse models. *PKM2* knockdown also reduced lactate and ATP production and glucose consumption by PTC cells.

Conclusions.—We conclude that overexpression of PKM2 provides a selective growth advantage for PTC cells through activation of glycolysis. Aberrant PKM2 overexpression may serve as a novel biomarker and a potential treatment target for PTC. The *BRAF* mutation may contribute to alterations in the expression pattern of glycolytic enzymes such as PKM2 (Table 2).

▶ The Warburg effect is a phenomenon described in cancer cells that predominantly use aerobic glycolysis with reduced mitochondrial oxidative phosphorylation for glucose metabolism.[1] This property is known to support the energetic requirement for the high proliferative rate of tumor cells. One necessary factor for aerobic glycolysis is the M2 isoform of pyruvate kinase (PKM2). Expression of this metabolic phenotype provides a selective growth advantage for tumor cells and is known to be aberrantly overexpressed in various kinds of human cancers.[2] The aim of the present study was to investigate whether a PKM2-induced alteration in glucose metabolism enables papillary thyroid carcinoma (PTC) cells to sustain rapid production of energy for cell proliferation.

TABLE 2.—Correlation of PKM2 Expression in Human PTC With Clinical Aggressiveness and the *BRAF* Mutation

Clinical Features	No.	Staining of PKM2, n (%) Negative	Weakly Positive	Positive	IRS (mean ± SD)	*P* Value[a]
Age						.08
<45 y	41	1 (2)	4 (10)	36 (88)	6.6 ± 3.6	
≥45 y	39	0 (0)	2 (8)	37 (95)	8.1 ± 4.0	
Sex						.14
Male	20	0 (0)	3 (15)	17 (85)	6.3 ± 3.7	
Female	60	1 (2)	3 (5)	56 (93)	7.7 ± 3.8	
Multifocality						.71
No	63	1 (2)	4 (6)	58 (92)	7.5 ± 3.9	
Yes	17	0 (0)	2 (12)	15 (88)	7.9 ± 3.7	
Lymph node metastasis						.003
No	41	1 (2)	6 (15)	34 (83)	6.1 ± 3.8	
Yes	39	0 (0)	0 (0)	39 (100)	8.4 ± 3.5	
Stages						.01
I/II	62	1 (2)	6 (10)	55 (88)	6.7 ± 3.7	
III/IV	18	0 (0)	0 (0)	18 (100)	9.4 ± 3.8	
BRAF gene						<.001
Wild type	34	1 (3)	5 (15)	28 (82)	4.5 ± 2.5	
T1799A mutation	46	0 (0)	1 (2)	45 (98)	9.5 ± 3.2	

[a]Comparisons between the IRS values in two groups.

Performing immunohistochemistry, Feng and colleagues demonstrated an overexpression of PKM2 in PTC tissue as well as in metastatic lymph node tissue of PTC (Fig 1 in the original article). The intensity of PKM2 staining significantly correlated with the aggressive features of PTC (lymph node metastasis and advanced tumor stages) as well as with the occurrence of the T1799A BRAF mutation (Table 2). Using 2 PKM2-positive PTC tumor cell lines (BCPAP and K1), knockdown of PKM2 by siRNA approved the role of PKM2 for cell proliferation because PKM2 knockdown inhibited cell growth (Fig 3 in the original article). Furthermore, alteration of PKM2 expression in PTC cells affected glucose metabolism, as shown by reduced lactate and ATP production in tumor cells after PKM2 knockdown (Fig 4 in the original article). Some limitations of this study are because of the experimental setting. Although the study's results suggests potential for PKM2 as a biomarker for diagnosing indeterminate thyroid nodules, further studies are needed because follicular thyroid tumors were not stained by Feng and colleagues. Furthermore, whether there is a direct linkage between PKM2 expression and disease prognosis could not be determined because long-term follow-up data from patients with PTC were not obtained in this study. Additionally, the mechanism through which PKM2 expression is regulated in PTC is unknown and should be investigated. In summary, Feng and colleagues showed that PKM2 is upregulated in PTC. This PKM2 expression was associated with clinical aggressiveness, leading to the suggestion that overexpression of PKM2 provides a selective growth advantage for PTC cells through activation of aerobic glycolysis. In addition, PKM2 overexpression correlates with the presence of the *BRAF* mutation.

M. Ehlers, PhD

M. Schott, MD, PhD

References

1. Warburg O, Wind F, Negelein E. The Metabolism of Tumors in the Body. *J Gen Physiol.* 1927;8:519-530.
2. Christofk HR, Vander Heiden MG, Harris MH, et al. The M2 splice isoform of pyruvate kinase is important for cancer metabolism and tumour growth. *Nature.* 2008;452:230-233.

S100A11 Overexpression Contributes to the Malignant Phenotype of Papillary Thyroid Carcinoma

Anania MC, Miranda C, Vizioli MG, et al (Fondazione IRCCS Istituto Nazionale dei Tumori, Milan, Italy)
J Clin Endocrinol Metab 98:E1591-E1600, 2013

Context.—Papillary thyroid carcinoma (PTC) is the most frequent thyroid tumor and is responsible for the overall increase in thyroid cancer incidence. S100A11 (calgizzarin), a member of the S100 Ca^{2+}-binding protein family, is involved in several different biological processes. S100A11 has been found up-regulated in PTC, both at the mRNA and protein levels.

Objective.—Through a combination of expression analysis and functional in vitro and in vivo studies, we have attempted to gain insight into the relevance of *S100A11* overexpression in PTC biology.

Design.—The expression of the *S100A11* gene in PTC was investigated in several gene expression data sets. The effect of *S100A11* silencing on the hallmarks of the malignant phenotype of several PTC-derived cell lines was investigated. In NIH3T3 cells, the cooperation of S100A11 with the different PTC-specific oncogenes was assessed.

Results.—We found that the *S100A11* gene expression is frequently up-regulated in PTC, anaplastic thyroid carcinoma, but not in follicular thyroid carcinoma. *S100A11* overexpression was also detected in PTC-derived cell lines, which were then used for functional studies. *S100A11* silencing in PTC-derived cell lines did not affect cell proliferation, whereas it reduced the loss of contact inhibition, anchorage-independent growth, and resistance to anoikis. Cotransfection experiments in NIH3T3 cells showed that overexpression of the *S100A11* gene was able to enhance the transforming capabilities of the different PTC-associated oncogenes by affecting the loss of contact inhibition, anchorage-independent growth, and in vivo tumor formation.

Conclusion.—Our data indicate that S100A11 overexpression exerts a protumoral functional role in PTC pathogenesis.

▶ Papillary thyroid carcinoma (PTC) is the most common thyroid malignancy. Although several elements are known to be associated with PTC (eg, rearrangement of the RET and NTRK1 tyrosine kinase receptors, mutations in the *BRAF* or *RAS* genes),[1] the molecular pathogenesis is partially unknown. Therefore, the impact of novel elements on the pathogenesis of PTC has to be investigated. One of these novel elements is S100A11, a Ca^{2+}-binding protein (also known as *calgizzarin*), that is known to be up-regulated in PTC with respect to normal thyroid and also to adenomas and goiter.[2] The aim of the study of Anania and colleagues was to investigate the impact of S100A11 overexpression on the PTC's pathogenesis. The aforementioned up-regulated gene expression of S100A11 was confirmed for PTC and anaplastic thyroid carcinoma compared with normal thyroid tissue and follicular thyroid carcinoma (Fig 1 in the original article). S100A11 knockdown did not affect the cell growth, whereas it played a role in conferring resistance to anoikis-mediated cell death, at least in PTC-derived cell lines (Fig 2 in the original article). In vivo, S100A11 knockdown had no effect on the tumorigenicity of a PTC cell line because S100A11 knocked-down tumor cells showed the same tumorigenicity as control cells (Fig 3 in the original article). At first glance, these results suggest that S100A11 regulates invasion and metastatic processes but not local tumor growth, although only a partial S100A11 knockdown cannot be excluded. Further investigation is needed to clearly describe the mechanism leading to the up-regulation of S100A11 in tumors, to define the role of S100A11 in PTC pathogenesis, and to predict the mechanism through which S100A11 regulates the phenotype of thyroid tumor cell in particular. The study by Anania suggests a protumoral functional role of S100A11 overexpression in PTC pathogenesis.

M. Ehlers, PhD
M. Schott, MD, PhD

References

1. Greco A, Borrello MG, Miranda C, Degl'Innocenti D, Pierotti MA. Molecular pathology of differentiated thyroid cancer. *Q J Nucl Med Mol Imaging*. 2009;5:440-453.
2. Stolf BS, Abreu CM, Mahler-Araújo MB, et al. Expression profile of malignant and non-malignant diseases of the thyroid gland reveals altered expression of a common set of genes in goiter and papillary carcinomas. *Cancer Lett*. 2005;227:59-73.

Frequent Somatic *TERT* Promoter Mutations in Thyroid Cancer: Higher Prevalence in Advanced Forms of the Disease

Landa I, Ganly I, Chan TA, et al (Memorial Sloan-Kettering Cancer Ctr, NY; et al)

J Clin Endocrinol Metab 98:E1562-E1566, 2013

Background.—TERT encodes the reverse transcriptase component of telomerase, which adds telomere repeats to chromosome ends, thus enabling cell replication. Telomerase activity is required for cell immortalization. Somatic *TERT* promoter mutations modifying key transcriptional response elements were recently reported in several cancers, such as melanomas and gliomas.

Objectives.—The objectives of the study were: 1) to determine the prevalence of *TERT* promoter mutations C228T and C250T in different thyroid cancer histological types and cell lines; and 2) to establish the possible association of *TERT* mutations with mutations of *BRAF, RAS*, or *RET/PTC*.

Methods.—*TERT* promoter was PCR-amplified and sequenced in 42 thyroid cancer cell lines and 183 tumors: 80 papillary thyroid cancers (PTCs), 58 poorly differentiated thyroid cancers (PDTCs), 20 anaplastic thyroid cancers (ATCs), and 25 Hurthle cell cancers (HCCs).

Results.—*TERT* promoter mutations were found in 98 of 225 (44%) specimens. *TERT* promoters *C228T* and *C250T* were mutually exclusive. Mutations were present in 18 of 80 PTCs (22.5%), in 40 of 78 (51%) advanced thyroid cancers (ATC + PDTC) ($P = 3 \times 10^{-4}$ vs PTC), and in widely invasive HCCs (4 of 17), but not in minimally invasive HCCs (0 of 8). *TERT* promoter mutations were seen more frequently in advanced cancers with *BRAF/RAS* mutations compared to those that were *BRAF/RAS* wild-type (ATC + PDTC, 67.3 vs 24.1%; $P < 10^{-4}$), whereas *BRAF*-mutant PTCs were less likely to have *TERT* promoter mutations than *BRAF* wild-type tumors (11.8 vs 50.0%; $P = .04$).

Conclusions.—*TERT* promoter mutations are highly prevalent in advanced thyroid cancers, particularly those harboring *BRAF* or *RAS* mutations, whereas PTCs with *BRAF* or *RAS* mutations are most often *TERT* promoter wild type. Acquisition of a *TERT* promoter mutation could extend survival of *BRAF*- or *RAS*-driven clones and enable accumulation of additional genetic defects leading to disease progression (Table 1).

► The *TERT* gene encodes the reverse transcriptase component of the telomerase complex, necessary for cell proliferation. High telomerase activity and *TERT* expression have been reported in thyroid tumors, mainly in advanced forms.[1] Furthermore, mutations in the promoter of *TERT* have been identified as a highly frequent event in metastatic forms of melanoma.[2] Neither the prevalence of *TERT* promoter mutations in different thyroid cancers (histologic tissues and cell lines) nor the possible association of *TERT* mutations with mutations of *BRAF, RAS,* or *RET/PTC* were known, and these were therefore the aims to

TABLE 1.—*TERT* Promoter Mutations in Thyroid Cancer Tumors and Cell Lines

Group	n	TERT Promoter Mutations, n (%) Wild- Type	C228T	C250T	C228T or C250T	*P* Value[a]
PTC (MSKCC)	29	21 (72.4)	5 (17.2)	3 (10.3)	8 (27.6)	
PTC (Japan)	51	41 (80.4)	5 (9.8)	5 (9.8)	10 (19.6)	
PTC (all)	80	62 (77.5)	10 (12.5)	8 (10.0)	18 (22.5)	
PDTC	58	28 (48.3)	18 (31.0)	12 (20.7)	30 (51.7)	.0005
ATC	20	10 (50.0)	10 (50.0)	0 (0.0)	10 (50.0)	.0241
Advanced thyroid cancers (PDTC + ATC)	78	38 (48.7)	28 (35.9)	12 (15.4)	40 (51.3)	.0003
HCC, minimally invasive (HCC-MIN)	8	8 (100.0)	0 (0.0)	0 (0.0)	0 (0.0)	
HCC, widely invasive (HCC-WIDE)	17	13 (76.5)	3 (17.6)	1 (5.9)	4 (23.5)	.2689
Thyroid cancer cell lines	42	6 (14.3)	26 (61.9)	10 (23.8)	36 (85.7)	<.0001

[a]*P* values were derived from Fisher's exact test, using "PTC (all)" as the reference group, with the exception of HCC, where "HCC-MIN" was used.

be investigated in this study. Comparing papillary thyroid cancers (PTC), advanced thyroid cancers (anaplastic thyroid cancer, poorly differentiated thyroid cancer), and widely invasive and minimally invasive Hurthle cell cancers, *TERT* promoter mutations were found significantly more often in advanced thyroid cancers compared with PTCs (Table 1). An association of *TERT* and *BRAF/RAS* mutations was also discovered (Fig 1 in the original article). Although diverse mechanisms may lead to increased activation of *TERT*, mutations of this gene may be relevant prognostic markers in thyroid cancer as the authors suggest.

In summary, Landa and colleagues report a high frequency of *TRET* promoter mutations in follicular cell-derived thyroid carcinomas. An overexpression of *TRET* promoter mutations in advanced thyroid cancers and an association with mutations in *BRAF* and *RAS* were found.

M. Ehlers, PhD
M. Schott, MD, PhD

References

1. Umbricht CB, Saji M, Westra WH, Udelsman R, Zeiger MA, Sukumar S. Telomerase activity: a marker to distinguish follicular thyroid adenoma from carcinoma. *Cancer Res.* 1997;57:2144-2147.
2. Horn S, Figl A, Rachakonda PS, et al. TERT promoter mutations in familial and sporadic melanoma. *Science.* 2013;339:959-961.

Development of p21 Activated Kinase-Targeted Multikinase Inhibitors That Inhibit Thyroid Cancer Cell Migration

Ma Y, McCarty SK, Kapuriya NP, et al (The Ohio State Univ Wexner Med Ctr, Columbus)
J Clin Endocrinol Metab 98:E1314-E1322, 2013

Context.—The p21 activated kinases (PAKs) are a family of serine/threonine kinases that are downstream effectors of small GTPase Cdc42 and Rac. PAKs regulate cell motility, proliferation, and cytoskeletal rearrangement. PAK isoform expression and activity have been shown to be enhanced in cancer and to function as an oncogene in vivo. PAKs also have been implicated in cancer progression.

Objective.—In thyroid cancer, we have previously determined that PAK overactivation is common in the invasive fronts of aggressive tumors and that it is functionally involved in thyroid cancer cell motility using molecular inhibitors. We report the development of two new PAK-inhibiting compounds that were modified from the structure OSU-03012, a previously identified multikinase inhibitor that competitively blocks ATP binding of both phosphoinositide-dependent kinase 1 (PDK1) and PAK1.

Results.—Seventeen compounds were created by combinatorial chemistry predicted to inhibit PAK activity with reduced anti-PDK1 effect. Two lead compounds were identified based on the ability to inhibit PAK1 activity in an ATP-competitive manner without discernible in vivo PDK1 inhibitory activity in thyroid cancer cell lines. Both compounds reduced thyroid cancer cell viability. Although they are not PAK-specific on a multikinase screening assay, the antimigration activity effect of the compounds in thyroid cancer cells was rescued by overexpression of a constitutively active PAK1, suggesting this activity is involved in this biological effect.

Conclusions.—We have developed 2 new multikinase inhibitors with anti-PAK activity that may serve as scaffolds for further compound development targeting this progression-related thyroid cancer target (Table 1).

▶ The p21-activated kinases (PAKs) are downstream effectors of small GTPase Cdc42 and Rac, participate in a wide range of physiologic processes (eg, cell motility, cytoskeletal rearrangement, proliferation, apoptosis, oncogenesis), and are known to be activated and overexpressed in aggressive papillary cancers and several other malignancies.[1] The PAK activity correlates with the baseline invasiveness of human breast cancers and breast cancer tumor grade as well as with Ras-mediated tumorigenesis in several tissue types, making PAK a potential therapeutic target for cancer therapy. OSU-03012, a multikinase inhibitor that blocks phosphoinositide-dependent kinase 1 (PDK1) has previously been described to also inhibit PAK in an adenosine triphosphate (ATP)-competitive manner.[2] The aim of the study was to develop OSU-03012 derivates that selectively inhibit PAK but not PDK1. Two of 17 compounds showed the property to block ATP binding to PAK1 leading to inhibition of PAK1 activity (Fig 2 in the original article) as shown by ATP competition assays. Both compounds were further shown to inhibit PAK without altering PDK1 in thyroid cancer cell lines in a concentration-dependent manner (Fig 4 in the original article). Additionally,

TABLE 1.—Potencies of Compounds for Reducing Viability of BCPAP, FTC133, and TPC1 Cells Versus DMSO Control[a]

Compound	IC_{50}, μmol/L BCPAP	FTC133	TPC1
OSU-03012	2.93 ± 1.05	2.93 ± 1.87	2.80 ± 1.33
1	2.01 ± 0.59	4.78 ± 4.53	2.60 ± 0.81
2	2.67 ± 0.82	4.83 ± 4.47	1.81 ± 1.24
3	2.34 ± 0.27	5.32 ± 4.05	3.17 ± 1.29
4	2.07 ± 0.06	2.68 ± 2.08	1.68 ± 0.32
5	>10	5.03 ± 0.25	>10
6	>10	>10	>10
7	3.71 ± 1.82	4.53 ± 2.57	3.67 ± 1.52
8	2.90 ± 2.35	3.08 ± 1.63	4.67 ± 4.16
9	4.04 ± 1.38	4.75 ± 2.47	2.42 ± 0.13
10	6.53 ± 2.16	8.95 ± 0.57	7.39 ± 1.90
11	4.50 ± 1.04	3.94 ± 2.29	4.98 ± 1.94
12	3.76 ± 1.20	7.55 ± 2.19	5.83 ± 1.73
13	2.76 ± 1.56	4.95 ± 3.21	3.62 ± 0.42
14	3.32 ± 1.09	5.42 ± 1.56	5.98 ± 0.28
15	1.49 ± 0.68	3.37 ± 3.31	2.66 ± 1.05
16	>10	>10	4.38 ± 2.18
17	>10	>10	8.96 ± 1.17

[a]The reported IC_{50} values are concentrations at which BCPAP, FTC133, and TPC1 cell viability by MTT assays are 50% of DMSO control after 72 hours of exposure. Data are presented as mean ± SD ($n = 3$).

inhibition of cell growth (Table 1) and migration could also be seen (Fig 5 in the original article). Further work is still needed, as the mechanism for OSU-03012 derivate–induced cell viability reduction is not identified. Additionally, because of technical limitations, only migration, and not invasion, was evaluated in these experiments. The other pathways may have a role in invasion and should be tested in the future. Furthermore, in vivo studies have to be performed to fully assess efficacy and toxicity of these OSU-03012 derivates. Ma and colleagues developed 2 new OSU-03012–like compounds that inhibited PAK but not PDK1 in an ATP-competitive manner. Nevertheless, further experiments are needed to devise more potent and selective inhibitors of PAK, the potential therapeutic target for thyroid cancer and other malignancies.

M. Schott, MD, PhD

M. Ehlers, PhD

References

1. Dummler B, Ohshiro K, Kumar R, Field J. Pak protein kinases and their role in cancer. *Cancer Metastasis Rev.* 2009;28:51-63.
2. Porchia LM, Guerra M, Wang YC, et al. 2-amino-N-{4-[5-(2-phenanthrenyl)-3-(trifluoromethyl)-1H-pyrazol-1-yl]-phenyl} acetamide (OSU-03012), a celecoxib derivative, directly targets p21-activated kinase. *Mol Pharmacol.* 2007;72:1124-1131.

Inhibition of AMPK and Krebs Cycle Gene Expression Drives Metabolic Remodeling of *Pten*-Deficient Preneoplastic Thyroid Cells

Antico Arciuch VG, Russo MA, Kang KS, et al (Albert Einstein College of Medicine, Bronx, NY)

Cancer Res 73:5459-5472, 2013

Rapidly proliferating and neoplastically transformed cells generate the energy required to support rapid cell division by increasing glycolysis and decreasing flux through the oxidative phosphorylation (OXPHOS) pathway, usually without alterations in mitochondrial function. In contrast, little is known of the metabolic alterations, if any, which occur in cells harboring mutations that prime their neoplastic transformation. To address this question, we used a *Pten*-deficient mouse model to examine thyroid cells where a mild hyperplasia progresses slowly to follicular thyroid carcinoma. Using this model, we report that constitutive phosphoinositide 3-kinase (PI3K) activation caused by PTEN deficiency in nontransformed thyrocytes results in a global downregulation of Krebs cycle and OXPHOS gene expression, defective mitochondria, reduced respiration, and an enhancement in compensatory glycolysis. We found that this process does not involve any of the pathways classically associated with the Warburg effect. Moreover, this process was independent of proliferation but contributed directly to thyroid hyperplasia. Our findings define a novel metabolic switch to glycolysis driven by PI3K-dependent AMPK inactivation with a consequent repression in the expression of key metabolic transcription regulators.

► Highly proliferative conditions require a complex reorganization of energy metabolism. A major feature of this metabolic remodeling is the switch from oxidative phosphorylation (OXPHOS) to aerobic glycolysis.[1] This phenomenon is well known for cancer cells with activated phosphoinositide 3-kinase (PI3K) playing a pivotal role. Without affecting the mitochondrial metabolism, the expression or activity of a variety of glycolytic enzymes is described to be increased.[2,3] In contrast, little is known of the mechanisms regulating energy metabolism in normal and preneoplastic cells. It is assumed that in normal cells, the glycolytic switch is linked to high proliferation rates. Investigating preneoplastic thyrocytes from young, tumor-free PTEN-deficient mice ($PTEN^{thyr-/-}$), Arciuch and colleagues aimed to discover the mechanism leading to the metabolic remodeling in nontransformed cells. As shown in Fig 1 of the original article, constitutive PI3K activation led to the downregulation of the expression of genes encoding members of the tricarboxylic acid (TCA) cycle and OXPHOS pathways, to extensive mitochondrial damage, and to severe impairment of mitochondrial function. This phenomenon was independent of mammalian target of rapamycin and the cellular proliferation rate (Fig 3 in the original article), leading to the discovery of a novel pathway for the glycolytic switch. Responsible for the repression of oxidative metabolism gene expression observed in $Pten^{thyr-/-}$ mice was the PI3K/AKT-mediated AMP-activated protein kinase (AMPK) inhibition (Figs 4 and 5 in the original article). A further consequence of the described constitutive PI3K activation in $Pten^{thyr-/-}$ mice (leading to the AMPK inhibition, further leading to the glycolytic switch) is the development of thyroid hyperplasia (Fig 5 in the original article). Investigating this mechanism in a human setting, the results suggest that the PI3K/AKT axis controls AMPK activity also in $PTEN^{-/-}$ human thyroid cancer cells (Fig 6 in the original article).

The study by Antico Arciuch and colleagues showed that, in response to PI3K activation and independent of cell proliferation, nontransformed thyroid epithelial cells increase metabolic flux through glycolysis. This metabolic reprogramming involved the inhibition of AMPK and the consequent downregulation of the expression of TCA cycle and OXPHOS genes, leading to the impairment of mitochondrial metabolism. Although further research is needed to investigate this phenomenon in humans, Antico Arciuch and colleagues discovered in their study a novel pathway responsible for the metabolic switch in normal and preneoplastic cells.

M. Ehlers, PhD
M. Schott, MD, PhD

References

1. Warburg O. On the origin of cancer cells. *Science.* 1956;123:309-314.
2. Raimundo N, Baysal BE, Shadel GS. Revisiting the TCA cycle: signaling to tumor formation. *Trends Mol Med.* 2011;17:641-649.
3. Koppenol WH, Bounds PL, Dang CV. Otto Warburg's contributions to current concepts of cancer metabolism. *Nat Rev Cancer.* 2011;11:325-337.

Identification of kinase fusion oncogenes in post-Chernobyl radiation-induced thyroid cancers

Ricarte-Filho JC, Li S, Garcia-Rendueles MER, et al (Memorial Sloan-Kettering Cancer Ctr, NY; Weill Cornell Med College, NY; et al)

J Clin Invest 123:4935-4944, 2013

Exposure to ionizing radiation during childhood markedly increases the risk of developing papillary thyroid cancer. We examined tissues from 26 Ukrainian patients with thyroid cancer who were younger than 10 years of age and living in contaminated areas during the time of the Chernobyl nuclear reactor accident. We identified nonoverlapping somatic driver

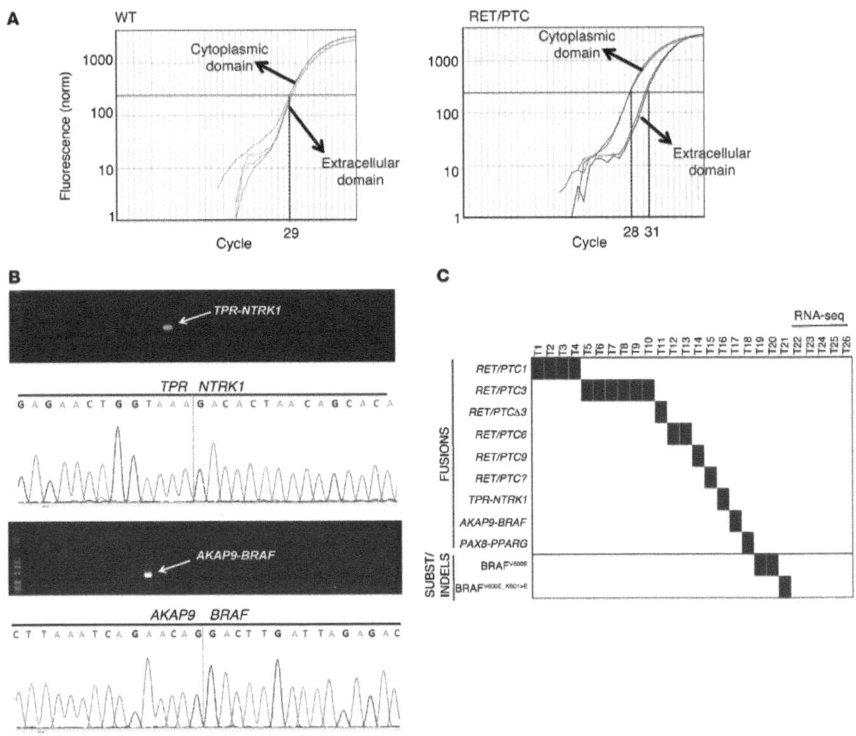

FIGURE 1.—Screen for genetic alterations in radiation-exposed pediatric thyroid cancer. (**A**) Analysis of RET unbalanced expression (exons 10 and 11/exons 12 and 13) to detect samples with *RET* fusion oncogenes. The figure shows representative CT plots from quantitative RT-PCR of exons 10 and 11 (encoding extracellular domain) and 12 and 13 (encoding cytoplasmic domain) of a sample without *RET* fusion oncogene (ratio ~1:1) (left) and a sample with *RET* fusion (right). (**B**) RT-PCR and Sanger sequencing for the identification and validation of *TPR-NTRK1* and *AKAP9-BRAF* fusion oncogenes in 2 radiation-exposed cancers. (**C**) Summary of genetic alterations found in 26 radiation-exposed pediatric thyroid cancers. All but 5 harbored one of the previously described oncogenic events. The 5 tumors with no identifiable defect on the candidate gene screen underwent RNA-seq. (Reprinted from Ricarte-Filho JC, Li S, Garcia-Rendueles MER, et al. Identification of kinase fusion oncogenes in post-Chernobyl radiation-induced thyroid cancers. *J Clin Invest.* 2013;123:4935-4944, © 2013, American Society of Clinical Investigation.)

mutations in all 26 cases through candidate gene assays and next-generation RNA sequencing. We found that 22 tumors harbored fusion oncogenes that arose primarily through intrachromosomal rearrangements. Altogether, 23 of the oncogenic drivers identified in this cohort aberrantly activate MAPK signaling, including the 2 somatic rearrangements resulting in fusion of transcription factor ETS variant 6 (*ETV6*) with neurotrophic tyrosine kinase receptor, type 3 (*NTRK3*) and fusion of acylglycerol kinase (*AGK*) with *BRAF.* Two other tumors harbored distinct fusions leading to overexpression of the nuclear receptor PPARγ. Fusion oncogenes were less prevalent in tumors from a cohort of children with pediatric thyroid cancers that had not been exposed to radiation but were from the same geographical regions. Radiation-induced thyroid cancers provide a paradigm of tumorigenesis driven by fusion oncogenes that activate MAPK signaling or, less frequently, a PPARγ-driven transcriptional program (Figs 1-3).

▶ One of the genetic components for the development of thyroid cancers is the existence of RET/PTC rearrangements. These fusion transcripts are generated by ionizing radiation in human thyroid cell lines and human fetal thyroid tissue xenografts[1] and lead to constitutive expression and activation of the kinase domain of the RET tyrosine kinase receptor. Individuals exposed to the ionizing radiation after the Chernobyl nuclear reactor accident are therefore at high risk for fusion oncogenes in thyroid cells.[2] In fact, many children who were exposed

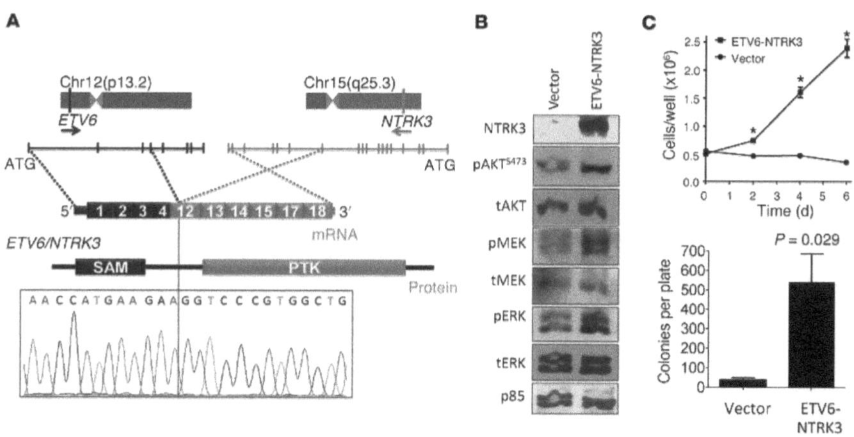

FIGURE 2.—Characterization of *ETV6-NTRK3* fusion oncogene in radiation-exposed pediatric thyroid cancer. (**A**) Genomic location, mRNA and protein structure, and validation by Sanger sequencing of *NTRK3* fusion oncogene. Exons 1–4 of *ETV6* are shown in blue and exons 12–18 of *NTRK3* are shown in red. PTK, protein tyrosine kinase; SAM, sterile α motif. (**B**) Western blot of NIH3T3 cells transiently transfected with empty vector or pMSCV-ETV6-NTRK3. Cells were depleted of serum for 24 hours prior to collection. ETV6-NTRK3–expressing cells had higher levels of pAKT, pMEK, pERK, and cyclin D1. tAKT, total AKT; tMEK, total MEK; tERK, total ERK. (C) Increased growth ($^*P < 3 \times 10^{-4}$ vs. vector transfected) and agar colony formation of NIH-3T3 cells expressing *ETV6-NTRK3*. Data represent mean ± SEM. (Reprinted from Ricarte-Filho JC, Li S, Garcia-Rendueles MER, et al. Identification of kinase fusion oncogenes in post-Chernobyl radiation-induced thyroid cancers. *J Clin Invest.* 2013;123:4935-4944, © 2013, American Society of Clinical Investigation.)

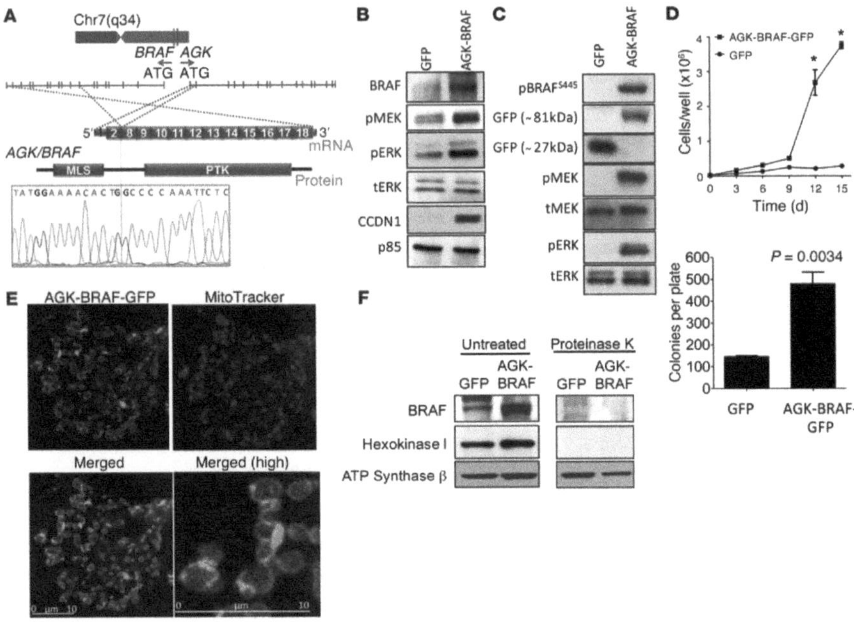

FIGURE 3.—Characterization of *AGK-BRAF* fusion oncogene in radiation-exposed pediatric thyroid cancer. (**A**) Genomic location, mRNA and protein structure, and validation by Sanger sequencing of *BRAF* fusion oncogenes. Exons 1 and 2 of *AGK* are shown in brown and exons 8–18 of *BRAF* are shown in green. (**B** and **C**) Western blot of serum-depleted (**B**) NIH3T3 or (**C**) COS7 cells transiently transfected with pLVX-AcGFP-N1 or pLVX-*AGK-BRAF*-GFP. *AGK-BRAF* expressing cells had robust induction of pMEK and pERK. (D) Increased growth ($^*P < 3 \times 10^{-3}$ vs. vector transfected) and agar colony formation of NIH-3T3 cells expressing *AGK-BRAF*. Data represent mean ± SEM. (**E**) Confocal fluorescence imaging of COS7 cells transfected with pLVX-*AGK-BRAF*-GFP and stained with MitoTracker. The distribution of green fluorescence overlaps but does not colocalize with that of MitoTracker (red). Merged images (bottom row) show mitochondria surrounded by a green fluorescent rim (original magnification, ×252 [top and bottom left]; ×840 [bottom right]). Scale bars: 10 μm. (**F**) The BRAF kinase domain faces the cytosol in cells transfected with *AGK-BRAF*. Western blotting of lysates of mitochondrial fractions of NIH3T3 cells stably transfected with pLVX-AcGFP-N1 (GFP) or pLVX-*AGK-BRAF*-GFP (*AGK-BRAF*) treated with or without proteinase K. Membranes were incubated with antibodies to BRAF, hexokinase 1, or ATP synthase β. All 3 proteins, including the *AGK-BRAF*-GFP fusion protein, are seen in intact mitochondrial lysates. *AGK-BRAF* is depleted by proteinase K, as is the outer mitochondrial-bound protein hexokinase 1, whereas the inner mitochondrial protein ATP synthase β is not. For Interpretation of the references to color in this figure legend, the reader is referred to web version of this article. (Reprinted from Ricarte-Filho JC, Li S, Garcia-Rendueles MER, et al. Identification of kinase fusion oncogenes in post-Chernobyl radiation-induced thyroid cancers. *J Clin Invest.* 2013;123:4935-4944, © 2013, American Society of Clinical Investigation.)

to the fallout developed papillary thyroid carcinoma (PTC). The aim of the study was to identify further driver translocations and novel fusions in post-Chernobyl cancer specimens indicating alternative mechanisms of thyroid cancer transformation. Investigating tissue from 26 patients with thyroid cancer who were younger than 10 years at the time of radiation exposure, somatic driver mutations were found in every case. Known oncogenic events were found in 21 patients, including driver mutations affecting rearrangements of *RET/PTC, TPR-NTRK1, PAX8-PPARG*, and *AKAP9-BRAF* and point mutations/indels of BRAF (Fig 1). In 5 patients, new somatic fusions were found with likely oncogenic properties including CREB3L2-PPARG, acylglycerol kinase—BRAF

(*AGK-BRAF*), and ETS variant 6—neurotrophic tyrosine kinase receptor type 3 (ETV6-NTRK3) (Fig 2). Functional analysis found that *CREB3L2-PPARG* leads to expression changes consistent with a known PPARG-driven transcriptional program, and *AGK-BRAF* and ETV6-NTRK3 activates MAPK and PI3K pathways and transforms NIH3T3 cells leading to cell growth and colony formation (Figs 2 and 3).

Ricarte-Filho and colleagues demonstrate the radiation-induced generation of fusion oncogenes, resulting mainly from intrachromosomal rearrangements and leading to activated MAPK pathway.

M. Schott, MD, PhD
M. Ehlers, PhD

References

1. Caudill CM, Zhu Z, Ciampi R, Stringer JR, Nikiforov YE. Dose-dependent generation of RET/PTC in human thyroid cells after in vitro exposure to gamma-radiation: a model of carcinogenic chromosomal rearrangement induced by ionizing radiation. *J Clin Endocrinol Metab*. 2005;4:2364-2369.
2. Fugazzola L, Pilotti S, Pinchera A, et al. Oncogenic rearrangements of the RET proto-oncogene in papillary thyroid carcinomas from children exposed to the Chernobyl nuclear accident. *Cancer Res*. 1995;23:5617-5620.

Comparative Analysis of the Thyrocytes and T Cells: Responses to H_2O_2 and Radiation Reveals an H_2O_2-Induced Antioxidant Transcriptional Program in Thyrocytes

Versteyhe S, Driessens N, Ghaddhab C, et al (Université Libre de Bruxelles, Brussels, Belgium)
J Clin Endocrinol Metab 98:E1645-E1654, 2013

Context.—Radiation is an established cause of thyroid cancer, and growing evidence supports a role for hydrogen peroxide (H_2O_2) in spontaneous thyroid carcinogenesis. Little is known about the molecular programs activated by these agents in thyrocytes.

Objective.—The purpose of this study was to compare the responses of thyrocytes and T cells to H_2O_2 and radiation.

Methods.—We profiled the DNA damage and cell death induced by γ-radiation (0.1—5 Gy) and H_2O_2 (0.0025—0.3 mM) in primary human thyrocytes and T cells. We next prepared thyroid and T-cell primary cultures from 8 donors operated for noncancerous thyroid pathological conditions and profiled their genome-wide transcriptional response 4 hours after (1) exposure to 1-Gy radiation, (2) treatment with H_2O_2 and (3) no treatment. Two H_2O_2 concentrations were investigated, calibrated in each cell type to elicit levels of single- and double-strand breaks equivalent to 1-Gy γ-radiation.

Results.—Although thyrocytes and T cells had comparable radiation responses, 3- to 10-fold more H_2O_2 was needed to induce detectable DNA damage in thyrocytes. At H_2O_2 and radiation doses inducing double-strand breaks, cell death occurred after 24 hours in T cells but not in thyrocytes. The transcriptional responses of thyrocytes and T cells to radiation were similar, involving DNA repair and cell death genes. In addition to this transcriptional program, H_2O_2 also up-regulated antioxidant genes in thyrocytes, including glutathione peroxidases and heme oxygenase at the double-strand breaks–inducing concentration. In contrast, a transcriptional storm involving thousands of genes was raised in T cells. Finally, we showed that inhibiting glutathione peroxidases activity increased the DNA damaging effect of H_2O_2 in thyrocytes.

Conclusion.—We propose that high H_2O_2 production in thyrocytes is matched with specific transcriptionally regulated antioxidant protection.

▶ Ionizing radiation is known to cause papillary thyroid carcinoma (PTC) while it is supposed for hydrogen peroxide (H_2O_2). H_2O_2 is produced by thyrocytes and is required for the iodine oxidation by thyroperoxidase, a key reaction in thyroid hormone synthesis. In dependency to the concentration, exogenous H_2O_2 exposure is known to have genotoxic properties causing single- and double-strand breaks in thyroid cell lines.[1] Given the long thyrocyte lifespan (7 years in adults),[2] the chronic exposure to H_2O_2 might produce the somatic mutations that could drive spontaneous PTC. The aim of this study was to characterize the response of thyrocytes to H_2O_2 from the perspective of DNA damage, cell death, and genomewide transcription. A dual comparative setup was performed. To gain thyrocyte-specific effects, all experiments were run in parallel in T cells; to compare the results with a proven etiologic agent of PTC, all experiments were replicated with radiation. Fig 1 in the original article shows thyrocytes being more resistant to H_2O_2 compared with T cells, as 3- to 10-fold more H_2O_2 was needed to induce DNA damage in thyrocytes. Furthermore, cell death occurred in T cells 24 hours after radiation and H_2O_2 exposure but not in thyrocytes. Radiation and H_2O_2 both induce transcriptional programs in T cells and thyrocytes related to DNA repair and apoptosis. Additionally, H_2O_2 induced an antioxidant program exclusively in thyrocytes by the induced up-regulation of heme oxygenase and glutathione peroxidases with the latter being found to prevent the DNA damaging effect of H_2O_2 in thyrocytes.

As discussed by the authors, this study has one fundamental limitation. The effects of radiation and H_2O_2 have overlapping toxicity profiles (eg, induction of single- and double-strand breaks in thyrocytes) and cannot be completely disentangled; radiolysis of water produces H_2O_2. Taken together, this study suggests a model of PTC susceptibility in which traits pertaining to DNA repair and H_2O_2 detoxification confer susceptibility to spontaneous as well as radiation-induced PTC. Conceivably, additional traits associated with H_2O_2 production and its cellular localization would confer susceptibility to spontaneous PTC only.

M. Ehlers, PhD
M. Schott, MD, PhD

References

1. Driessens N, Versteyhe S, Ghaddhab C, et al. Hydrogen peroxide induces DNA single- and double-strand breaks in thyroid cells and is therefore a potential mutagen for this organ. *Endocr Relat Cancer.* 2009;16:845-856.
2. Coclet J, Foureau F, Ketelbant P, Galand P, Dumont JE. Cell population kinetics in dog and human adult thyroid. *Clin Endocrinol (Oxf).* 1989;31:655-665.

Vandetanib in Children and Adolescents with Multiple Endocrine Neoplasia Type 2B Associated Medullary Thyroid Carcinoma

Fox E, Widemann BC, Chuk MK, et al (The Children's Hosp of Philadelphia, PA; Natl Cancer Inst, Bethesda, MA; et al)

Clin Cancer Res 19:4239-4248, 2013

Purpose.—Medullary thyroid carcinoma (MTC) is a manifestation of multiple endocrine neoplasia type 2 (MEN2) syndromes caused by germline, activating mutations in the *RET* (*REarranged during Transfection*) proto-oncogene. Vandetanib, a VEGF and EGF receptor inhibitor, blocks RET tyrosine kinase activity and is active in adults with hereditary MTC.

Experimental Design.—We conducted a phase I/II trial of vandetanib for children (5–12 years) and adolescents (13–18 years) with MTC to define a recommended dose and assess antitumor activity. The starting dose was 100 mg/m^2 administered orally, once daily, continuously for 28-day treatment cycles. The dose could be escalated to 150 mg/m^2/d after two cycles. Radiographic response to vandetanib was quantified using RECIST (v1.0), biomarker response was measured by comparing posttreatment serum calcitonin and carcinoembryonic antigen (CEA) levels to baseline, and a patient-reported outcome was used to assess clinical benefit.

Results.—Sixteen patients with locally advanced or metastatic MTC received vandetanib for a median (range) 27 (2–52) cycles. Eleven patients remain on protocol therapy. Diarrhea was the primary dose-limiting toxicity. In subjects with M918T *RET* germline mutations ($n = 15$) the confirmed objective partial response rate was 47% (exact 95% confidence intervals, 21%–75%). Biomarker partial response was confirmed for calcitonin in 12 subjects and for CEA in 8 subjects.

Conclusion.—Using an innovative trial design and selecting patients based on target gene expression, we conclude that vandetanib 100 mg/m^2/d is a well-tolerated and highly active new treatment for children and adolescents with MEN2B and locally advanced or metastatic MTC.

► Medullary thyroid carcinoma (MTC), a malignancy of the parafollicular C cells of the thyroid gland, accounts for approximately 5% of all thyroid cancers and presents either sporadically (75% of patients) or in a hereditary pattern. Neither radiotherapy nor chemotherapy has shown durable objective responses in patients with advanced MTC. Germline mutations in the *RET* (rearranged during transfection) proto-oncogene occur in virtually all patients with hereditary MTC. In this study, the authors designed a trial of vandetanib for children and adolescents with hereditary MTC to define the dose, toxicity profile, pharmacokinetics, and antitumor activity. This is the first clinical trial of a *RET* inhibitor in children and adolescents with MTC. Using intrapatient dose escalation meant that all patients with this very rare cancer were also evaluable for response, and a therapeutic effect could be used to define the recommended dose. As shown in Fig 3 of the original article, all 15 patients with M918T *RET* germline mutations experienced a decrease in tumor size. Two examples are shown in Fig 4 of the original article. Of course, patients also had diverse side effects as shown in Fig 2 of the original article. Nonetheless, this is the first study showing a prolonged progression-free survival in children and adolescents with hereditary MTC. Whether any effect is seen in terms of overall survival needs to be investigated in future trials.

M. Schott, MD

Targeted Next-Generation Sequencing Panel (ThyroSeq) for Detection of Mutations in Thyroid Cancer

Nikiforova MN, Wald AI, Roy S, et al (Univ of Pittsburgh Med Ctr, PA)

J Clin Endocrinol Metab 98:E1852-E1860, 2013

Objectives.—Next-generation sequencing (NGS) allows for high-throughput sequencing analysis of large regions of the human genome. We explored the use of targeted NGS for simultaneous testing for multiple mutations in thyroid cancer.

Design.—A custom panel (ThyroSeq) was designed to target 12 cancer genes with 284 mutational hot spots. Sequencing was performed to analyze DNA from 228 thyroid neoplastic and nonneoplastic samples including 105 frozen, 72 formalin-fixed, and 51 fine-needle aspiration samples representing all major types of thyroid cancer.

Results.—Only 5–10 ng of input DNA was sufficient for successful analysis of 99.6% of samples. The analytical accuracy for mutation detection was 100% with the sensitivity of 3%–5% of mutant allele. ThyroSeq DNA assay identified mutations in 19 of 27 of classic papillary thyroid carcinomas (PTCs) (70%), 25 of 30 follicular variant PTCs (83%), 14 of 18 conventional (78%) and 7 of 18 oncocytic follicular carcinomas (39%), 3 of 10 poorly differentiated carcinomas (30%), 20 of 27 anaplastic (ATCs) (74%), and 11 of 15 medullary thyroid carcinomas (73%). In contrast, 5 of 83 benign nodules (6%) were positive for mutations. Most tumors had a single mutation, whereas several ATCs and PTCs demonstrated two or three mutations. The most common mutations detected were *BRAF* and *RAS* followed by *PIK3CA, TP53, TSHR, PTEN, GNAS, CTNNB1*, and *RET.* The *BRAF* mutant allele frequency was 18%–48% in PTCs and was lower in ATCs.

Conclusions.—The ThyroSeq NGS panel allows simultaneous testing for multiple mutations with high accuracy and sensitivity, requires a small amount of DNA and can be performed in a variety of thyroid tissue and fine-needle aspiration samples, and provides quantitative assessment of mutant alleles. Using this approach, the point mutations were detected in 30%–83% of specific types of thyroid cancer and in only 6% of benign thyroid nodules and were shown to be present in the majority of cells within the cancer nodule.

► Thyroid cancer is the most common malignancy of endocrine organs. Ultrasound-guided fine-needle aspiration (FNA) of the thyroid nodule followed by cytologic examination is a common diagnostic approach that allows detection of cancer or establishment of a diagnosis of a benign nodule in most cases. However, in approximately 25% of nodules, the diagnosis cannot be reliably established using FNA cytology. Molecular techniques, that is, a panel of most common mutations in thyroid cancer (BRAF, RAS, RET/PTC, PAX8/PPARdelta) and the Affirma Gene Expression Classifier, offer significant diagnostic improvement over FNA cytology, although the accuracy of cancer detection with both approaches needs further enhancement. In the present study, the authors evaluated targeted next-generation sequencing as a new approach for testing a broad spectrum of point mutations that occur in thyroid cancer and validated the use of a next-generation sequencing mutational panel (ThyroSeq) in various types of thyroid samples obtained from malignant and benign thyroid nodules. Fig 2 in the original article shows the mutational profiles of various types of thyroid cancer. Fig 3 in the original article shows some examples of mutations identified by ThyroSeq. In general, the ThyroSeq next-generation sequencing panel allows simultaneous testing for multiple mutations with high accuracy and sensitivity. Importantly, it requires only a small amount of DNA and can be performed in a variety of thyroid tissue and FNA samples. It is expected that this method further improves the accuracy of cancer diagnosis and prognostication in thyroid nodules.

M. Schott, MD, PhD

Thyroid Nodules

Comparison of Elastographic Strain Index and Thyroid Fine-Needle Aspiration Cytology in 631 Thyroid Nodules

Magri F, Chytiris S, Capelli V, et al (Univ of Pavia, Italy)

J Clin Endocrinol Metab 98:4790-4797, 2013

Context.—Ultrasound (US) elastography (USE) was recently been reported as a sensitive, noninvasive tool for identifying thyroid cancer. However, the accuracy of this technique is hampered by the intra- and interoperator variability, some US features of the nodule, and the coexistence of autoimmune thyroid disease (ATD).

Objectives.—The purpose of this article was to assess the accuracy of USE findings in the differential diagnosis of thyroid nodules compared with other US features to evaluate its feasibility in the presence of ATDs and identify the strain index (SI) cutoff with the highest diagnostic performance. Design: We evaluated 528 consecutive patients for a total of 661 thyroid nodules. All nodules underwent fine-needle aspiration cytology (FNAC) and USE evaluation. The SI was calculated as a ratio of the nodule strain divided by the strain of the softest part of the surrounding normal tissue.

Results.—The median SI value was significantly higher in THY4 and THY5 than in THY2 nodules in ATD-positive, ATD-negative, and ATD-unknown patients. The cutoff of SI for malignancy was estimated to be 2.905 by receiver operating characteristic curve analysis in a screening set (379 FNACresults), and then tested in a replication set (252 FNACresults). In all cases, a SI value of ≥2.905 conferred to the nodule a significantly greater probability of being malignant. This SI cutoff had the greatest area under the curve, sensitivity, and negative predictive value, compared with the conventional US features of malignancy.

Conclusion.—The elastographic SI has a high sensitivity, specificity, and negative predictive value for the diagnosis of thyroid malignancy both in the presence and in the absence of ATD. If our data on USE are also confirmed in THY3 nodules, FNAC could be avoided in a number of thyroid nodules with certain features.

▶ Ultrasound elastography (USE) was recently introduced as a technique that, by assessing tissue elasticity, might differentiate malignant (usually hard) from benign lesions. With this technique, tissue elasticity is evaluated by measuring the local displacement of nodular tissue being compressed by an external force: the softer the nodule, the larger the displacement and vice versa. The resulting elastogram is an image of relative stiffness compared with the extranodular tissue. The aim of the study by Magri et al was to assess the diagnostic accuracy of USE in predicting thyroid malignancy by identifying the optimal cutoff value for the strain index, evaluating the feasibility of USE in patients with coexistent autoimmune thyroid disease (ATD), and comparing USE findings with conventional US signs of thyroid malignancy.

Within this study, cytologic samples were classified into 5 classes (n = 24): THY1 (nondiagnostic), THY2 (benign), THY3 (indeterminate follicular lesion), THY4 (suspicious for malignancy), and THY5 (malignant). All THY4 and THY5 results (n = 35) were confirmed as malignant lesions by histologic examination of surgical specimens. The median strain index (SI) value was significantly higher in THY4 and THY5 than in THY2 nodules in ATD-positive, ATD-negative, and ATD-unknown patients (Fig 1 in the original article). The cutoff of SI for malignancy was estimated to be 2.905 by receiver operating characteristic curve analysis in a screening set. The main limitation of this study stems from the exclusion of cytologically indeterminate (THY3) nodules, which gave contradictory results in previous studies. Rago et al,[1] who specifically studied indeterminate nodules by USE in a large series of patients, reported that greater nodular stiffness was associated with malignancy in these nodules. Thus, these authors concluded that USE could serve as a useful tool in the differential diagnosis of malignancy even in indeterminate nodules. The elastographic SI had a high negative predictive value for malignant thyroid nodules. Its diagnostic accuracy was not hampered by coexistent ATD and was higher than that obtained with any conventional US sign of malignancy. As stated by the authors, further studies will be needed to assess the diagnostic value of USE in THY3 nodules. If the current data on USE are confirmed in this subgroup of nodules, fine-needle aspiration cytology could be avoided in a number of thyroid nodules with certain features.

M. Schott, MD, PhD

Reference

1. Rago T, Scutari M, Santini F, et al. Real-time elastosonography: useful tool for refining the presurgical diagnosis in thyroid nodules with indeterminate or nondiagnostic cytology. *J Clin Endocrinol Metab*. 2010;95:5274-5280.

Thyrotoxicosis

Analysis of 754 Cases of Antithyroid Drug-Induced Agranulocytosis Over 30 Years in Japan

Nakamura H, Miyauchi A, Miyawaki N, et al (Kuma Hosp, Chuo-ku, Japan; Nihonbashi-Muromachi 2-Chome, Chuo-ku, Tokyo, Japan)
J Clin Endocrinol Metab 98:4776-4783, 2013

Background.—Agranulocytosis is a rare but serious complication of antithyroid drug (ATD) therapy. Characteristics of agranulocytosis have been reported in only a small number of patients.

Method.—We studied 754 cases of ATD-induced agranulocytosis reported over 30 years. The age distribution and sex ratio were compared with those in 12 503 untreated Graves' patients at Kuma Hospital. The annual number of new Graves' patients in Japan was estimated from the Japan Medical Data Center Data Mart-Pharmacovigilance health insurance receipt database.

Results.—Agranulocytosis developed within 90 days after starting ATD therapy in most patients (84.5%). The methimazole dose given at onset was 25.2 ± 12.8 mg/d (mean ± SD). The mean age was 43.4 ± 15.2 years, and the male to female ratio was 1:6.3. When compared with patients at Kuma Hospital, patients with agranulocytosis were older ($P < .001$) and more females ($P < .0001$). Of 211 patients with more than 1 granulocyte measurement before onset, 131 (62%) showed normal counts (>1000/μL) within 2 weeks before onset, demonstrating real sudden onset of agranulocytosis. In contrast, some of the 20 patients with more than 4 measurements showed gradual decreases in granulocyte counts. Analysis of physician reports for 30 fatal cases revealed that some deaths might have been prevented. The number of new Graves' patients treated with ATD was estimated at about 35 000 per year, and the incidence rate of agranulocytosis was 0.1% to 0.15% in Japan.

Conclusion.—This is the largest study of agranulocytosis. Agranulocytosis tends to occur abruptly within 3 months after initiation of ATD therapy, although it develops gradually in some patients. Providing every patient with sufficient information on agranulocytosis is critical.

▶ Antithyroid drug (ATD) therapy is associated with several adverse reactions. Among them, agranulocytosis is the most serious life-threatening event. It can occur abruptly, and prediction and prevention are very difficult. Agranulocytosis is a rare event, occurring in 0.1% to 0.5% of Graves' patients. The authors of this study studied 754 reports of ATD-induced agranulocytosis. In accordance with the frequency of hyperthyroidism, there is a clear peak of ATD-induced agranulocytosis in the third up to the fifth decade (Fig 1 in the original article). The mean onset of agranulocytosis is between the 20th and about the 40th day after initiation of ATD therapy (Fig 2 in the original article). Importantly, only a few patients died from agranulocytosis during the follow-up since 1986 (Fig 3 in the original article). As stated by the authors, limitations of this study are that data are completely dependent on physician reports, and necessary data are missing in a considerable number of reports. The distinction between agranulocytosis and pancytopenia was not necessarily rigorous, and, in some cases, it was unclear whether symptoms or even death were caused by agranulocytosis. Despite these limitations, the authors believe that this study, the largest to date in patients with agranulocytosis, provides important and thought-provoking information.

M. Schott, MD, PhD

Thyroid Disease in Pregnancy

Effect of inadequate iodine status in UK pregnant women on cognitive outcomes in their children: results from the Avon Longitudinal Study of Parents and Children (ALSPAC)

Bath SC, Steer CD, Golding J, et al (Univ of Surrey, Guildford, UK; Univ of Bristol, UK)

Lancet 382:331-337, 2013

Background.—As a component of thyroid hormones, iodine is essential for fetal brain development. Although the UK has long been considered iodine replete, increasing evidence suggests that it might now be mildly iodine deficient. We assessed whether mild iodine deficiency during early pregnancy was associated with an adverse effect on child cognitive development.

Methods.—We analysed mother-child pairs from the Avon Longitudinal Study of Parents and Children (ALSPAC) cohort by measuring urinary iodine concentration (and creatinine to correct for urine volume) in stored samples from 1040 first-trimester pregnant women. We selected women on the basis of a singleton pregnancy and availability of both a urine sample from the first trimester (defined as ≤13 weeks' gestation; median 10 weeks [IQR 9–12]) and a measure of intelligence quotient (IQ) in the offspring at age 8 years. Women's results for iodine-to-creatinine ratio were dichotomised to less than 150 μg/g or 150 μg/g or more on the basis of WHO criteria for iodine deficiency or sufficiency in pregnancy. We assessed the association between maternal iodine status and child IQ at age 8 years and reading ability at age 9 years. We included 21 socioeconomic, parental, and child factors as confounders.

Findings.—The group was classified as having mild-to-moderate iodine deficiency on the basis of a median urinary iodine concentration of 91·1 μg/L (IQR 53·8–143; iodine-to-creatinine ratio 110 μg/g, IQR 74–170). After adjustment for confounders, children of women with an iodine-to-creatinine ratio of less than 150 μg/g were more likely to have scores in the lowest quartile for verbal IQ (odds ratio 1·58, 95% CI 1·09–2·30; $P = 0·02$), reading accuracy (1·69, 1·15–2·49; $P = 0·007$), and reading comprehension (1·54, 1·06–2·23; $P = 0·02$) than were those of mothers with ratios of 150 μg/g or more. When the less than 150 μg/g group was subdivided, scores worsened ongoing from 150 μg/g or more, to 50–150 μg/g, to less than 50 μg/g.

Interpretation.—Our results show the importance of adequate iodine status during early gestation and emphasise the risk that iodine deficiency can pose to the developing infant, even in a country classified as only mildly iodine deficient. Iodine deficiency in pregnant women in the UK should be treated as an important public health issue that needs attention (Fig 1).

▶ The World Health Organization considers iodine deficiency to be the single most important preventable cause of brain damage worldwide. Although iodine deficiency is often thought to be a problem of developing countries, industrialized countries are not immune. Indeed, concern is emerging that iodine deficiency might be widespread in industrialized countries. The aim of this study was to investigate whether women with low iodine status in early pregnancy would have children with poorer cognitive outcomes than would those with higher status. A previous Avon Longitudinal Study of Parents and Children (ALSPAC) found a positive association between maternal seafood consumption and child intelligence quotient (IQ), which the authors suggest could at least partly have been driven by the high iodine content of seafood.[1]

As shown in Fig 1 there was a significant difference in the verbal IQ, the total IQ, and reading comprehension in children of iodine-deficient mothers compared with children of mothers with normal iodine intake.

As discussed by the authors, this study has several limitations. First, because it is observational, residual confounding by factors that the authors either have not measured or not considered is a possibility; however, adjustment for up to 21 variables mostly made little difference to overall effect sizes. The authors did not control for potential iodine deficiency in the child, but this deficiency is likely to be less of an issue than in pregnancy because the iodine requirement in childhood is substantially lower and more likely to be met by children's high consumption of milk. Second, use of one spot-urine sample has limitations for measurement of iodine status in an individual. However, these limitations were minimized by correcting for urinary volume with use of iodine-to-creatinine ratio and by broad grouping of women into 2 categories of iodine

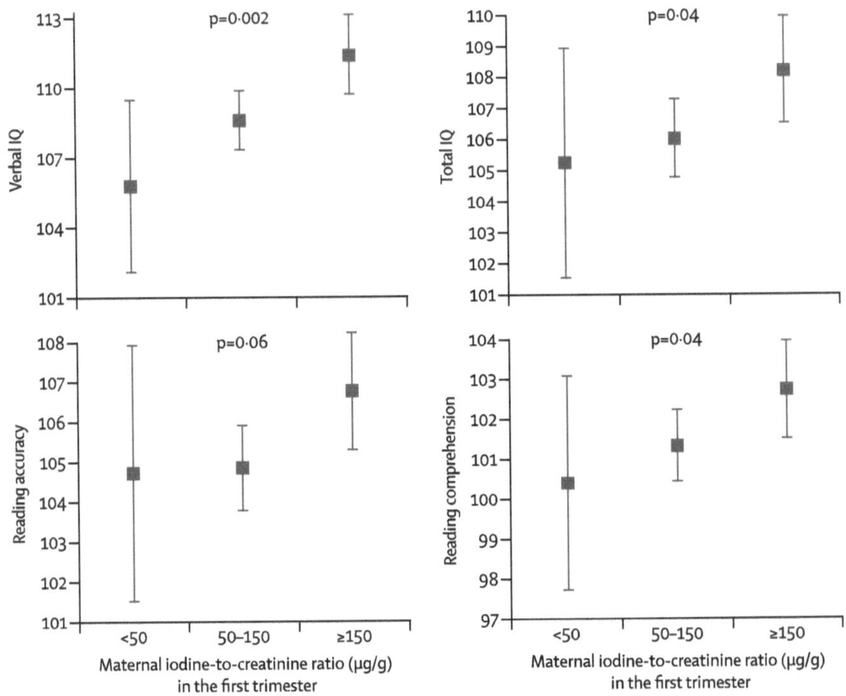

FIGURE 1.—Means (95% CIs) for child cognitive outcomes according to maternal iodine status in the first trimester Values are adjusted for the effect of confounders (model three). Child verbal and total IQ were assessed at age 8 years and reading accuracy and comprehension at age 9 years. IQ = intelligence quotient. (Reprinted from Bath SC, Steer CD, Golding J, et al. Effect of inadequate iodine status in UK pregnant women on cognitive outcomes in their children: results from the Avon Longitudinal Study of Parents and Children (ALSPAC). *Lancet.* 2013;382:331-337, Copyright 2013, with permission from Elsevier.)

status, effectively giving 2 populations and reducing the effect of any misclassification of status. Third, measurement of iodine status at one time point in pregnancy might not represent dietary iodine intake during the entire pregnancy and does not give specific information about maternal thyroid function, of which the authors have no measure.

Because of the observational nature of this study, these findings need to be replicated by others. Evidence from a randomized placebo-controlled trial of the effect of iodine supplementation in pregnancy on child cognition is needed from regions of mild-to-moderate iodine deficiency because existing evidence from trials in such regions is weak.

M. Schott, MD

Reference

1. Hibbeln JR, Davis JM, Steer C, et al. Maternal seafood consumption in pregnancy and neurodevelopmental outcomes in childhood (ALSPAC study): an observational cohort study. *Lancet.* 2007;369:578-585.

Hypothyroxinemia and TPO-Antibody Positivity Are Risk Factors for Premature Delivery: The Generation R Study

Korevaar TIM, Schalekamp-Timmermans S, De Rijke YB, et al (Erasmus Med Ctr, Rotterdam, The Netherlands; et al)

J Clin Endocrinol Metab 98:4382-4390, 2013

Context.—Premature delivery is an important risk factor for child mortality and psychiatric, metabolic, and cardiovascular disease later in life. In the majority of cases, the cause of prematurity cannot be identified. Currently, it remains controversial whether abnormal maternal thyroid function during pregnancy increases the risk of premature delivery. Therefore, we investigated the relation between maternal serum thyroid parameters and the risk of premature delivery in a large prospective population-based study.

Design.—Serum TSH, free T_4 (FT_4), T_4, and TPO antibodies (TPOAbs) were determined during early pregnancy in 5971 pregnant women from the Generation R study. Data were available on maternal age, parity, smoking, socioeconomic status, ethnicity, maternal anthropometrics, and urinary iodine levels.

Results.—Of all women, 5.0% had a premature delivery (<37 weeks), 4.4% had a spontaneous premature delivery, and 1.4% had a very premature delivery (<34 weeks). High TSH levels and subclinical hypothyroidism were associated with premature delivery but not with spontaneous premature delivery. Maternal hypothyroxinemia was associated with a 2.5-fold increased risk of premature delivery, a 3.4-fold increased risk of spontaneous premature delivery, and a 3.6-fold increased risk of very premature delivery (all $P < .01$). TPOAb positivity was associated with a 1.7-fold increased risk of premature delivery ($P = .01$), a 2.1-fold increased risk of spontaneous premature delivery ($P = .02$), and a 2.5-fold increased risk of very premature delivery ($P = .04$). These effects remained similar after correction for TSH and FT4 levels.

Conclusions.—Hypothyroxinemia and TPOAb positivity are associated with an increased risk of premature delivery. The increased risk in TPOAb-positive women seems to be independent of thyroid function (Table 3).

► Premature delivery is associated with various adverse effects on child health and survival. In this study, the authors show that pregnant women with low LT4 levels in the first or second trimester have an increased risk of a premature delivery, which is independent of their thyroid-stimulating hormone (TSH) level, thyroid peroxidase antibody (TPOAb) status, or concomitant comorbidities. Details are given in Table 3. Women with an elevated TSH level or subclinical hypothyroidism also had an increased risk of a premature delivery, but this association did not persist after exclusion of TPOAb-positive women or women with comorbidities. Finally, the authors show that TPOAb positivity is also associated with an increased risk of premature delivery, and this association is independent of thyroid function.

In line with previous studies, these data showed an association of an elevated TSH level and of subclinical hypothyroidism with an increased risk of premature

TABLE 3.—Hypothyroxinemia and the Risk of Prematurity

		Spontaneous and Iatrogenic Deliveries (n = 5971)				Only Spontaneous Deliveries (n = 4446)			
		Prematurity <37 wk		Prematurity <34 wk		Prematurity <37 wk		Prematurity <34 wk	
	Prematurity % (n)	aOR (95% CI)[a]	*P*	aOR (95% CI)[a]	*P*	aOR (95% CI)[a]	*P*	aOR (95% CI)[a]	*P*
Hypothyroxinemia	10.3 (15/145)	2.54 (1.42–4.54)	<.01	3.56 (1.50–8.43)	<.01	3.44 (1.76–6.70)	<.01	4.21 (1.34 –13.3)	.01
Euthyroid (reference)[b]	4.7 (235/4970)								

[a]Analysis were adjusted for gestational age at blood sampling, maternal age, smoking, SES, parity, ethnicity, maternal BMI, maternal height, and child sex.
[b]Defined as TSH and FT_4 levels within the 2.5th to 97.5th percentiles.

delivery. However, this correlation no longer persisted after exclusion of women with concomitant comorbidities, and there was no association with spontaneous premature delivery. Furthermore, the association between subclinical hypothyroidism and premature delivery disappeared after the exclusion of TPOAb-positive women. This finding supports previous suggestions that the association with a premature delivery is caused by a high prevalence of TPOAb-positive women among women with subclinical hypothyroidism (32% in this study). The about 50% reduction in risk after the exclusion of TPOAb-positive women or women with comorbidities suggests independent direct effects on both thyroid function and premature delivery. Taken together, these data do not support the concept that subclinical hypothyroidism is an independent risk factor for premature delivery.

M. Schott, MD

Five-Year Follow-Up for Women With Subclinical Hypothyroidism in Pregnancy

Shields BM, Knight BA, Hill AV, et al (Univ of Exeter, UK)
J Clin Endocrinol Metab 98:E1941-E1945, 2013

Context.—Increasing numbers of women are being treated with L-thyroxine in pregnancy for mild thyroid dysfunction because of its association with impaired neuropsychological development in their offspring and other adverse obstetric outcomes. However, there are limited data to indicate whether treatment should be continued outside of pregnancy.

Objectives.—We aimed to determine whether subclinical hypothyroidism and maternal hypothyroxinemia resolve postdelivery.

Design, Setting, and Participants.—A total of 523 pregnant healthy women with no known thyroid disorders were recruited during routine antenatal care and provided blood samples at 28 weeks of pregnancy and at a mean of 4.9 years postpregnancy.

Main Outcome Measures.—TSH, free T_4, free T_3, and thyroid peroxidase antibody levels were measured in serum taken in pregnancy and at follow-up.

Results.—Subclinical hypothyroidism in pregnancy (TSH >3 mIU/L) was present in 65 of 523 (12.4%) women. Of these, 49 (75.4%) women had normal thyroid function postpregnancy; 16 of 65 (24.6%) had persistent high TSH (TSH >4.5 mIU/L postpregnancy) with 3 women receiving L-thyroxine treatment. A total of 44 of 523 (8.4%) women had isolated maternal hypothyroxinemia in pregnancy (free T_4 <10th centile and TSH $\leq$3 mIU/L). Only 2 of 44 (4.5%) had TSH >4.5 mIU/L outside pregnancy. Of the women with subclinical hypothyroidism in pregnancy with antibody measurements available, those with thyroid peroxidase antibodies in pregnancy were more likely to have persistently elevated TSH or be receiving L-thyroxine replacement after pregnancy (6 of 7 [86%] vs 10 of 57 [18%], $P < .001$).

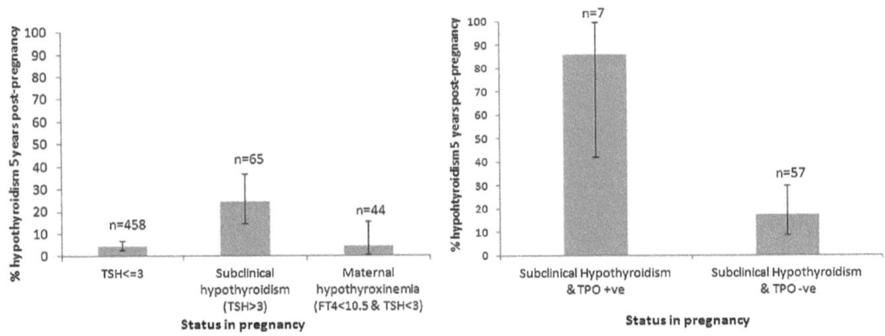

FIGURE 1.—Prevalence of hypothyroidism 5 years postpregnancy. Bar charts show the prevalence of hypothyroidism 5 years postpregnancy in (A) women with TSH ≤3 mIU/L, subclinical hypothyroidism (TSH >3 mIU/L), or maternal hypothyroxinemia in pregnancy (FT4 <10.5 pmol/L and TSH ≤3 mIU/L) ($P < .0001$ (by χ^2 test) for comparison between those with TSH ≤3 mIU/L and TSH >3 mIU/L) and (B) women with subclinical hypothyroidism in pregnancy with (+ve) and without (-ve) TPO-Abs ($P < .001$). Error bars represent 95% confidence intervals. One TPO-Ab result for a patient with subclinical hypothyroidism was unavailable. (Reprinted from Shields BM, Knight BA, Hill AV, et al. Five-Year follow-Up for women with subclinical hypothyroidism in pregnancy. *J Clin Endocrinol Metab*. 2013;98:E1941-E1945, Copyright 2013, with permission from the Author[s] and The Endocrine Society.)

Conclusions.—The majority of cases of subclinical hypothyroidism in pregnancy are transient, so treatment with L-thyroxine in these patients should be reviewed because it may not be warranted after pregnancy (Fig 1, Table 2).

▶ Increasing numbers of clinicians and hospitals are testing thyroid function in pregnancy to detect and treat mild thyroid dysfunction. The use of trimester-specific reference ranges in routine clinical practice results in milder forms of thyroid dysfunction (subclinical hypothyroidism and isolated maternal hypothyroxinemia) being diagnosed in as many as 15% of pregnant women.[1,2] The aim of the study by Shields and coworkers was to investigate the natural history of mild thyroid hormone deficiency during pregnancy and after delivery. The authors performed the first systematic follow-up study of subclinical hypothyroidism in pregnancy. They found that the majority (75%) of women identified as having subclinical hypothyroidism in pregnancy had normal thyroid-stimulating hormone (TSH) levels after pregnancy, and only 2 of 44 (4.4%) women with maternal hypothyroxinemia had high TSH levels outside pregnancy (Fig 1). The biggest risk factor for raised TSH levels after pregnancy was the presence of thyroid peroxidase antibodies. A TSH level > 5 mIU/L in pregnancy was also a risk factor, but a history of cesarean delivery was not (Table 2). This study has a number of limitations. First, the authors only measured thyroid function at a single time point during and after pregnancy. However, this is not likely to have a significant impact on the conclusions of this study because it has been demonstrated that variations in an individual's thyroid function over a short duration tends to be narrow both in and outside pregnancy. Irrespective of the limitations, these results highlight the need for reassessment of the thyroid status of pregnant women after pregnancy.

M. Schott, MD, PhD

TABLE 2.—Thyroid Function Test Results for Women at 28 Weeks of Pregnancy Split by Whether They Had Subclinical Hypothyroidism in Pregnancy (TSH >3 mIU/L) or Not (TSH ≤3 mIU/L)

	Pregnancy			Postpregnancy		
	TSH ≤3 mIU/L (n = 458)	TSH >3 mIU/L (n = 65)	*P*	TSH ≤4.5 mIU/L (n = 486)	TSH >4.5 mIU/L (n = 28)	*P*
TSH, mIU/L	1.7 (1.32, 2.15)	3.57 (3.24, 4.23)	<.0001	1.84 (1.28, 2.44)	5.35 (4.76, 6.77)	<.0001
FT_4, pmol/L	12.13 (11.16, 13.06)	11.9 (11.18, 12.64)	.29	14.8 (13.6, 16)	14.0 (12.45, 15.25)	.02
FT_3, pmol/L	4.12 (3.85, 4.42)	4.16 (3.88, 4.44)	.52	4.5 (4.2, 4.8)	4.45 (4.1, 4.8)	.67
TPO-Ab positive	48/458 (10)	16/65 (25)	.001	47/486 (10)	11/28 (39)	<.0001

Similar results were presented for postpregnancy thyroid function test results (split by women with TSH >4.5 mIU/L or with TSH ≤4.5 mIU/L), excluding those taking L-thyroxine and those with Graves disease (n = 9). Data are presented as median (interquartile range) or n (%).

References

1. Blatt AJ, Nakamoto JM, Kaufman HW. National status of testing for hypothyroidism during pregnancy and postpartum. *J Clin Endocrinol Metab.* 2012;97:777-784.
2. Altomare M, La Vignera S, Asero P, et al. High prevalence of thyroid dysfunction in pregnant women. *J Endocrinol Invest.* 2013;36:407-411.

Miscellaneous

Histidines in Potential Substrate Recognition Sites Affect Thyroid Hormone Transport by Monocarboxylate Transporter 8 (MCT8)

Braun D, Lelios I, Krause G, et al (Charité-Universitätsmedizin Berlin, Germany; Forschungsinstitut für Molekulare Pharmakologie, Berlin, Germany)
Endocrinology 154:2553-2561, 2013

Mutations in monocarboxylate transporter 8 (MCT8; *SLC16A2*) cause the Allan-Herndon-Dudley syndrome, a severe X-linked psychomotor retardation syndrome. MCT8 belongs to the major facilitator superfamily of 12 transmembrane-spanning proteins and transports thyroid hormones across the blood-brain barrier and into neurons. How MCT8 distinguishes thyroid hormone substrates from structurally closely related compounds is not known. The goal of this study was to identify critical amino acids along the transport channel cavity, which participate in thyroid hormone recognition. The fact that T_3 is bound between a His-Arg clamp in the crystal structure of the T_3 receptor/T_3 complex prompted us to investigate whether such a motif might potentially be relevant for T_3 recognition in MCT8. We therefore replaced candidate histidines and arginines by site-directed mutagenesis and performed activity assays in MDCK-1 cells and *Xenopus* oocytes. Histidines were replaced by alanine, phenylalanine, and glutamine to probe for molecular properties like aromatic ring structure and H-bonding properties. It was found that some mutations in His192 and His415 significantly changed substrate transport kinetics. Arg301 at the intracellular end of the substrate channel is at an ideal distance to His415 to participate in a His-Arg clamp and mutation to alanine-abrogated hormone transport. Molecular modeling demonstrates a perfect fit of T_3 poised into the substrate channel between His415 and Arg301 and observing the same geometry as in the T_3 receptor.

▶ Monocarboxylate transporter 8 (MCT8), a transmembrane protein, is known to transport iodothyronines (eg, triiodothyronine [T_3], thyroxine [T_4]) along their concentration gradients across the plasma membrane.[1] How MCT8 distinguishes thyroid hormone substrates from structurally closely related compounds is not known and was aimed to be investigated in this study. Previous work investigating the cocrystal structures of T_3 receptor β/T_3 showed a histidine-arginine (His-Arg) clamp, separated by about 15 β/T3, that bound T_3.[2] In analogy to these data, Braun and colleagues investigated whether such a motif might be relevant for T_3 recognition in MCT8 by using Madin-Darby canine kidney (MDCK)-1 cells and Xenopus oocytes. As shown in Fig 1 of the original article, 2 potential His-Arg clamp motifs, separated by 15 to 17 β/T3 were found in MCT8 (His192-Arg445 and His415-Arg301). Performing transport activity assays, Braun and colleagues showed both histidines (His192 and His415) being critical for the functionality of MCT8 (Figs 2 and 4 in the original article), as mutations at these positions significantly changed substrate transport kinetics. Furthermore, Arg301 was shown to be essential for the hormone transport (Fig 3 in the original article).

From the clinical point of view, mutations in MCT8 are known to lead to a severe psychomotor retardation syndrome called *Allan-Herndon-Dudley syndrome*. Whether the described site-specific mutations in His192, His415, and Arg301 play a role for the pathogenesis of Allan-Herndon-Dudley syndrome still needs to be clarified.

Braun and colleagues gave an insight into how MCT8 specifically recognizes its ligand and showed the impact of a spatial His-Arg clamp motif in analogy to the T_3 receptor.

M. Ehlers, PhD
M. Schott, MD, PhD

References

1. Friesema EC, Ganguly S, Abdalla A, Manning Fox JE, Halestrap AP, Visser TJ. Identification of monocarboxylate transporter 8 as a specific thyroid hormone transporter. *J Biol Chem*. 2003;278:40128-40135.
2. Kleinau G, Schweizer U, Kinne A, et al. Insights into molecular properties of the human monocarboxylate transporter 8 by combining functional with structural information. *Thyroid Res*. 2011;4:S4.

Embryonic exposure to excess thyroid hormone causes thyrotrope cell death

Tonyushkina KN, Shen M-C, Ortiz-Toro T, et al (Baystate Med Ctr, Springfield, MA; Univ of Massachusetts, Amherst)
J Clin Invest 124:321-327, 2014

Central congenital hypothyroidism (CCH) is more prevalent in children born to women with hyperthyroidism during pregnancy, suggesting a role for thyroid hormone (TH) in the development of central thyroid regulation. Using the zebrafish embryo as a model for thyroid axis development, we have characterized the ontogeny of negative feedback regulation of thyrotrope function and examined the effect of excess TH on thyrotrope development. We found that thyroid-stimulating hormone β subunit (*tshb*) and type 2 deiodinase (*dio2*) are coexpressed in zebrafish thyrotropes by 48 hours after fertilization and that TH-driven negative feedback regulation of *tshb* transcription appears in the thyroid axis by 96 hours after fertilization. Negative feedback regulation correlated with increased systemic TH levels from the developing thyroid follicles. We used a transgenic zebrafish that expresses GFP under the control of the *tshb* promoter to follow thyrotrope fates in vivo. Time-lapse imaging revealed that early exposure to elevated TH leads to thyrotrope cell death. Thyrotrope numbers slowly recovered following the removal of excess TH. These data

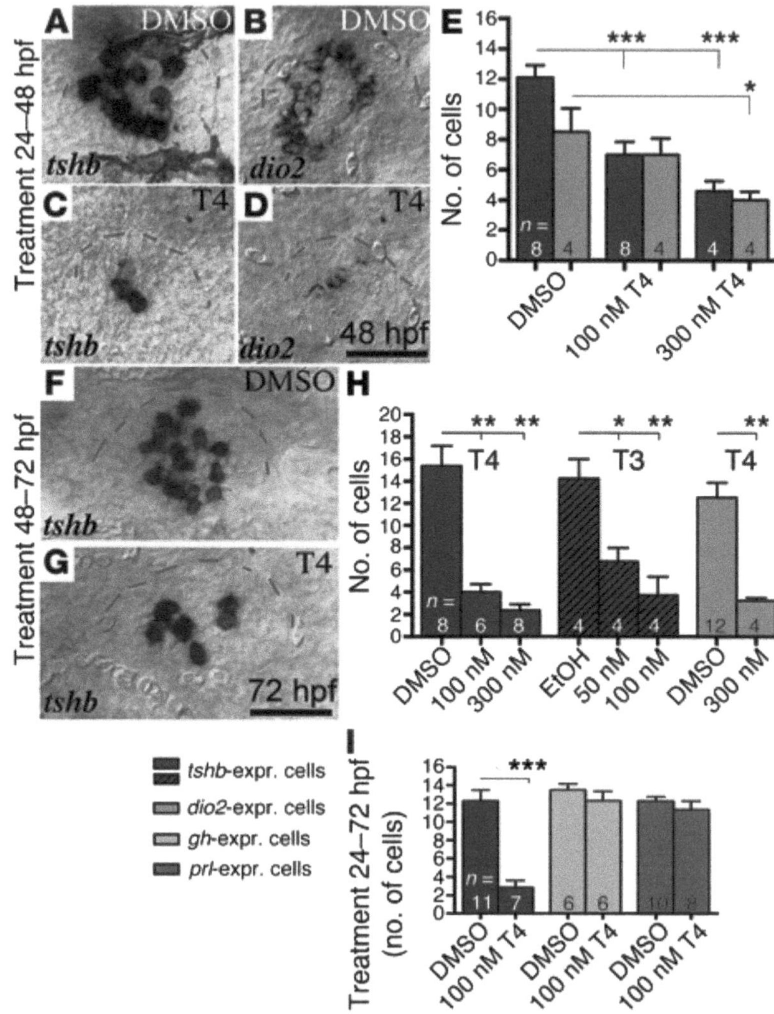

FIGURE 2.—Embryonic exposure to elevated T4 reduces the number of cells expressing *tshb* and *dio2*. (**A–D**) *tshb*- and *dio2*-expressing thyrotropes by 48 hpf following exposure to 300 nM T4 or DMSO (carrier) starting at 24 hpf, as visualized by ISH. (**E**) Graph showing decreases in *tshb*- (blue) and *dio2*-labeled (green) cells. (**F** and **G**) *tshb*-expressing thyrotropes by 72 hpf following a 24-hour exposure to 300 nM T4 or DMSO. (**H**) Graph showing decreases in *tshb*- (blue) and *dio2*-labeled (green) cells after a 24-hour exposure to T4 and T3. (**I**) Graph showing a decrease in *tshb*-labeled (blue) cells and no changes in *gh*- and *prl*-labeled cells after a 48-hour exposure to 100 nM T4 or DMSO (carrier) started 24 hpf. $^{*}P < 0.05$; $^{**}P < 0.01$; $^{***}P < 0.001$. (**A–D**, **F**, and **G**) Ventral views of the left anterior head; red dashed lines outline the left half of the pituitary placode. Scale bars: 25 µm. For Interpretation of the references to color in this figure legend, the reader is referred to web version of this article. (Reprinted from Tonyushkina KN, Shen M-C, Ortiz-Toro T, et al. Embryonic exposure to excess thyroid hormone causes thyrotrope cell death. *J Clin Invest.* 2014;124:321-327, © 2014, American Society of Clinical Investigation.)

demonstrate that transient TH exposure profoundly impacts the thyrotrope population during a critical period of pituitary development and may have long-term implications for the functional reserve of thyroid-stimulating hormone (TSH) production and the TSH set point later in life (Figs 2-4).

▶ Thyroid hormone (TH) is essential for normal development of the brain, liver, heart, intestine, blood, and bone, both before and after birth. In the present

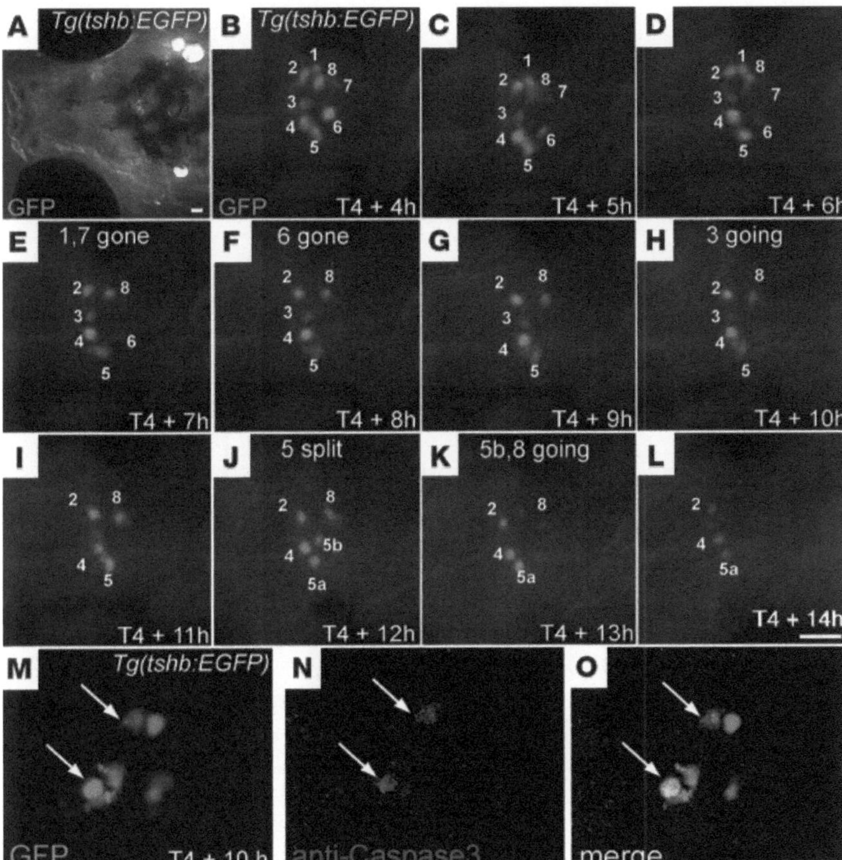

FIGURE 3.—Early embryonic exposure to high T4 levels leads to thyrotrope cell death. (**A**) Ventral view of the zebrafish head in a 6-dpf *Tg(tshb:EGFP)* embryo showing GFP-labeled thyrotropes in the pituitary. (B–L) Single frames from a time-lapse movie (see Supplemental Video 1) of GFP-expressing thyrotropes (numbered) in a *Tg(tshb:EGFP)* embryo 4–14 hours after the application of 300 nM T4 48 hpf. (**B**) Eight GFP-expressing thyrotropes were present 4 hours after application of T4. (**D** and **E**) GFP-expressing thyrotropes began to disappear 6–7 hours after T4 application. (**L**) Only 3 cells remained 14 hours after application of T4. (**M–O**) Example of anti–activated caspase 3 labeling of 2 GFP-expressing thyrotropes (arrows) in a *Tg(tshb:EGFP)* embryo 10 hours after the application of 300 nM T4. Single focal plane images show GFP (**M**), caspase 3 (**N**), and merged channels (**O**). All panels show ventral views of the left anterior forebrain between the eyes. Scale bars: 25 µm. (Reprinted from Tonyushkina KN, Shen M-C, Ortiz-Toro T, et al. Embryonic exposure to excess thyroid hormone causes thyrotrope cell death. *J Clin Invest.* 2014;124:321-327, © 2014, American Society of Clinical Investigation.)

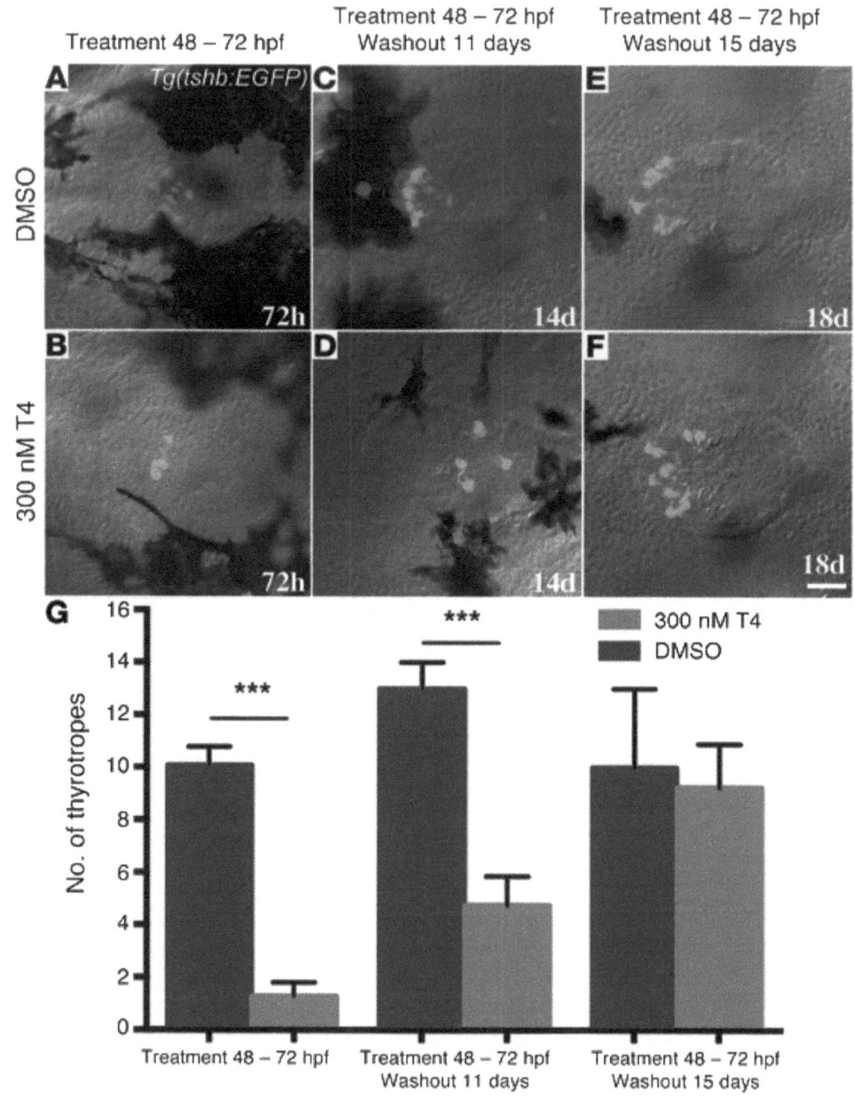

FIGURE 4.—Lasting effects of T4 exposure on thyrotrope numbers. (**A**) Approximately 10 thyrotropes were present in the pituitary by 72 hpf in DMSO-treated control embryos, as visualized by GFP fluorescence in the *Tg(tshb:EGFP)* line. (**B**) Example of decreased thyrotrope numbers by 72 hpf immediately following a 24-hour exposure to 300 nM T4. (**C**) Approximately 13 thyrotropes were present by 14 dpf in DMSO-treated control embryos. (**D**) Example of a 14-dpf larva with 4 thyrotropes that was treated with 300 nM T4 from 48 to 72 hpf, followed by an 11-day washout period. (E) Approximately 10 thyrotropes were present in the pituitary by 18 dpf in DMSO-treated control embryos. (F) Example of a larva with normal thyrotrope numbers that was treated with 300 nM T4 from 48 to 72 hpf, followed by a 15-day washout period. (**G**) Graph showing thyrotrope numbers, with a minimum of 20 embryos scored for each treatment. $^{***}P < 0.001$. (**A–F**) Ventral views of pituitary in the left anterior forebrain. Scale bar: 25 μm. (Reprinted from Tonyushkina KN, Shen M-C, Ortiz-Toro T, et al. Embryonic exposure to excess thyroid hormone causes thyrotrope cell death. *J Clin Invest.* 2014;124:321-327, © 2014, American Society of Clinical Investigation.)

study, the authors report the impact of excess TH on early thyrotrope development and define the onset of negative regulation of TSH transcription by TH in thyrotropes. To image thyrotropes in live embryos, the authors generated a zebrafish transgenic line in which the GFP was inserted into the genome under *tshb* promoter regulation. Unexpectedly, the authors found that elevated TH levels trigger thyrotrope cell death before, but not after, the onset of negative feedback regulation of *tshb* expression. As shown in Fig 2, embryonic exposure to elevated T4 reduces the number of cells expressing *tshb* and *dio2*. Figs 3 and 4 show that early embryonic exposure to high T4 levels leads to thyrotrope cell death. This study identifies an important developmental window of TH action and uncovers thyrotrope cell death as a potential mechanism underlying central congenital hypothyroidism and altered set points in mammalian neonates exposed to high levels of maternal TH during embryogenesis, as occurs in poorly controlled Graves' disease in humans.

M. Schott, MD, PhD

5 Calcium and Bone Metabolism

Introduction

A significant number of excellent clinical studies were published in calcium and bone disorders during the last year. Due to continued strong clinical interest regarding calcium and vitamin D metabolism, the first group of selections in this chapter focuses on evaluation of the effect of vitamin D on the long-term outcomes of interest in patients with calcium and bone disorders. The second group focuses on a variety of important studies describing the pathophysiology of osteoporosis. Findings of major clinical trials published in the area of osteoporosis are the focus of the third group, and the fourth group describes a number of advances in the treatment or understanding of metabolic bone disease.

The studies selected are intended to focus attention on the major advances in our understanding of calcium and bone disorders reported during the last year. These studies are already significantly impacting the clinical practice of endocrinology. As with any review of selected publications garnered from the recent literature, there were many other significant papers published this past year that could not be included in this chapter.

Mineral and Vitamin D Metabolism

The first two studies focus on the effect of serum vitamin D levels on long-term outcomes of interest in patients with calcium and bone disorders. "Serum 25-hydroxyvitamin D and Risk of Major Osteoporotic Fractures in Older U.S. Adults" evaluates the effect of serum vitamin D on long-term major osteoporotic fracture (hip, spine, wrist, and shoulder fracture) outcomes in older US adults. This study correlated serum 25-hydroxyvitamin D levels with fracture risk in adults 65 years or older. "Association between Serum 25-hydroxyvitamin D Level and Subclinical Cardiovascular Disease in Primary Hyperparathyroidism" evaluated whether serum 25-hydroxyvitamin D predicts cardiovascular disease in patients with mild primary hyperparathyroidism, as has been reported in other populations.

Epidemiology and Pathophysiology of Osteoporosis

The next group of seven studies reports significant findings from studies focusing on the pathophysiology of osteoporosis. "Abdominal Fat Is Associated with Lower Bone Formation and Inferior Bone Quality in Healthy Premenopausal Women: A Transiliac Bone Biopsy Study" reported that abdominal adiposity is associated with lower bone formation and reduced bone quality in premenopausal women, as assessed by transiliac bone biopsy.

"Relationship of Weight, Height, and Body Mass Index with Fracture Risk at Different Sites in Postmenopausal Women: The Global Longitudinal Study of Osteoporosis in Women" reports that body weight, height, and body mass index (BMI) predicted differential fracture risk at different skeletal sites in a large international clinical practice cohort, the Global Longitudinal Study of Osteoporosis in Women (GLOW).

"In Vivo Assessment of Bone Quality in Postmenopausal Women with Type 2 Diabetes" reported for the first time that postmenopausal women with type 2 diabetes mellitus, many of whom are obese, have reduced bone material strength (BMS) as measured by *in vivo* tibial microindentation. "Fracture Risk Following Bariatric Surgery: A Population-Based Study" reported that bariatric surgery to treat medically complicated obesity led to increased post-surgical fracture risk compared to the general population. These findings suggest that bariatric surgery, while beneficial for inducing weight loss, may increase fracture risk for multiple reasons. "Gonadal Steroids and Body Composition, Strength, and Sexual Function in Men" evaluated the effect of gonadal steroids on body composition, strength, and sexual function in men. The study showed that the amount of testosterone required to maintain lean mass, fat mass, muscle strength, or sexual function varied widely in men, and that lean mass, muscle size, and muscle strength were determined primarily by testosterone, fat mass by estrogen, and sexual function by both testosterone and estrogen.

The next group of four selections further clarifies our understanding of increased fracture risk in different populations. "Cortical Porosity Identifies Women with Osteopenia at Increased Risk for Forearm Fractures" evaluated the effect of cortical porosity measured by high-resolution quantitative CT scanning (HRpQCT) on forearm fracture risk in postmenopausal women with osteopenia or osteoporosis. The findings suggest that fracture risk can be further stratified beyond DXA by assessment of cortical porosity in postmenopausal women with osteopenia. "A Distal Forearm Fracture in Childhood Is Associated with an Increased Risk for Future Fragility Fractures in Adult Men, But Not Women" evaluated the effect of childhood forearm fractures on future fragility fractures in adults. The study showed that distal forearm fractures in childhood predicted future fragility fractures in adult men, but not adult women. "Rapid Cortical Bone Loss in Patients with Chronic Kidney Disease" evaluated bone loss in 58 patients with chronic kidney disease (CKD) stage 2 to 5D and reported that rapid cortical bone loss was responsible for most of the decrease in BMD seen in this cohort followed over 18 months. "Hepatitis

C Co-Infection and Severity of Liver Disease as Risk Factors for Osteoporotic Fractures among HIV-Infected Patients" demonstrated that hepatitis C virus co-infection and liver disease severity are both risk factors for osteoporotic fractures among patients with HIV infection.

OSTEOPOROSIS THERAPY

The next group of seven selections further evaluates the treatment effects of currently approved medications for osteoporosis. "Zoledronic Acid Acutely Increases Sclerostin Serum Levels in Women with Postmenopausal Osteoporosis" gives further insight into the mechanism of action of zoledronic acid on the skeleton. The study showed that a single 5-mg dose of zoledronic acid given intravenously in 40 postmenopausal women with osteoporosis resulted in an increase in serum sclerostin that peaked 7 days after infusion and remained increased over the next year before returning to baseline.

"Duration of Antiresorptive Effects of Low-Dose Zoledronate in Osteopenic Postmenopausal Women: A Randomized, Placebo-Controlled Trial" re-analyzes a previous dose-ranging clinical trial for therapeutic effect of low-dose zoledronic acid in postmenopausal women. The study showed that a single 1-mg or 2.5-mg dose of zoledronic acid had anti-resorptive effect persistent for up to two years.

"Effects of Pioglitazone on Bone in Postmenopausal Women with Impaired Fasting Glucose or Impaired Glucose Tolerance: A Randomized, Double-Blind, Placebo-Controlled Study" showed that the anti-diabetic agent pioglitazone had no effect on BMD or bone turnover in postmenopausal women with impaired fasting glucose or impaired glucose tolerance.

"Femoral and Vertebral Strength Improvements in Postmenopausal Women with Osteoporosis Treated with Denosumab" showed that denosumab, the monoclonal antibody to receptor-activator of nuclear factor kappa B ligand (RANKL), reduces fracture risk, in part by causing increased strength in femoral and vertebral bone during treatment. "RANKL Inhibition with Denosumab Does Not Influence 3-Year Progression of Aortic Calcification or Incidence of Adverse Cardiovascular Events in Postmenopausal Women with Osteoporosis and High Cardiovascular Risk" assessed whether denosumab could limit progression of aortic calcification or prevent development of cardiovascular events in postmenopausal women at high risk of cardiovascular disease.

"Teriparatide for Idiopathic Osteoporosis in Premenopausal Women: A Pilot Study" reported that teriparatide (PTH 1-34) worked well to treat idiopathic osteoporosis in premenopausal women in a pilot study.

"Risk Factors for Treatment Failure with Antiosteoporosis Medication: The Global Longitudinal Study of Osteoporosis in Women (GLOW)" attempted to determine risk factors for treatment failure with osteoporosis medication in a multinational practice cohort of 26,918 women ≥55 years who had sustained two or more fractures while on anti-osteoporosis medication.

"Effects of Odanacatib on BMD and Safety in the Treatment of Osteoporosis in Postmenopausal Women Previously Treated with Alendronate: A

Randomized Placebo-Controlled Trial" reports that the new antiresorptive drug odanacatib caused a further small increase in BMD when given to postmenopausal women over two years who were previously treated with alendronate for at least 3 years.

"Romosozumab in Postmenopausal Women with Low Bone Mineral Density" evaluated the effect of the anti-sclerostin monoclonal antibody romosozumab on BMD in postmenopausal women with osteopenia. Sclerostin is produced by osteocytes in the skeleton and reduces new bone formation by inhibiting the Wnt-signaling pathway. Romosozumab inhibits sclerostin from limiting the Wnt-signaling pathway, thereby leading to significant new bone formation.

Metabolic Bone Disease

The next group of five selections describes new findings in patients with metabolic bone disease. "Persistent Hyperparathyroidism Is a Major Risk Factor for Fractures in the Five Years after Kidney Transplantation" demonstrated for the first time that persistent hyperparathyroidism increased the risk of fractures during the first 5 years after renal transplantation.

"Normocalcemic Hyperparathyroidism and Hypoparathyroidism in Two Community-Based Nonreferral Populations" evaluated the risk of normocalcemic primary hyperparathyroidism and hypoparathyroidism in two community-based non-referral populations. This study is important because the prevalence of these newly-described entities remains unclear.

"Efficacy and Safety of Recombinant Human Parathyroid Hormone (1-84) in Hypoparathyroidism (REPLACE): A Double-Blind, Placebo-Controlled, Randomised, Phase 3 Study" reports the results of a phase III clinical trial using PTH 1-84 to treat patients with hypoparathyroidism. These patients are usually treated with high-dose calcium and active vitamin D supplementation with variable serum calcium levels and significant consequent hypercalciuria.

"Incidence and Prevalence of Primary Hyperparathyroidism in a Racially Mixed Population" is the first study to evaluate the incidence and prevalence of primary hyperparathyroidism in a racially mixed population. The study investigated the epidemiology of primary hyperparathyroidism in the 3.5-million-member Kaiser Permanente Southern California database between 1995 and 2010. "Primary Hyperparathyroidism Is Associated with Abnormal Cortical and Trabecular Microstructure and Reduced Bone Stiffness in Postmenopausal Women" described changes in bone microstructure and stiffness in postmenopausal women with primary hyperparathyroidism.

Conclusion

In conclusion, these selected papers reflect a sample of the wide variety of excellent clinical studies published in the area of calcium and bone disorders over the last year. Many other significant papers could not be included in this perspective due to space limitations. Most of the studies discussed here add incrementally to current knowledge regarding calcium and bone disorders, based on previous studies and clinical experience, whereas others demonstrate significant advances or clarification of understanding of physiological functions of the skeleton. Future clinical investigation will continue to advance our knowledge regarding skeletal function in health and disease.

Bart L. Clarke, MD

Mineral and Vitamin D Metabolism

Serum 25-Hydroxyvitamin D and Risk of Major Osteoporotic Fractures in Older U.S. Adults

Looker AC (Natl Ctr for Health Statistics, Hyattsville, MD)
J Bone Miner Res 28:997-1006, 2013

Results from previous prospective studies linking serum 25-hydroxyvitamin D (25OHD) with fracture risk have been inconsistent. The present study examined the relationship between serum 25OHD and risk of incident major osteoporotic fracture (hip, spine, radius, and humerus) in older U.S. adults. The study used a pooled cohort of 4749 men and women ages 65 years and older from the third National Health and Nutrition Examination Survey (NHANES III, 1988–1994) and NHANES 2000–2004. Incident fractures were identified using linked mortality and Medicare records that were obtained for participants from both surveys. Serum 25OHD values were measured by radioimmunoassay in both surveys. Cox proportional hazards models were used to estimate the relative risk (RR) of fracture by serum 25OHD level. There were 525 incident major osteoporotic fractures (287 hip fractures) in the sample. Serum 25OHD was a significant linear predictor of major osteoporotic fracture and significant quadratic predictor of hip fracture in the total sample and among those with less than 10 years of follow-up, but it was not related to risk of either fracture type among those with ≥10 years of follow-up. Major osteoporotic fracture risk was increased by 26% to 27% for each SD decrease in serum 25OHD among those with less than 10 years of follow-up. Serum 25OHD was significantly related to risk of major osteoporotic fractures as a group and to hip fracture alone in this cohort of older U.S. adults from NHANES III and NHANES 2000–2004. However, the predictive utility of serum 25OHD diminished after 10 years. In addition, the relationship appeared to be linear when major osteoporotic fracture risk was considered but quadratic when hip fracture risk was assessed.

▶ Significant controversy continues to exist regarding the effect of serum vitamin D on prevention of fractures. Just over half of previous studies have shown a protective effect of serum 25-hydroxyvitamin D on fractures occurring at 1 or more sites examined.[1-4] However, several studies have shown no benefit.[5-7]

This study evaluated the relationship between serum 25-hydroxyvitamin D and fractures of the hip, spine, wrist, and shoulder in a large pooled cohort of men and women of all races who were 65 years and older at the time of the third National Health and Nutrition Examination Survey (NHANES III) and NHANES 2002–2004. Incident fractures were captured from linked mortality and Medicare records. Serum 25-hydroxyvitamin D was measured by radioimmunoassay rather than tandem mass spectroscopy. There were 525 incident major osteoporotic fractures, including 287 hip fractures, in the cohort over the observation interval. Serum 25-hydroxyvitamin D was a significant linear predictor of major osteoporotic fractures and significant quadratic predictor of hip fractures in those with less than 10 years of follow-up, but it did not predict fractures of either type in those with more than 10 years of follow-up. Major osteoporotic fractures were increased by 26% to 27% for each standard deviation decrease in serum 25-hydroxyvitamin D in subjects with less than 10 years of follow-up. The ability of serum 25-hydroxyvitamin D to predict fractures decreased after 10 years of follow-up.

These interesting findings suggest that serum 25-hydroxyvitamin D may be protective against fractures over short-term follow-up. Most previous studies of the effect of vitamin D on fracture risk have had less than 10 years of follow-up or not reported the effect of vitamin D on fracture risk by follow-up time. Further studies of other cohorts with larger numbers of fractures are necessary to replicate these results.

B. L. Clarke, MD

References

1. Cauley JA, LaCroix AZ, Wu L, et al. Serum 25-hydroxyvitamin D concentrations and risk for hip fractures. *Ann Intern Med.* 2008;149:242-250.
2. Cauley JA, Parimi N, Ensrud KE, et al. Osteoporotic Fractures in Men (MrOS) Research Group. Serum 25-Hydroxyvitamin D and the risk of hip and nonspine fractures in older men. *J Bone Miner Res.* 2010;25:545-553.
3. Cauley JA, Danielson ME, Boudreau R, et al. Serum 25-hydroxyvitamin D and clinical fracture risk in a multiethnic cohort of women: the Women's Health Initiative (WHI). *J Bone Miner Res.* 2011;26:2378-2388.
4. van Schoor NM, Visser M, Pluijm SM, Kuchuk N, Smit JH, Lips P. Vitamin D deficiency as a risk factor for osteoporotic fractures. *Bone.* 2008;42:260-266.
5. Barbour KE, Houston DK, Cummings SR, et al. the Health ABC Study. Calciotropic hormones and the risk of hip and nonspine fractures in older adults: the Health ABC Study. *J Bone Miner Res.* 2012;27:1177-1185.
6. Cummings SR, Browner WS, Bauer D, et al. Endogenous hormones and the risk of hip and vertebral fractures among older women. *N Engl J Med.* 1998;339:733-738.
7. Garnero P, Munoz F, Sornay-Rendu E, Delmas PD. Associations of vitamin D status with bone mineral density, bone turnover, bone loss and fracture risk in healthy postmenopausal women. The OFELY Study. *Bone.* 2007;40:716-722.

Association Between Serum 25-Hydroxyvitamin D Level and Subclinical Cardiovascular Disease in Primary Hyperparathyroidism

Walker MD, Cong E, Kepley A, et al (Columbia Univ, NY; et al)
J Clin Endocrinol Metab 99:671-680, 2014

Context.—Vitamin D (25OHD) deficiency may be a modifiable cardiovascular (CV) risk factor. 25OHD insufficiency (20–29 ng/mL) and deficiency (<20 ng/mL) are common in primary hyperparathyroidism (PHPT), but their association with CV disease in PHPT has not been systematically investigated.

Objective.—This study evaluated whether low 25OHD is associated with subclinical CV disease in PHPT.

Design.—This is a cross-sectional analysis of PHPT patients with and without low 25OHD.

Settings and Participants.—We studied 110 PHPT patients in a university hospital setting.

Outcome Measures.—We measured carotid intima-media thickness; carotid plaque presence/thickness; carotid strain and stiffness; left ventricular mass index; cardiac systolic and diastolic function; and mitral annular calcification.

Results.—Low 25OHD levels (<30 ng/mL) were observed in 28%, but only 9% had 25OHD deficiency (<20 ng/mL). In the whole group, 25OHD levels negatively correlated with body mass index ($r = -0.33$, $P = .0005$), PTH ($r = -0.30$, $P = .001$), calcium ($r = -0.29$, $P = .002$), renal function, and PHPT duration. CV indices were normal except for carotid intima-media thickness, stiffness, and plaque thickness, which were increased, regardless of 25OHD status. Isovolumic relaxation time was the only CV measure associated with 25OHD ($r = -0.26$, $P = .01$). Those with 25OHD less than 20 ng/mL had more severe PHPT and a higher rate of nephrolithiasis. Those with 25OHD less than 30 ng/mL were younger, had higher body mass index, had lower serum phosphate, and were more likely to be male, nonwhite, and Hispanic. Other than lower tissue Doppler e′ and higher isovolumic relaxation time within normal range in those with 25OHD less than 30 vs greater than 30 ng/mL, there were no differences in CV indices using either 25OHD threshold.

Conclusions.—Patients with mild PHPT have subclinical carotid abnormalities, but low 25OHD is not associated with abnormal carotid or cardiac measures. To the extent that PTH levels differentiated those with 25OHD less than 20 but not 30 ng/mL, these data support a 25OHD threshold of 20 ng/mL as clinically relevant in PHPT.

▶ Vitamin D has significant effects on calcium and bone metabolism and the skeleton, but it also appears to have pleiotropic effects on other tissues, including the cardiovascular system.[1,2] Vitamin D deficiency may increase the risk of cardiovascular disease, including myocardial infarction, peripheral arterial disease, combined cardiovascular events, and cardiovascular mortality independent of traditional risk factors.[3-7] No previous studies have evaluated serum 25-hydroxyvitamin D deficiency as a risk factor for cardiovascular disease in patients with primary hyperparathyroidism.

This study evaluated relationships between serum 25-hydroxyvitamin D deficiency and subclinical cardiovascular disease endpoints in 110 patients with primary hyperparathyroidism. Thirty-seven percent of the study subjects had vitamin D deficiency (9%) or insufficiency (28%). Cardiovascular indices assessed were normal except for carotid intima-media thickness, stiffness, and plaque thickness, which were increased regardless of serum 25-hydroxyvitamin D level. Isovolumic relaxation time was the only cardiovascular measure inversely associated with serum 25-hydroxyvitamin D. Subjects with 25-hydroxyvitamin D less than 20 ng/mL had more severe primary hyperparathyroidism and a higher rate of kidney stones. Those with serum 25-hydroxyvitamin D less than 30 ng/mL were younger, had higher body mass index, had lower serum phosphate, and were more likely to be male, nonwhite, and Hispanic. Other than lower tissue Doppler Ei and higher isovolumic relaxation time within the normal range in those with serum 25-hydroxyvitamin D less than 30 ng/mL, there were no differences in cardiovascular indices regardless of the vitamin D level.

These findings suggest that patients with mild primary hyperparathyroidism have subclinical carotid abnormalities. Even though vitamin D deficiency contributes to more severe primary hyperparathyroidism, vitamin D deficiency does not appear to contribute significantly to cardiovascular risk in patients with mild primary hyperparathyroidism. Further studies will be necessary to determine whether treatment of vitamin D deficiency will affect skeletal health and risk of nephrolithiasis.

B. L. Clarke, MD

References

1. Scragg R, Jackson R, Holdaway IM, Lim T, Beaglehole R. Myocardial infarction is inversely associated with plasma 25-hydroxyvitamin D3 levels: a community-based study. *Int J Epidemiol.* 1990;19:559-563.
2. Scragg R. Seasonality of cardiovascular disease mortality and the possible protective effect of ultra-violet radiation. *Int J Epidemiol.* 1981;10:337-341.
3. Artaza JN, Mehrotra R, Norris KC. Vitamin D and the cardiovascular system. *Clin J Am Soc Nephrol.* 2009;4:1515-1522.
4. Dobnig H, Pilz S, Scharnagl H, et al. Independent association of low serum 25-hydroxyvitamin D and 1,25-dihydroxyvitamin D levels with all-cause and cardiovascular mortality. *Arch Intern Med.* 2008;168:1340-1349.
5. Melamed ML, Michos ED, Post W, Astor B. 25-Hydroxyvitamin D levels and the risk of mortality in the general population. *Arch Intern Med.* 2008;168:1629-1637.
6. Pilz S, März W, Wellnitz B, et al. Association of vitamin D deficiency with heart failure and sudden cardiac death in a large cross-sectional study of patients referred for coronary angiography. *J Clin Endocrinol Metab.* 2008;93:3927-3935.
7. Wang TJ, Pencina MJ, Booth SL, et al. Vitamin D deficiency and risk of cardiovascular disease. *Circulation.* 2008;117:503-511.

Epidemiology and Pathophysiology of Osteoporosis

Abdominal fat is associated with lower bone formation and inferior bone quality in healthy premenopausal women: a transiliac bone biopsy study

Cohen A, Dempster DW, Recker RR, et al (Columbia Univ, NY; Helen Hayes Hosp, West Haverstraw, NY; Creighton Univ, Omaha, NE; et al)
J Clin Endocrinol Metab 98:2562-2572, 2013

Context.—The conventional view that obesity is beneficial for bone strength has recently been challenged by studies that link obesity, particularly visceral obesity, to low bone mass and fractures. It is controversial whether effects of obesity on bone are mediated by increased bone resorption or decreased bone formation.

Objective.—To evaluate bone microarchitecture and remodeling in healthy premenopausal women of varying weight.

Design.—We measured bone density and trunk fat by DXA in 40 women, and by quantitative computed tomography (QCT) in a subset. Bone microarchitecture, stiffness, remodeling and marrow fat were assessed in labeled transiliac bone biopsies.

Results.—Body mass index (BMI) ranged from 20.1 to 39.2 kg/m^2. DXA-trunk fat was directly associated with BMI ($r = 0.78$, $p < 0.001$) and visceral fat by QCT ($r = 0.79$, $p < 0.001$). Compared to women in the lowest tertile of trunk fat, those in the highest tertile had inferior bone quality: lower trabecular bone volume (20.4 ± 5.8 versus 29.1 ± 6.1%; $p = 0.001$) and stiffness (433 ± 264 versus 782 ± 349 MPa; $p = 0.01$), higher cortical porosity (8.8 ± 3.5 versus 6.3 ± 2.4%; $p = 0.049$). Bone formation rate (0.004 ± 0.002 versus 0.011 ± 0.008 mm^2/mm/year; $p = 0.006$) was 64% lower in the highest tertile. Trunk fat was inversely associated with trabecular bone volume ($r = -0.50$; $p < 0.01$) and bone formation rate ($r = -0.50$; $p < 0.001$). The relationship between trunk fat and bone volume remained significant after controlling for age and BMI.

Conclusions.—At the tissue level, premenopausal women with more central adiposity had inferior bone quality and stiffness, and markedly lower bone formation. Given the rising levels of obesity, these observations require further investigation.

► Obesity is a significant public health problem in the United States, affecting 36% of US adults, and around the world.[1] Obesity increases the risk of cardiovascular disease, hypertension, and type 2 diabetes mellitus[2] but is thought to be protective against bone loss and fractures.[3,4] However, more recent studies have shown that obesity, especially abdominal obesity, may be associated with decreased bone mineral density (BMD).[5,6] Visceral adipose tissue is the fat depot most strongly associated with decreased BMD and compromised bone structure.[7] A number of epidemiologic studies have shown increased fracture risk in obese cohorts.[8]

Although most studies have used noninvasive imaging to measure bone marrow fat and bone quality, this study used tetracycline-labeled transiliac bone biopsies in 40 healthy premenopausal women to assess relationships between body fat and bone microstructure and remodeling at the bone tissue level. The key findings were that women with central adiposity had decreased bone quality and stiffness and greatly reduced bone formation, suggesting that obesity causes adverse effects on the skeleton even in premenopausal women who are estrogen replete.

This is the first study to characterize relationships between body fat distribution and trabecular bone microarchitecture, stiffness, and remodeling in healthy premenopausal women. Given that the findings are similar to those in children, men, and postmenopausal women, it is difficult to ignore the adverse influence of abdominal obesity in premenopausal women with normal gonadal sex steroid levels and normal menstrual function. Additional studies are required to demonstrate increased fracture risk in premenopausal women with increased truncal fat.

B. L. Clarke, MD

References

1. Flegal KM, Carroll MD, Kit BK, Ogden CL. Prevalence of obesity and trends in the distribution of body mass index among US adults, 1999–2010. *JAMA*. 2012;307:491-497.
2. Nejat EJ, Polotsky AJ, Pal L. Predictors of chronic disease at midlife and beyond—the health risks of obesity. *Maturitas*. 2010;65:106-111.
3. Klein KO, Larmore KA, de Lancey E, Brown JM, Considine RV, Hassink SG. Effect of obesity on estradiol level, and its relationship to leptin, bone maturation, and bone mineral density in children. *J Clin Endocrinol Metab*. 1998;83:3469-3475.
4. Reid IR, Plank LD, Evans MC. Fat mass is an important determinant of whole body bone density in premenopausal women but not in men. *J Clin Endocrinol Metab*. 1992;75:779-782.
5. Bredella MA, Torriani M, Ghomi RH, et al. Determinants of bone mineral density in obese premenopausal women. *Bone*. 2011;48:748-754.
6. Bredella MA, Torriani M, Ghomi RH, et al. Vertebral bone marrow fat is positively associated with visceral fat and inversely associated with IGF-1 in obese women. *Obesity (Silver Spring)*. 2011;19:49-53.
7. Gilsanz V, Chalfant J, Mo AO, Lee DC, Dorey FJ, Mittelman SD. Reciprocal relations of subcutaneous and visceral fat to bone structure and strength. *J Clin Endocrinol Metab*. 2009;94:3387-3393.
8. Compston JE, Watts NB, Chapurlat R, et al. Obesity is not protective against fracture in postmenopausal women: GLOW. *Am J Med*. 2011;124:1043-1050.

Relationship of Weight, Height, and Body Mass Index With Fracture Risk at Different Sites in Postmenopausal Women: The Global Longitudinal Study of Osteoporosis in Women (GLOW)

Compston JE, for the GLOW Investigators (Cambridge Univ Hosps Natl Health Service (NHS) Foundation Trust, UK)

J Bone Miner Res 29:487-493, 2014

Low body mass index (BMI) is a well-established risk factor for fracture in postmenopausal women. Height and obesity have also been associated with increased fracture risk at some sites. We investigated the relationships of weight, BMI, and height with incident clinical fracture in a practice-based cohort of postmenopausal women participating in the Global Longitudinal study of Osteoporosis in Women (GLOW). Data were collected at baseline and at 1, 2, and 3 years. For hip, spine, wrist, pelvis, rib, upper arm/shoulder, clavicle, ankle, lower leg, and upper leg fractures, we modeled the time to incident self-reported fracture over a 3-year period using the Cox proportional hazards model and fitted the best linear or nonlinear models containing height, weight, and BMI. Of 52,939 women, 3628 (6.9%) reported an incident clinical fracture during the 3-year follow-up period. Linear BMI showed a significant inverse association with hip, clinical spine, and wrist fractures: adjusted hazard ratios (HRs) (95% confidence intervals [CIs]) per increase of 5 kg/m^2 were 0.80 (0.71–0.90),

0.83 (0.76–0.92), and 0.88 (0.83–0.94), respectively (all $p < 0.001$). For ankle fractures, linear weight showed a significant positive association: adjusted HR per 5-kg increase 1.05 (1.02–1.07) ($p < 0.001$). For upper arm/shoulder and clavicle fractures, only linear height was significantly associated: adjusted HRs per 10-cm increase were 0.85 (0.75–0.97) ($p = 0.02$) and 0.73 (0.57–0.92) ($p = 0.009$), respectively. For pelvic and rib fractures, the best models were for nonlinear BMI or weight ($p = 0.05$ and 0.03, respectively), with inverse associations at low BMI/body weight and positive associations at high values. These data demonstrate that the relationships between fracture and weight, BMI, and height are site-specific. The different associations may be mediated, at least in part, by effects on bone mineral density, bone structure and geometry, and patterns of falling.

▶ Obesity has recently been associated with increased fracture risk at certain skeletal sites in men and women. Fracture risk in obese postmenopausal women has been reported to be increased at the ankle, upper leg, lower leg, and proximal humerus,[1-5] whereas these individuals have been reported to have lower risk of hip, pelvis, and wrist fractures.[1,3,5] Obesity is currently defined as body mass index (BMI) of > 30 kg/m^2. In contrast to patients with obesity, individuals with BMI < 20 have increased risk of fracture, particularly hip fracture.[6,7]

This prospective longitudinal practice-based cohort study of almost 60 000 women in 10 countries sought to assess the relationship of body weight, height, and BMI to incident fractures in postmenopausal women over 3 years. Almost 7% of these patients reported an incident clinical fracture during the follow-up period. A significant linear inverse association was reported between BMI and hip, clinical spine, and wrist fractures, whereas a significant linear positive association was reported between BMI and ankle fracture. Arm/shoulder and clavicular fractures were significantly associated with linear height, and pelvic and rib fractures were associated with nonlinear BMI or weight, with inverse associations at low BMI/body weight and positive associations at high BMI/body weight. The study concluded that relationships among fracture and weight, height, and BMI are site-specific, with the observed associations mediated by effects on bone mineral density, bone structure and geometry, and patterns of falling.

This important study has further clarified the associations between body weight, height, BMI, and fracture risk. The relationships are complex and vary between skeletal sites, with higher body weight being protective against hip, clinical spine, and wrist fractures. For most fractures the relationships were linear, but for rib and pelvic fractures, the relationships were nonlinear with increased risk at both extremes of BMI and weight, although the risk was much higher at low BMI and weight. No association was seen between weight, height, or BMI and upper or lower leg fractures. These findings are consistent with previous studies showing that obesity increases the risk of fracture at certain sites but is protective at other sites. Because the incidence of obesity is rapidly increasing in certain countries, the distribution of fractures observed at various sites may also change over time.

B. L. Clarke, MD

References

1. Armstrong ME, Spencer EA, Cairns BJ, et al. Million Women Study Collaborators. Body mass index and physical activity in relation to the incidence of hip fracture in postmenopausal women. *J Bone Miner Res.* 2011;26:1330-1338.
2. Bergkvist D, Hekmat K, Svensson T, Dahlberg L. Obesity in orthopedic patients. *Surg Obes Relat Dis.* 2009;5:670-672.
3. Compston JE, Watts NB, Chapurlat R, et al. GLOW Investigators. Obesity is not protective against fracture in postmenopausal women: GLOW. *Am J Med.* 2011; 124:1043-1050.
4. Gnudi S, Sitta E, Lisi L. Relationship of body mass index with main limb fragility fractures in postmenopausal women. *J Bone Miner Metab.* 2009;27:479-484.
5. King CM, Hamilton GA, Cobb M, Carpenter D, Ford LA. Association between ankle fractures and obesity. *J Foot Ankle Surg.* 2012;51:543-547.
6. Prieto-Alhambra D, Premaor MO, Fina Avilés F, et al. The association between fracture and obesity is site-dependent: a population-based study in postmenopausal women. *J Bone Miner Res.* 2012;27:294-300.
7. De Laet C, Kanis JA, Odén A, et al. Body mass index as a predictor of fracture risk: a meta-analysis. *Osteoporos Int.* 2005;16:1330-1338.

In Vivo Assessment of Bone Quality in Postmenopausal Women with Type 2 Diabetes

Farr JN, Drake MT, Amin S, et al (Mayo Clinic, Rochester, MN)
J Bone Miner Res 29:787-795, 2014

While patients with type 2 diabetes (T2D) are at significant risk for well recognized diabetic complications, including macrovascular disease, retinopathy, nephropathy, and neuropathy, it is also clear that T2D patients are at increased risk for fragility fractures. Furthermore, fragility fractures in patients with T2D occur at higher bone mineral density (BMD) values compared to non-diabetic controls, suggesting abnormalities in bone material strength (BMS) and/or bone microarchitecture (bone "quality"). Thus, we performed *in vivo* microindentation testing of the tibia to directly measure BMS in 60 postmenopausal women (age range, 50–80 yrs) including 30 patients diagnosed with T2D for >10 yrs and 30 age-matched, non-diabetic controls. Regional BMD was measured by DXA; cortical and trabecular bone microarchitecture was assessed from HRpQCT images of the distal radius and tibia. Compared to controls, T2D patients had significantly lower BMS: unadjusted (−11.7%; $p < 0.001$); following adjustment for BMI (−10.5%; $p < 0.001$); and following additional adjustment for age, hypertension, nephropathy, neuropathy, retinopathy, and vascular disease (−9.2%; $p = 0.022$). By contrast, after adjustment for confounding by BMI, T2D patients had bone microarchitecture and BMD that were not significantly different than controls; however, radial cortical porosity tended to be higher in the T2D patients. In addition, patients with T2D had significantly reduced serum markers of bone turnover (all $p < 0.001$) compared to controls. Of note, in patients with T2D, the average glycated hemoglobin level over the previous 10 yrs was negatively correlated with BMS ($r = -0.41$; $p = 0.026$). In conclusion, these findings represent the first demonstration of compromised bone material strength in patients with T2D. Furthermore, our results confirm previous studies demonstrating low bone turnover in patients with T2D and highlight the potential detrimental effects of prolonged hyperglycemia on bone quality. Thus, the skeleton needs to be recognized as another important target tissue subject to diabetic complications.

► Patients with type 2 diabetes mellitus have an increased risk of fragility fractures at the hip, spine, and wrist,[1-5] despite having normal or increased bone mineral density (BMD) normalized for body mass index (BMI).[6,7] Data from 3 large prospective observational studies in the United States have recently shown that BMD and the Fracture Risk Assessment Tool (FRAX) underestimate fracture risk for a given femoral neck T-score and age in patients with type 2 diabetes mellitus.[8,9] These observations suggest that an underlying skeletal microstructural or bone material strength abnormalities may be present to explain the increased fracture risk in type 2 diabetes mellitus, but no abnormalities have been identified to date.

This study used *in vivo* microindentation testing of the tibia to assess bone material strength (BMS), dual-energy x-ray absorptiometry (DXA) BMD, and high-resolution peripheral quantitative computed tomography (HRpQCT) scanning to assess microstructural abnormalities in 60 postmenopausal women, 30 of whom had type 2 diabetes mellitus, and 30 of whom were healthy age-matched nondiabetic controls. Patients with type 2 diabetes mellitus had 11.7% lower BMS, 10.5% lower BMS after adjustment for BMI, and 9.2% lower BMS after further adjustment for age, hypertension, nephropathy, neuropathy, retinopathy, and vascular disease compared with the healthy controls. In contrast, DXA BMD and bone microstructure were not different in the diabetics compared with the controls, with radial cortical porosity nonsignificantly mildly increased in the diabetics. Serum markers of bone turnover were all decreased in the diabetics. Average glycated hemoglobin over the preceding 10 years was inversely correlated with BMS.

These findings represent the first demonstration of reduced bone material strength in postmenopausal women with type 2 diabetes mellitus. The study confirms previous findings of low serum markers of bone turnover in adults with type 2 diabetes mellitus, and the findings suggest that prolonged hyperglycemia may have detrimental effects on the skeleton. Further studies will be required to assess whether abnormalities in bone material strength alone completely explain the increased fracture risk seen in patients with type 2 diabetes mellitus.

B. L. Clarke, MD

References

1. Schwartz AV, Sellmeyer DE, Ensrud KE, et al. Older women with diabetes have an increased risk of fracture: a prospective study. *J Clin Endocrinol Metab.* 2001;86: 32-38.
2. Strotmeyer ES, Cauley JA, Schwartz AV, et al. Nontraumatic fracture risk with diabetes mellitus and impaired fasting glucose in older white and black adults: the health, aging, and body composition study. *Arch Intern Med.* 2005;165:1612-1617.

3. Bonds DE, Larson JC, Schwartz AV, et al. Risk of fracture in women with type 2 diabetes: the Women's Health Initiative Observational Study. *J Clin Endocrinol Metab*. 2006;91:3404-3410.
4. Melton LJ, Leibson CL, Achenbach SJ, Therneau TM, Khosla S. Fracture risk in type 2 diabetes: update of a population-based study. *J Bone Miner Res*. 2008; 23:1334-1342.
5. Janghorbani M, Van Dam RM, Willett WC, Hu FB. Systematic review of type 1 and type 2 diabetes mellitus and risk of fracture. *Am J Epidemiol*. 2007;166:495-505.
6. Vestergaard P. Discrepancies in bone mineral density and fracture risk in patients with type 1 and type 2 diabetes—a meta-analysis. *Osteoporos Int*. 2007;18:427-444.
7. Strotmeyer ES, Cauley JA, Schwartz AV, et al. Diabetes is associated independently of body composition with BMD and bone volume in older white and black men and women: The Health, Aging, and Body Composition Study. *J Bone Miner Res*. 2004;19:1084-1091.
8. Schwartz AV, Vittinghoff E, Bauer DC, et al. Association of BMD and FRAX score with risk of fracture in older adults with type 2 diabetes. *JAMA*. 2011;305: 2184-2192.
9. Dawson-Hughes B, Tosteson AN, Melton LJ 3rd, et al. Implications of absolute fracture risk assessment for osteoporosis practice guidelines in the USA. *Osteoporos Int*. 2008;19:449-458.

Fracture risk following bariatric surgery: a population-based study

Nakamura KM, Haglind EGC, Clowes JA, et al (Mayo Clinic, Rochester, MN)
Osteoporos Int 25:151-158, 2014

The effects of bariatric surgery on skeletal health are poorly understood.We found that bariatric surgery patients are more prone to fracture when compared to the general population. While further studies of fracture risk in this population are needed, bone health should be discussed in bariatric surgery clinics.

Introduction.—Bariatric surgery is an increasingly common treatment for medically complicated obesity. Adverse skeletal changes after bariatric surgery have been reported, but their clinical importance remains unknown. We hypothesized that bariatric surgery patients are at increased risk of fracture.

Methods.—We conducted a historical cohort study of fracture incidence among 258 Olmsted County, Minnesota, residents who underwent a first bariatric surgery in 1985–2004. Relative fracture risk was expressed as standardized incidence ratios (SIRs), while potential risk factors were evaluated by hazard ratios (HR) obtained from a time-to-fracture regression model.

Results.—The mean (±SD) body mass index at bariatric surgery was 49.0 ± 8.4 kg/m^2, with an average age of 44 ± 10 years and 82 % (212) females. Gastric bypass surgery was performed in 94 % of cases. Median follow-up was 7.7 years (range, 6 days to 25 years), during which 79 subjects experienced 132 fractures. Relative risk for any fracture was increased 2.3-fold (95 % confidence interval (CI), 1.8–2.8) and was elevated for a first fracture at the hip, spine, wrist, or humerus (SIR, 1.9; 95 % CI, 1.1–2.9), as well as for a first fracture at any other site (SIR, 2.5; 95 % CI, 2.0–3.2). Better preoperative activity status was associated with a lower age-adjusted risk

(HR, 0.4; 95 % CI, 0.2–0.8) while prior fracture history was not associated with postoperative fracture risk.

Conclusions.—Bariatric surgery, which is accompanied by substantial biochemical, hormonal, and mechanical changes, is associated with an increased risk of fracture.

▶ Bariatric surgery is increasingly frequently recommended as treatment for obesity in patients with body mass index ≥ 40 kg/m^2, or ≥35 kg/m^2 when complicated by type 2 diabetes mellitus or other disorders.[1-3] In the United States in 2009, 220 000 bariatric surgeries were performed, representing a greater than 10-fold increase over those performed in the previous decade.[4] Long-term skeletal outcomes of bariatric surgery are not well defined. Two previous studies reported increased fracture risk after bariatric surgery,[5,6] whereas evaluation of a large population-based cohort in the United Kingdom showed no evidence of increased fractures after this type of surgery.[7] Malabsorption of calcium, vitamin D, and other nutrients after bariatric surgery could potentially lead to bone loss and increased fractures.

This study was done to assess fracture risk after bariatric surgery in a population-based study of 258 patients in Olmsted County, Minnesota. Most subjects had gastric bypass procedures. Over a median follow-up of 7.7 years, with a range of 6 days to 25 years, 79 patients in the study had 132 fractures. These observations led to an estimate of a 2.3-fold increased first fracture risk after surgery, with increased fractures of the hip, spine, wrist, and humerus observed. First fractures at other sites were also increased by 2.5-fold. More than half of the fractures identified occurred more than 5 years after the surgical procedure. Lesser preoperative physical activity and vitamin D deficiency were associated with increased age-adjusted risk of fracture, whereas presurgical fracture history did not increase postsurgical fracture risk. The study concluded that bariatric surgery led to an increase in fracture risk.

These findings provide further evidence that bariatric surgery may cause adverse skeletal outcomes years after the procedure. The pathophysiologic mechanisms causing the increased fracture risk appeared to be activated early after surgery, and appeared to be sustained over many years, given the relatively uniform divergence in cumulative fracture incidence after surgery compared with expected fracture incidence in the general population. This is the only population-based study to estimate fracture incidence during a long period of follow-up in women and men who have undergone bariatric surgery.

B. L. Clarke, MD

References

1. Centers for Disease Control and Prevention. *Overweight and Obesity*, http://www.cdc.gov/obesity; 2011. Accessed February 21, 2014.
2. Sjöström L, Lindroos AK, Peltonen M, et al. Lifestyle, diabetes, and cardiovascular risk factors 10 years after bariatric surgery. *N Engl J Med.* 2004;351:2683-2693.
3. Adams TD, Gress RE, Smith SC, et al. Long-term mortality after gastric bypass surgery. *N Engl J Med.* 2007;357:753-761.
4. American Society for Metabolic and Bariatric Surgery. *Fact Sheet: Metabolic and Bariatric Surgery*, http://asmbs.org/; 2010. Accessed February 21, 2014.

5. Berarducci A, Haines K, Murr MM. Incidence of bone loss, falls, and fractures after Roux-en-Y gastric bypass for morbid obesity. *Appl Nurs Res*. 2009;22:35-41.
6. Abu-Lebdeh HS, Paat JJ. Are post bariatric surgery fractures different from fractures in severely obese subjects? In: IOF World Congress on Osteoporosis. Florence, Italy. 2010.
7. Lalmohamed A, de Vries F, Bazelier MT, et al. Risk of fracture after bariatric surgery in the United Kingdom: population based, retrospective cohort study. *BMJ*. 2011;345:e5085.

Gonadal Steroids and Body Composition, Strength, and Sexual Function in Men

Finkelstein JS, Lee H, Burnett-Bowie S-AM, et al (Massachusetts General Hosp, Boston)
N Engl J Med 369:1011-1022, 2013

Background.—Current approaches to diagnosing testosterone deficiency do not consider the physiological consequences of various testosterone levels or whether deficiencies of testosterone, estradiol, or both account for clinical manifestations.

Methods.—We provided 198 healthy men 20 to 50 years of age with goserelin acetate (to suppress endogenous testosterone and estradiol) and randomly assigned them to receive a placebo gel or 1.25 g, 2.5 g, 5 g, or 10 g of testosterone gel daily for 16 weeks. Another 202 healthy men received goserelin acetate, placebo gel or testosterone gel, and anastrozole (to suppress the conversion of testosterone to estradiol). Changes in the percentage of body fat and in lean mass were the primary outcomes. Subcutaneous- and intraabdominal-fat areas, thigh-muscle area and strength, and sexual function were also assessed.

Results.—The percentage of body fat increased in groups receiving placebo or 1.25 g or 2.5 g of testosterone daily without anastrozole (mean testosterone level, 44 ± 13 ng per deciliter, 191 ± 78 ng per deciliter, and 337 ± 173 ng per deciliter, respectively). Lean mass and thigh-muscle area decreased in men receiving placebo and in those receiving 1.25 g of testosterone daily without anastrozole. Leg-press strength fell only with placebo administration. In general, sexual desire declined as the testosterone dose was reduced.

Conclusions.—The amount of testosterone required to maintain lean mass, fat mass, strength, and sexual function varied widely in men. Androgen deficiency accounted for decreases in lean mass, muscle size, and strength; estrogen deficiency primarily accounted for increases in body fat; and both contributed to the decline in sexual function. Our findings support changes in the approach to evaluation and management of hypogonadism in men. (Funded by the National Institutes of Health and others; ClinicalTrials.gov number, NCT00114114.)

▶ Hypogonadism in men remains difficult to define. In most cases, a low serum testosterone level and clinical symptoms of hypogonadism are required to make the diagnosis, and much emphasis is placed on the serum testosterone level, especially in older men.[1,2] Usually serum total testosterone more than 2 standard deviations below the mean value in normal young men is considered deficient. Because more than 80% of circulating estradiol in men is derived from aromatization of testosterone,[3] estradiol levels decrease as testosterone levels decline.[4,5] Testosterone treatment is usually given to treat nonspecific symptoms, such as fatigue, lack of energy, or sexual dysfunction, when the serum testosterone level is less than the laboratory reference range.

This study evaluated the relative degree of testosterone deficiency, estradiol deficiency, or both at which undesirable changes in body composition, strength, and sexual function occurred and whether these changes were caused by androgen or estrogen deficiency or both. About 400 men were given the GnRH agonist goserelin acetate to suppress endogenous testosterone and estradiol production. They were then randomly selected to receive different doses of testosterone gel or placebo, with or without anastrozole to inhibit aromatization of testosterone into estradiol, for 16 weeks. Changes in the percentage of body fat, lean mass, subcutaneous and intra-abdominal fat, thigh muscle area and strength, and sexual function were assessed at baseline and at the end of treatment. The study found that lean mass, muscle size, and muscle strength were regulated by androgens, fat accumulation was stimulated by estrogen deficiency, and sexual function was regulated by both androgens and estrogens. However, the amount of testosterone required for an effect varied widely among men.

The findings of this significant study suggest that testosterone replacement alone may not adequately treat the full syndrome of testosterone deficiency. Goal levels of serum testosterone during therapy should likely be individualized based on symptoms in response to treatment. Definition of the degrees of hypogonadism at which each adverse consequence develops and of the relative roles of androgens and estrogens in each outcome will help develop more logical approaches to the diagnosis and treatment of hypogonadism in men.

B. L. Clarke, MD

References

1. Liverman CT, Blazer DG. *Testosterone and Aging: Clinical Research Directions*. Washington, DC: National Academy of Sciences; 2004.
2. Harman SM, Metter EJ, Tobin JD, Pearson J, Blackman MR. Longitudinal effects of aging on serum total and free testosterone levels in healthy men. *J Clin Endocrinol Metab*. 2001;86:724-731.
3. Longcope C, Kato T, Horton R. Conversion of blood androgens to estrogens in normal adult men and women. *J Clin Invest*. 1969;48:2191-2201.
4. Khosla S, Melton LJ III, Atkinson EJ, O'Fallon WM, Klee GG, Riggs BL. Relationship of serum sex steroid levels and bone turnover markers with bone mineral density in men and women: a key role for bioavailable estrogen. *J Clin Endocrinol Metab*. 1998;83:2266-2274.
5. van den Beld AW, de Jong FH, Grobbee DE, Pols HA, Lamberts SW. Measures of bioavailable serum testosterone and estradiol and their relationships with muscle strength, bone density, and body composition in elderly men. *J Clin Endocrinol Metab*. 2000;85:3276-3282.

Cortical Porosity Identifies Women with Osteopenia at Increased Risk for Forearm Fractures

Bala Y, Zebaze R, Ghasem-Zadeh A, et al (Univ of Melbourne, Australia; et al)
J Bone Miner Res 29:1356-1362, 2014

Background.—Most fragility fractures arise among the many women with osteopenia, not the smaller number with osteoporosis at high risk for fracture. Thus, most women at risk for fracture assessed only by measuring areal bone mineral density (aBMD) will remain untreated.

Methods.—We measured cortical porosity and trabecular bone volume/total volume (BV/TV) of the ultradistal radius (UDR) using high-resolution peripheral quantitative computed tomography, aBMD using densitometry, and 10-year fracture probability using the country-specific FRAX tool in 68 postmenopausal women with forearm fractures and 70 age-matched community controls in Olmsted County, Minnesota.

Results.—Women with forearm fractures had 0.4 standard deviations (SD) higher cortical porosity and 0.6 SD lower trabecular BV/TV. Compact-appearing cortical porosity predicted fracture independent of aBMD; odds ratio [OR] 1.92 (95%CI, 1.10-3.33). In women with osteoporosis at the UDR, cortical porosity did not distinguish those with, from those without, fractures because high porosity was present in 92% and 86% of each group respectively. By contrast, in women with osteopenia at the UDR, high porosity of the compact-appearing cortex conferred an OR for fracture of 4.00 (95%CI, 1.15-13.90).

Conclusion.—In women with osteoporosis, porosity is captured by aBMD and so measuring UDR cortical porosity does not improve diagnostic sensitivity. However, in women with osteopenia, cortical porosity was associated with forearm fractures.

► Patients with osteopenia have a lower risk of fracture than patients with osteoporosis, but about 50% of all fractures, and 50% of recurrent fractures, in the population occur in patients with osteopenia.[1-4] The challenge is to identify which patients with osteopenia will fracture. One approach is to use FRAX[5,6] or similar fracture risk prediction models; another is to characterize microstructural deterioration in patients. High-resolution peripheral quantitative CT (HRpQCT) scanning allows quantification of cortical bone loss at the distal wrist and tibia, and StrAx1.0, a new method of image analysis that permits quantification of cortical porosity, may predict fracture risk.[7,8]

This study evaluated cortical porosity and trabecular bone volume of the ultradistal radius using HRpQCT, dual-energy x-ray absorptiometry (DXA) bone mineral density (BMD) and estimated 10-year absolute fracture risk using FRAX in 68 postmenopausal women with forearm fractures and 70 age-matched community controls. The findings showed that postmenopausal women with osteopenia at the ultradistal radius who had increased cortical porosity had increased fracture risk, independent of DXA BMD measurement, whereas those without increased cortical porosity did not. Women with osteoporosis at the ultradistal radius did not benefit from measurement of cortical porosity. The study concluded that measurement of ultradistal radius cortical porosity was predictive of fractures independent of DXA BMD measurement in postmenopausal women with osteopenia.

This important study describes a new way to assess fracture risk in postmenopausal women with osteopenia. In postmenopausal women with osteoporosis, DXA BMD measurement predicts fracture risk with sufficiently high sensitivity that cortical porosity measurement is not necessary. However, in postmenopausal women with osteopenia, measurement of ultradistal radius cortical porosity adds additional information that predicts fracture risk independent of DXA BMD.

B. L. Clarke, MD

References

1. Sanders KM, Nicholson GC, Watts JJ, et al. Half the burden of fragility fractures in the community occur in women without osteoporosis. When is fracture prevention cost-effective? *Bone.* 2006;38:694-700.
2. Schuit SC, van der Klift M, Weel AE, et al. Fracture incidence and association with bone mineral density in elderly men and women: the Rotterdam Study. *Bone.* 2004;34:195-202.
3. Siris ES, Chen YT, Abbott TA, et al. Bone mineral density thresholds for pharmacological intervention to prevent fractures. *Arch Intern Med.* 2004;164: 1108-1112.
4. Langsetmo L, Goltzman D, Kovacs CS, et al. Repeat low-trauma fractures occur frequently among men and women who have osteopenic BMD. *J Bone Miner Res.* 2009;24:1515-1522.
5. Kanis JA, Johnell O, Oden A, Johansson H, McCloskey E. FRAX and the assessment of fracture probability in men and women from the UK. *Osteoporos Int.* 2008;19:385-397.
6. Moriwaki K, Komaba H, Noto S, et al. Cost-effectiveness of alendronate for the treatment of osteopenic postmenopausal women in Japan. *J Bone Miner Res.* 2013;28:395-403.
7. Zebaze RM, Ghasem-Zadeh A, Bohte A, et al. Intracortical remodelling and porosity in the distal radius and post-mortem femurs of women: a cross-sectional study. *Lancet.* 2010;375:1729-1736.
8. Zebaze R, Ghasem-Zadeh A, Mbala A, Seeman E. A new method of segmentation of compact-appearing, transitional and trabecular compartments and quantification of cortical porosity from high resolution peripheral quantitative computed tomographic images. *Bone.* 2013;54:8-20.

A Distal Forearm Fracture in Childhood Is Associated With an Increased Risk for Future Fragility Fractures in Adult Men, but Not Women

Amin S, Melton LJ III, Achenbach SJ, et al (Mayo Clinic, Rochester, MN)

J Bone Miner Res 28:1751-1759, 2013

Distal forearm fractures are among the most common fractures during childhood, but it remains unclear whether they predict an increased fracture risk later in life. We studied a population–based cohort of 1776 children ≤18 years of age, from Olmsted County, MN, USA, who had a distal forearm fracture in 1935–1992. Incident fractures occurring at age ≥35 years were identified through review of complete medical records using the linkage system of the Rochester Epidemiology Project. Observed nonpathologic fractures resulting from no more than moderate trauma (fragility fractures) were compared with expected numbers estimated from fracture site–specific incidence rates, based on age, sex, and calendar year, for Olmsted County (standardized incidence ratios [SIR]). In 1086 boys (mean ± SD age; 11 ± 4 years) and 690 girls (10 ± 4 years) followed for 27,292 person–years after the age of 35 years, subsequent fragility fractures were observed in 144 (13%) men and 74 (11%) women. There was an increased risk for future fragility fractures in boys who had a distal forearm fracture (SIR, 1.9; 95% CI, 1.6–2.3) but not girls (SIR, 1.0; 95% CI, 0.8–1.2). Fragility fractures at both major osteoporotic (hip, spine, wrist, and shoulder) sites (SIR, 2.6; 95% CI, 2.1–3.3) and remaining sites (SIR, 1.7; 95% CI, 1.3–2.0) were increased in men, irrespective of age at distal forearm fracture as boys. A distal forearm fracture in boys, but not girls, is associated with an increased risk for fragility fractures as older adults. It is necessary to determine whether the increased fractures observed in men is due to persistent deficits of bone strength, continued high fracture risk activity, or both. Until then, men should be asked about a childhood distal forearm fracture and, if so, warrant further screening and counseling on measures to optimize bone health and prevent fractures.

▶ Distal forearm fractures are common in childhood, accounting for up to one-third of all pediatric fractures.[1] More than 40% of girls and more than 50% of boys have at least one fracture during childhood and adolescence.[2] Distal forearm fractures in childhood are increasing in incidence,[3,4] particularly in girls.[3] Previous studies have found lower bone mineral density and weaker bone structure in boys and girls with distal forearm fractures compared with controls.[5] Even though distal forearm fractures in adults are considered predictive of future fractures, it is not clear that a childhood distal forearm fracture would be similarly predictive of adult fracture risk. This is the first study to attempt to determine whether distal forearm fractures in childhood predict adult fragility fractures.

The study evaluated moderate trauma fractures during adulthood in a population-based cohort of children who had sustained distal forearm fractures during childhood. Boys in the study with childhood distal forearm fractures had increased risk of osteoporotic fractures later in life, whereas girls did not. Fractures of all types were increased in the men with childhood distal forearm fractures, including hip, spine, wrist, shoulder, and other fractures. Fracture risk did not depend on age of the childhood distal forearm fracture. The study did not determine whether the increased fracture risk in men was caused by persistent bone deficits or continued high fracture risk activity, or both.

These findings imply that men with childhood distal forearm fractures should be further evaluated for fracture risk and advised regarding measures to optimize their bone health and prevent future fractures. Further studies are needed to determine whether increased fracture risk in these men is caused by persistent bone deficits or continued high-fracture-risk behavior and to clarify the most effective means of preventing future fracture.

B. L. Clarke, MD

References

1. Hedström EM, Svensson O, Bergström U, Michno P. Epidemiology of fractures in children and adolescents. *Acta Orthop*. 2010;81:148-153.
2. Jones IE, Williams SM, Dow N, Goulding A. How many children remain fracture-free during growth? a longitudinal study of children and adolescents participating in the Dunedin Multidisciplinary Health and Development Study. *Osteoporos Int*. 2002;13:990-995.
3. Khosla S, Melton LJ 3rd, Dekutoski MB, Achenbach SJ, Oberg AL, Riggs BL. Incidence of childhood distal forearm fractures over 30 years: a population-based study. *JAMA*. 2003;290:1479-1485.
4. Mäyränpää MK, Mäkitie O, Kallio PE. Decreasing incidence and changing pattern of childhood fractures: a population-based study [Erratum appears in J Bone Miner Res. 2011 Feb;26(2):439]. *J Bone Miner Res*. 2010;25:2752-2759.
5. Goulding A, Cannan R, Williams SM, Gold EJ, Taylor RW, Lewis-Barned NJ. Bone mineral density in girls with forearm fractures. *J Bone Miner Res*. 1998;13:143-148.

Rapid Cortical Bone Loss in Patients With Chronic Kidney Disease

Nickolas TL, Stein EM, Dworakowski E, et al (Columbia Univ Med Ctr, NY; et al)

J Bone Miner Res 28:1811-1820, 2013

Chronic kidney disease (CKD) patients may have high rates of bone loss and fractures, but microarchitectural and biochemical mechanisms of bone loss in CKD patients have not been fully described. In this longitudinal study of 53 patients with CKD Stages 2 to 5D, we used dual-energy X-ray absorptiometry (DXA), high-resolution peripheral quantitative computed tomography (HRpQCT), and biochemical markers of bone metabolism to elucidate effects of CKD on the skeleton. Median follow-up was 1.5 years (range 0.9 to 4.3 years); bone changes were annualized and compared with baseline. By DXA, there were significant declines in areal bone mineral density (BMD) of the total hip and ultradistal radius: −1.3% (95% confidence interval [CI] −2.1 to −0.6) and −2.4% (95% CI −4.0 to −0.9), respectively. By HRpQCT at the distal radius, there were significant declines in cortical area, density, and thickness and increases in porosity: −2.9% (95% CI −3.7 to −2.2), −1.3% (95% CI −1.6 to −0.6), −2.8% (95% CI −3.6 to −1.9), and +4.2% (95% CI 2.0 to 6.4), respectively. Radius trabecular area increased significantly: +0.4% (95% CI 0.2 to 0.6), without significant changes in trabecular density or microarchitecture. Elevated time-averaged levels of parathyroid hormone (PTH) and bone turnover markers predicted cortical deterioration. Higher levels of serum 25-hydroxyvitamin D predicted decreases in trabecular network heterogeneity. These data suggest that significant cortical loss occurs with CKD, which is mediated by hyperparathyroidism and elevated turnover. Future investigations are required to determine whether these cortical losses can be attenuated by treatments that reduce PTH levels and remodeling rates.

▶ Later-stage chronic kidney disease (CKD) typically causes bone disease. Abnormal calcium-phosphate metabolism, decreased serum 1,25-dihydroxyvitamin D, and increased parathyroid hormone (PTH) result in renal osteodystrophy, in part and in combination. Fractures are increased as a result of the bone disease associated with late-stage CKD. Hip[1-3] and spine[4] fractures are increased 2- to 4-fold compared with the general population, and mortality after hip fracture is 60% greater.[5] The biochemical and microarchitectural basis of increased skeletal fragility in CKD is not well understood.

This longitudinal study of 53 patients with moderate (stage 2) to severe (stage 5D) CKD evaluated the extent and pathogenesis of bone loss in this population over a median of 1.5 years of follow-up. Bone mineral density (BMD) by dual-energy X-ray absorptiometry showed significant decreases of 1.3% and 2.4% in areal BMD of the total hip and ultradistal radius, respectively. High-resolution peripheral quantitative CT scanning of the distal radius showed decreases in cortical area by 2.9%, in density by 1.3%, and in thickness by 2.8%, and increases in cortical porosity of 4.2%. Radius trabecular area increased by 0.4%, without significant changes in trabecular density or microarchitecture. Increased PTH and markers of bone turnover predicted cortical bone loss. The study concluded that CKD is associated with significant cortical bone loss caused by hyperparathyroidism and increased bone turnover.

This important study quantitated skeletal changes in patients with moderate to severe CKD over 1.5 years of follow-up. The findings indicate that CKD is associated with predominantly cortical bone loss driven by hyperparathyroidism and increased bone turnover. The impact of these findings on the central skeleton and vertebral and hip fractures remains to be determined. Future studies will be required to assess the skeletal impact of treatments that decrease PTH levels or lower bone turnover in CKD.

B. L. Clarke, MD

References

1. Ball AM, Gillen DL, Sherrard D, et al. Risk of hip fracture among dialysis and renal transplant recipients. *JAMA*. 2002;288:3014-3018.
2. Nickolas TL, McMahon DJ, Shane E. Relationship between moderate to severe kidney disease and hip fracture in the United States. *J Am Soc Nephrol*. 2006; 17:3223-3232.
3. Fried LF, Biggs ML, Shlipak MG, et al. Association of kidney function with incident hip fracture in older adults. *J Am Soc Nephrol*. 2007;18:282-286.
4. Kaji H, Yamauchi M, Yamaguchi T, Shigematsu T, Sugimoto T. Mild renal dysfunction is a risk factor for a decrease in bone mineral density and vertebral fractures in Japanese postmenopausal women. *J Clin Endocrinol Metab*. 2010;95: 4635-4642.
5. Nitsch D, Mylne A, Roderick PJ, Smeeth L, Hubbard R, Fletcher A. Chronic kidney disease and hip fracture-related mortality in older people in the UK. *Nephrol Dial Transplant*. 2009;24:1539-1544.

Hepatitis C Co-infection and Severity of Liver Disease as Risk Factors for Osteoporotic Fractures Among HIV-Infected Patients

Maalouf NM, Zhang S, Drechsler H, et al (Univ of Texas Southwestern Med Ctr, Dallas; et al)

J Bone Miner Res 28:2577-2583, 2013

Osteoporosis is increasingly reported in the aging HIV-positive population, and co-infection with hepatitis C virus (HCV) may further increase the risk of osteoporosis. However, it remains unclear whether HCV-related increased fracture risk is a function of the severity of liver disease. We calculated the time-updated alanine aminotransferase to platelet ratio index (APRI) score (an indirect marker of hepatic fibrosis) in all HIV-infected patients enrolled in the Veterans Affairs' Clinical Case Registry between 1984 and 2009. The association between HCV co-infection and incident osteoporotic fracture (defined as closed wrist, vertebral, or hip fracture) was assessed in univariate and multivariate Cox survival models adjusting for traditional risk factors for osteoporosis and APRI score or the presence of cirrhosis. A total of 772 osteoporotic fractures were identified among 56,660 HIV-infected patients (98.1% male; 31.3% HCV co-infected; median age 44.0 years) contributing 305,237 patient-years of follow-up. Fracture rates were significantly higher among HIV/HCV patients than HIV-only patients (2.57 versus 2.07/1000 patient-years, relative risk = 1.24, $p < 0.0001$). In a Cox multivariable model including age, race, smoking, drug use, body mass index, and antiretroviral therapy, HCV co-infection remained an independent predictor of osteoporotic fractures after controlling for presence of cirrhosis (hazard ratio [HR] = 1.32; $p < 0.001$) or APRI score (HR = 1.30; $p = 0.003$). Among HIV/HCV co-infected patients, cirrhosis strongly predicted osteoporotic fractures (HR = 1.65; 95% confidence interval [CI] 1.11–2.44; $p = 0.012$), but APRI score was a weaker predictor (HR = 1.008; 95% CI 1.002–1.014; $p = 0.015$). In conclusion, among HIV-infected patients, severity of liver disease partly explains the HCV-associated increased risk of osteoporotic fractures. Other determinants of this increased risk remain to be defined.

▶ Osteoporosis and osteoporotic fractures are now recognized as common among the aging HIV-infected population.[1-4] Both HIV infection and its treatment with highly active antiretroviral therapy are associated with increased bone loss and fracture risk.[5,6] Approximately 30% of HIV-infected patients are also infected with hepatitis C virus (HCV), which may further increase the risk of osteoporosis and osteoporotic fractures.[7,8] There is currently little information on whether HCV coinfection increases fracture risk in HIV-infected patients while controlling for cumulative exposure to any antiretroviral therapy or highly active antiretroviral therapy. This study assessed the impact of HCV coinfection on fracture risk in HIV-infected individuals in a large national Veterans Affairs database and evaluated the impact of liver cirrhosis and severity of liver fibrosis on fracture risk in this cohort.

The study showed that HIV/HCV-infected patients had significantly higher fracture rates than patients infected with HIV alone. Multivariate analysis showed that HCV coinfection remained an independent predictor of osteoporotic fractures after controlling for cirrhosis. Among HCV/HIV coinfected patients, cirrhosis strongly predicated osteoporotic fractures. The study concluded that severity of liver disease partly explains the HCV-associated increased risk of osteoporotic fractures among HIV-infected patients.

This study indicates that HCV coinfection increases the risk of osteoporotic fractures in HIV-infected patients and that this risk is partly dependent on HCV-associated liver cirrhosis. Other independent risk factors of osteoporotic fracture remain to be identified in this population.

B. L. Clarke, MD

References

1. Triant VA, Brown TT, Lee H, Grinspoon SK. Fracture prevalence among human immunodeficiency virus (HIV)-infected versus non-HIV-infected patients in a large U.S. healthcare system. *J Clin Endocrinol Metab.* 2008;93:3499-3504.
2. McComsey GA, Tebas P, Shane E, et al. Bone disease in HIV infection: a practical review and recommendations for HIV care providers. *Clin Infect Dis.* 2010;51: 937-946.
3. Young B, Dao CN, Buchacz K, Baker R, Brooks JT. Increased rates of bone fracture among HIV-infected persons in the HIV Outpatient Study (HOPS) compared with the US general population, 2000–2006. *Clin Infect Dis.* 2011;52:1061-1068.
4. Kühne CA, Heufelder AE, Hofbauer LC. Bone and mineral metabolism in human immunodeficiency virus infection. *J Bone Miner Res.* 2001;16:2-9.
5. Brown TT, Qaqish RB. Antiretroviral therapy and the prevalence of osteopenia and osteoporosis: a meta-analytic review. *AIDS.* 2006;20:2165-2174.
6. Tebas P, Powderly WG, Claxton S, et al. Accelerated bone mineral loss in HIV-infected patients receiving potent antiretroviral therapy. *AIDS.* 2000;14:F63-F67.
7. Bedimo R, Maalouf NM, Zhang S, Drechsler H, Tebas P. Osteoporotic fracture risk associated with cumulative exposure to tenofovir and other antiretroviral agents. *AIDS.* 2012;26:825-831.
8. Hansen AB, Gerstoft J, Kronborg G, et al. Incidence of low and high-energy fractures in persons with and without HIV infection: a Danish population-based cohort study. *AIDS.* 2012;26:285-293.

Current Issues in Osteoporosis Therapy

Zoledronic Acid Acutely Increases Sclerostin Serum Levels in Women with Postmenopausal Osteoporosis

Catalano A, Morabito N, Basile G, et al (Univ of Messina, Italy)
J Clin Endocrinol Metab 98:1911-1915, 2013

Context.—Sclerostin is a circulating inhibitor of the Wnt-signaling pathway produced by osteocytes, which acts as a negative regulator of bone formation. Effects of zoledronic acid on sclerostin serum levels in postmenopausal osteoporosis are unknown.

Objective.—The purpose of this study was to evaluate sclerostin serum levels after zoledronic acid administration and correlate variations with bone turnover markers.

Design and Setting.—We conducted a prospective intervention study in an ambulatory care setting.

Participants and Intervention.—Forty women (mean age 62.6 ± 4.9 years) with postmenopausal osteoporosis were enrolled in this study and randomized into 2 groups to receive zoledronic acid (5 mg) or placebo.

Main Outcomes Measures.—At baseline and then at 2, 7, 30, and 360 days after zoledronic acid or placebo administration, serum levels of sclerostin, bone-specific alkaline phosphatase (BSAP), as a bone formation marker, and serum C-telopeptide of type 1 collagen (CTX), as a bone resorption marker, were measured.

Results.—Sclerostin serum levels increased by day 2, reached a peak at day 7 (3-fold baseline, $P < .001$), and then decreased at day 30 and returned near to baseline after 360 days in the zoledronic acid group. Both CTX and BSAP were reduced, and a significant negative correlation was observed between the percentage changes of sclerostin and the variation in BSAP and CTX at all time points in the zoledronic acid group ($P < .05$). No changes were observed in the placebo group.

Conclusions.—Our data demonstrate that zoledronic acid increases sclerostin serum levels and that sclerostin could play a role in coupling bone resorption to bone formation.

► Sclerostin is an inhibitor of the Wnt-signaling pathway expressed almost exclusively within osteocytes in bone.[1] Activation of the Wnt/β-catenin pathway in osteoblasts leads to increased proliferation and differentiation of osteoblast precursor cells, decreases apoptosis of mature osteoblasts, and stimulates the ability of mature osteoblasts to inhibit osteoclast differentiation.[2] Osteoclasts, osteoblasts, and bone lining cells do not produce sclerostin in humans. Bone marrow plasma and peripheral blood serum sclerostin levels are strongly correlated, suggesting that osteocytes are the major source of sclerostin production.[3] Sclerostin binds competitively to the Wnt coreceptor low-density lipoprotein receptor—related proteins 5 and 6 and prevents the binding of Wnt ligands to the 7-transmembrane domain spanning frizzled receptors.[1] This study was performed to assess the variation in serum sclerostin in response to infusion of zoledronic acid or placebo for postmenopausal osteoporosis and to determine correlations with changes in bone turnover markers. Forty postmenopausal women were evaluated at different time points after zoledronic acid infusion. The study showed that serum sclerostin increased by the second day after infusion, peaked at 3-fold baseline at 7 days, decreased by 30 days, and then returned to baseline by 360 days. Serum bone-specific alkaline phosphatase, a marker of bone formation, and serum C-telopeptide of type 1 collagen, a marker of bone resorption, both decreased as expected after zoledronic acid infusion.

These findings show that zoledronic acid increases serum sclerostin for up to 1 year after infusion and suggest that sclerostin could play a role in coupling bone resorption to bone formation. Sclerostin may contribute to inhibition of bone formation after zoledronic acid infusion. Two other bisphosphonates, neridronate and risedronate; parathyroid hormone; calcitonin; and denosumab all have similar effects, whereas estrogens, raloxifene, and strontium ranelate reduce serum sclerostin, and alendronate has no apparent effect. The differences in the effects on serum sclerostin among these agents used to treat osteoporosis remain unclear, but blunting of this effect could lead to enhanced response to anabolic agents.

B. L. Clarke, MD

References

1. Bonewald LF. The amazing osteocyte. *J Bone Miner Res.* 2011;26:229-238.
2. Glass DA 2nd, Bialek P, Ahn JD, et al. Canonical Wnt signaling in differentiated osteoblasts controls osteoclast differentiation. *Dev Cell.* 2005;8:751-764.
3. Drake MT, Srinivasan B, Mödder UI, et al. Effects of parathyroid hormone treatment on circulating sclerostin levels in postmenopausal women. *J Clin Endocrinol Metab.* 2010;95:5056-5062.

Duration of Antiresorptive Effects of Low-Dose Zoledronate in Osteopenic Postmenopausal Women: A Randomized, Placebo-Controlled Trial

Grey A, Bolland M, Mihov B, et al (Univ of Auckland, New Zealand)
J Bone Miner Res 29:166-172, 2014

Annual intravenous administration of 5 mg zoledronate decreases fracture risk, but the optimal dosing regimen for zoledronate has not been determined. We set out to evaluate the antiresorptive effects of a single administration of lower doses of zoledronate. A total of 180 postmenopausal women with osteopenia enrolled in a double-blind, randomized, placebo-controlled trial over 2 years at an academic research center. Participants were randomized to a single baseline administration of intravenous zoledronate in doses of 1 mg, 2.5 mg, or 5 mg, or placebo. The primary endpoint was change in bone mineral density (BMD) at the lumbar spine. Secondary endpoints were change in BMD at the proximal femur and total body, and changes in biochemical markers of bone turnover. After 2 years, the change in spine BMD was greater in each of the zoledronate groups than in the placebo group; values are mean (95% confidence interval [CI]) difference versus placebo: zoledronate 1 mg 4.4% [2.7% to 6.1%]; 2.5 mg 5.5% [3.9% to 7.2%]; 5 mg 5.3% [3.8% to 6.7%], $p < 0.001$ for each dose). Change in BMD at the total hip was greater in each of the zoledronate groups than the placebo group (mean [95% CI] difference versus placebo: zoledronate 1 mg 2.6% [1.5% to 3.7%]; 2.5 mg 4.4% [3.5% to 5.3%]; 5 mg 4.7% [3.7% to 5.7%], $p < 0.001$ for each dose). Each of the bone turnover markers, β-C-terminal telopeptide of type I collagen (β-CTX) and procollagen type-I N-terminal propeptide (P1NP), was lower in each of the 2.5-mg and 5-mg zoledronate groups than the placebo group throughout the trial ($p < 0.001$ versus placebo for each marker for each dose at each time point). For each endpoint, changes were similar in the 2.5-mg and 5-mg zoledronate groups, whereas those in the 1-mg group were smaller than those in the other zoledronate groups. These data demonstrate that single administrations of zoledronate 1 mg or 2.5 mg produce antiresorptive effects that persist for at least 2 years.

Trials assessing the antifracture efficacy of intermittent low doses of zoledronate, in particular the 2.5-mg dose, are justified.

▶ Zoledronic acid is approved by the US Food and Drug Administration (FDA) for treatment of osteoporosis at 5 mg intravenously over 15 minutes once a year.[1,2] This dose effectively reduces fracture risk and also reduces mortality after hip fracture.[2] The optimal dosing regimen has not yet been determined. Antiresorptive effect of a single dose of zoledronic acid may persist for at least 5 years.[3] Similar effects on bone mineral density (BMD) and markers of bone turnover were observed after 2 years in a trial comparing the effect of a single dose of 5 mg versus 2 yearly 5-mg doses.[4] Another recent study found that a single 5-mg dose caused fracture risk reduction comparable to 3 yearly 5-mg doses.[5] This study reports the results of further analysis of the previously reported phase II dose-ranging trial with zoledronic acid.[6] The trial included 180 postmenopausal women randomly assigned to receive single baseline intravenous doses of 1 mg, 2.5 mg, 5 mg, or placebo, with follow-up over 2 years. All doses increased both lumbar spine and total hip BMD compared with placebo over 2 years. Serum markers of bone turnover were reduced compared with placebo for each dose throughout the trial. Statistical analysis suggested that changes were similar with the 2.5 and 5-mg doses but reduced with the 1-mg dose. The study concluded that the antiresorptive effect of single doses of 1 mg and 2.5 mg zoledronic acid persist for up to 2 years, with the 2.5-mg dose effect similar to that of the 5-mg dose effect at 2 years. The 1-mg dose effect was similar to the higher doses at year and then gradually was lost over time.

The findings of this study are important, as they suggest that lower-dose zoledronic acid may be as efficacious, or nearly as efficacious, as the FDA-approved treatment dose of 5 mg once yearly. This suggests that lower-dose zoledronic acid could be used with equal efficacy in patients, particularly those with conditions limiting the use of higher-dose zoledronic acid, such as chronic kidney disease or older age. Further trials will be required to show efficacy and safety with lower-dose zoledronic acid in these populations.

B. L. Clarke, MD

References

1. Black DM, Delmas PD, Eastell R, et al. Once-yearly zoledronic acid for treatment of postmenopausal osteoporosis. *N Engl J Med.* 2007;356:1809-1822.
2. Lyles KW, Colón-Emeric CS, Magaziner JS, et al. Zoledronic acid and clinical fractures and mortality after hip fracture. *N Engl J Med.* 2007;357:1799-1809.
3. Grey A, Bolland MJ, Horne A, et al. Five years of anti-resorptive activity after a single dose of zoledronate—results from a randomized double-blind placebo controlled trial. *Bone.* 2012;50:1389-1393.
4. McClung M, Miller P, Recknor C, Mesenbrink P, Bucci-Rechtweg C, Benhamou CL. Zoledronic acid for the prevention of bone loss in postmenopausal women with low bone mass: a randomized controlled trial. *Obstet Gynecol.* 2009; 114:999-1007.
5. Reid IR, Black DM, Eastell R, et al. Reduction in the risk of clinical fractures after a single dose of zoledronic acid 5 mg. *J Clin Endocrinol Metab.* 2013;98:557-563.
6. Reid IR, Brown JP, Burckhardt P, et al. Intravenous zoledronic acid in postmenopausal women with low bone mineral density. *N Engl J Med.* 2002;346:653-661.

Effects of Pioglitazone on Bone in Postmenopausal Women With Impaired Fasting Glucose or Impaired Glucose Tolerance: A Randomized, Double-Blind, Placebo-Controlled Study

Bone HG, Lindsay R, McClung MR, et al (Michigan Bone and Mineral Clinic, Detroit; Helen Hayes Hosp, West Haverstraw, NY; Oregon Osteoporosis Ctr, Portland; et al)

J Clin Endocrinol Metab 98:4691-4701, 2013

Context.—Meta-analyses of clinical studies have suggested an increased incidence of peripheral fractures in postmenopausal women with type 2 diabetes mellitus taking pioglitazone. The mechanism behind this apparent increase is unknown.

Objective.—The objective of the study was to examine the effects of pioglitazone on bone mineral density (BMD) and turnover.

Design and Setting.—Twenty-five sites (in the United States) enrolled participants in this randomized, double-blind, placebo-controlled study.

Participants.—Postmenopausal women (n = 156) with impaired fasting glucose or impaired glucose tolerance participated in the study.

Interventions.—The intervention consisted of pioglitazone 30 mg/d (n = 78) or placebo (n = 78), increased to 45 mg/d after 1 month, for 12 months of treatment total, followed by 6 months of washout/follow-up.

Main Outcome Measures.—Percentage changes from baseline to month 12 and from month 12 to month 18 in BMD in total proximal femur (primary end point), total body, femoral neck, lumbar spine, and radius were measured.

Results.—Least squares mean changes from baseline to month 12 in total proximal femur BMD were −0.69% for pioglitazone and −0.14% for placebo (*P* =.170). No statistically significant between-group differences were observed for any BMD or bone remodeling marker end point. We observed improved glycemic control and insulin sensitivity with pioglitazone treatment. In addition, pioglitazone appeared to increase body fat, which may affect bone density measurements, especially in the lumbar spine. One pioglitazone-treated and three placebo-treated women experienced confirmed fractures. Over 18 months, one pioglitazone-treated (1.3%) and eight placebo-treated women (10.3%) developed overt type 2 diabetes mellitus. The pattern and incidence of adverse events with pioglitazone were consistent with clinical experience with thiazolidinediones.

Conclusions.—Maximal-dose pioglitazone had no effects on BMD or bone turnover, while improving glycemic control as expected, in postmenopausal women with impaired fasting glucose or impaired glucose tolerance.

▶ Several meta-analyses of clinical trials have indicated that pioglitazone or rosiglitazone therapy in postmenopausal women and older men with type 2 diabetes mellitus may increase the risk of peripheral fractures.[1-6] Patients with type 2 diabetes mellitus have an increased risk of fracture despite normal or increased bone mineral density (BMD).[7] Thiazolidinedione therapy stimulates peroxisome proliferator–activated receptor-γ activation, which shifts the differentiation of mesenchymal stem cells toward adipocytes and away from osteoblasts.[8] These findings collectively suggest that thiazolidinedione therapy may have adverse effects on the skeleton.

This study evaluated the effect of maximal dose pioglitazone vs placebo for 12 months on BMD and serum markers of bone turnover in postmenopausal women with impaired fasting glucose or impaired glucose tolerance. No significant effects on BMD or serum markers of bone turnover were seen. Pioglitazone improved glycemic control and insulin sensitivity in study subjects as expected and also increased body fat. Confirmed fractures were seen in 1 woman on pioglitazone and 3 women on placebo.

These findings indicated that pioglitazone at maximal doses for 12 months had no detectable effects on BMD or bone turnover in postmenopausal women with impaired fasting glucose or impaired glucose tolerance. Glucose control and insulin sensitivity improved as expected. Further studies are required to clarify the apparent increase in fracture risk seen with long-term thiazolidinedione therapy.

B. L. Clarke, MD

References

1. Kahn SE, Haffner SM, Heise MA, et al. Glycemic durability of rosiglitazone, metformin, or glyburide monotherapy. *N Engl J Med.* 2006;355:2427-2443.
2. Kahn SE, Zinman B, Lachin JM, et al. Rosiglitazone-associated fractures in type 2 diabetes: an Analysis from A Diabetes Outcome Progression Trial (ADOPT). *Diabetes Care.* 2008;31:845-851.
3. Home PD, Pocock SJ, Beck-Nielsen H, et al. Rosiglitazone evaluated for cardiovascular outcomes in oral agent combination therapy for type 2 diabetes (RECORD): a multicentre, randomised, open-label trial. *Lancet.* 2009;373:2125-2135.
4. Meymeh RH, Wooltorton E. Diabetes drug pioglitazone (Actos): risk of fracture. *CMAJ.* 2007;177:723-724.
5. Dormandy J, Bhattacharya M, van Troostenburg de Bruyn AR. Safety and tolerability of pioglitazone in high-risk patients with type 2 diabetes: an overview of data from PROactive. *Drug Saf.* 2009;32:187-202.
6. Loke YK, Singh S, Furberg CD. Long-term use of thiazolidinediones and fractures in type 2 diabetes: a meta-analysis. *CMAJ.* 2009;180:32-39.
7. Forsén L, Meyer HE, Midthjell K, Edna TH. Diabetes mellitus and the incidence of hip fracture: results from the Nord-Trøndelag health survey. *Diabetologia.* 1999;42:920-925.
8. Rzonca SO, Suva LJ, Gaddy D, Montague DC, Lecka-Czernik B. Bone is a target for the antidiabetic compound rosiglitazone. *Endocrinology.* 2004;145:401-406.

Femoral and Vertebral Strength Improvements in Postmenopausal Women With Osteoporosis Treated With Denosumab

Keaveny TM, McClung MR, Genant HK, et al (Univ of California Berkeley; Oregon Osteoporosis Ctr, Portland; Univ of California San Francisco; et al)
J Bone Miner Res 29:158-165, 2014

In the randomized, placebo-controlled FREEDOM study of women aged 60 to 90 years with postmenopausal osteoporosis, treatment with denosumab once every 6 months for 36 months significantly reduced hip and new vertebral fracture risk by 40% and 68%, respectively. To gain further insight into this efficacy, we performed a nonlinear finite element analysis (FEA) of hip and spine quantitative computed tomography (QCT) scans to estimate hip and spine strength in a subset of FREEDOM subjects ($n = 48$ placebo; $n = 51$ denosumab) at baseline, 12, 24, and 36 months. We found that, compared with baseline, the finite element estimates of hip strength increased from 12 months (5.3%; $p < 0.0001$) and through 36 months (8.6%; $p < 0.0001$) in the denosumab group. For the placebo group, hip strength did not change at 12 months and decreased at 36 months (−5.6%; $p < 0.0001$). Similar changes were observed at the spine: strength increased by 18.2% at 36 months for the denosumab group ($p < 0.0001$) and decreased by −4.2% for the placebo group ($p = 0.002$). At 36 months, hip and spine strength increased for the denosumab group compared with the placebo group by 14.3% ($p < 0.0001$) and 22.4% ($p < 0.0001$), respectively. Further analysis of the finite element models indicated that strength associated with the trabecular bone was lost at the hip and spine in the placebo group, whereas strength associated with both the trabecular and cortical bone improved in the denosumab group. In conclusion, treatment with denosumab increased hip and spine strength as estimated by FEA of QCT scans compared with both baseline and placebo owing to positive treatment effects in both the trabecular and cortical bone compartments. These findings provide insight into the mechanism by which denosumab reduces fracture risk for postmenopausal women with osteoporosis.

▶ Denosumab is a fully human monoclonal antibody that inhibits receptor-activator of nuclear factor kappa B ligand from stimulating osteoclast formation, function, and survival.[1-4] The FREEDOM phase III clinical trial showed that denosumab 60 mg subcutaneously every 6 months given to 7808 postmenopausal women aged 60 to 90 years for 3 years reduced vertebral and hip fractures by 68% and 40%, respectively.[5] This reduction in fracture risk was associated with an 8.8% increase in areal bone mineral density (BMD) at the lumbar spine and a 6.4% increase in areal BMD at the total hip,[6] as well as rapid and marked reductions in serum bone markers of bone resorption with a return toward baseline at the end of each 6-month dosing interval.[5,7]

This study applied nonlinear finite element analysis to spine and hip quantitative computed tomography scans obtained in a subset of the FREEDOM trial subjects to noninvasively assess changes in spine and hip strength associated with denosumab treatment over the 36 months of the trial. These scans were obtained in 51 subjects treated with denosumab and calcium and vitamin D supplementation, and 48 treated with placebo and calcium and vitamin D supplementation. The study found that spine strength increased by 18.2% over 36 months in the denosumab-treated group and decreased by 4.2% in the placebo group over this interval. Total hip strength increased by 8.6% in the denosumab-treated group and decreased by 5.6% in the placebo group. Strength associated with both cortical and trabecular bone increased at both the spine and hip in the denosumab-treated group, whereas strength associated with trabecular bone decreased at both the spine and hip in the placebo group.

These findings suggest that denosumab significantly reduces fracture risk at the spine and hip by strengthening both the cortical and trabecular compartments at both the spine and hip compared with calcium and vitamin D supplementation alone. The changes in strength at both the spine and hip were relatively large compared with baseline and placebo treatment with calcium and vitamin D supplementation alone. Denosumab is efficacious for the treatment of postmenopausal osteoporosis.

B. L. Clarke, MD

References

1. Lacey DL, Tan HL, Lu J, et al. Osteoprotegerin ligand modulates murine osteoclast survival in vitro and in vivo. *Am J Pathol.* 2000;157:435-448.
2. Lacey DL, Timms E, Tan HL, et al. Osteoprotegerin ligand is a cytokine that regulates osteoclast differentiation and activation. *Cell.* 1998;93:165-176.
3. Udagawa N, Takahashi N, Yasuda H, et al. Osteoprotegerin produced by osteoblasts is an important regulator in osteoclast development and function. *Endocrinology.* 2000;141:3478-3484.
4. Yasuda H, Shima N, Nakagawa N, et al. Osteoclast differentiation factor is a ligand for osteoprotegerin/osteoclastogenesis-inhibitory factor and is identical to TRANCE/RANKL. *Proc Natl Acad Sci U S A.* 1998;95:3597-3602.
5. Cummings SR, San Martin J, McClung MR, et al. Denosumab for prevention of fractures in postmenopausal women with osteoporosis. *N Engl J Med.* 2009; 361:756-765.
6. Bolognese MA, Teglbjærg CS, Zanchetta JR, et al. Denosumab significantly increases DXA BMD at both trabecular and cortical sites: results from the FREEDOM study. *J Clin Densitom.* 2013;16:147-153.
7. Eastell R, Christiansen C, Grauer A, et al. Effects of denosumab on bone turnover markers in postmenopausal osteoporosis. *J Bone Miner Res.* 2011;26:530-537.

RANKL Inhibition With Denosumab Does Not Influence 3-Year Progression of Aortic Calcification or Incidence of Adverse Cardiovascular Events in Postmenopausal Women With Osteoporosis and High Cardiovascular Risk

Samelson EJ, Miller PD, Christiansen C, et al (Hebrew Senior Life and Harvard Med School, Boston, MA; Colorado Ctr for Bone Res, Lakewood; Ctr for Clinical and Basic Res, Ballenrup, Denmark; et al)

J Bone Miner Res 29:450-457, 2014

Atherosclerosis and osteoporosis are chronic diseases that progress with age, and studies suggest aortic calcification, an indicator of atherosclerosis, is inversely associated with bone mineral density (BMD). The osteoprotegerin (OPG)/receptor activator of NF-κB (RANK)/RANK ligand (RANKL) system has been proposed as a shared regulatory system for bone and vasculature. Denosumab (DMAb), a monoclonal antibody against RANKL, improved BMD and reduced fracture risk in the Fracture Reduction Evaluation of Denosumab in Osteoporosis Every 6 Months (FREEDOM) trial. We evaluated whether or not treatment with DMAb influenced progression of aortic calcification (AC) and incidence of cardiovascular (CV) adverse events. We included 2363 postmenopausal women with osteoporosis (1142 placebo, 1221 DMAb), selected from 7808 participants in the FREEDOM trial (3906 placebo, 3902 DMAb), at high risk of CV events according to modified Raloxifene Use for the Heart (RUTH) criteria. CV adverse events were reported by participants. AC scores were assessed using a semiquantitative method from lateral spine X-rays. Change in AC score from baseline to 12 ($n = 1377$), 24 ($n = 1231$), and 36 months ($n = 1045$) was calculated as AC score at follow-up minus AC score at baseline. AC progression was defined as change in AC score >0. Baseline characteristics, CV risk factors, and AC scores were similar between treatment groups. Mean age of participants was 74 years (range, 60–90), 88% were white, and 77% had AC score >0 at baseline. Frequency of AC progression over 3 years did not differ between women in placebo (22%) and DMAb (22%) groups ($p = 0.98$). AC progression did not differ between treatment groups when analyzed by baseline estimated glomerular filtration rate or by baseline AC scores. Frequency of CV adverse events did not differ between placebo (40%) and DMAb (38%) groups ($p = 0.26$). In conclusion, DMAb treatment had no effect on progression of AC or incidence of CV adverse events compared to placebo.

▶ Aortic calcification strongly predicts cardiovascular events.[1] Several epidemiologic studies also show that aortic calcification is associated with decreased bone mineral density (BMD), greater bone loss, and fractures.[2-5] The osteoprotegerin/receptor-activator of nuclear factor kappa B ligand (RANKL) system has been suggested as the link between bone remodeling and vascular calcification.[6]

This study assessed progression of aortic calcification and incidence of cardiovascular events in participants in the FREEDOM phase III clinical trial with denosumab versus placebo. Denosumab is a fully human monoclonal antibody to RANKL. A total of 2363 postmenopausal women at high risk of cardiovascular events were selected from the 7808 study subjects in the trial. Cardiovascular adverse events were reported by study participants, and lateral spine x-rays were used to assess aortic calcification. Baseline characteristics, cardiovascular risk factors, and aortic calcification scores were similar between treatment groups. Frequency of aortic calcification progression over 3 years was not different between the denosumab and placebo groups. The analysis did not change when subjects were stratified by baseline estimated glomerular filtration rate of aortic calcification score. The frequency of cardiovascular events also did not differ between the treatment groups.

These findings indicate that denosumab did not prevent progression of aortic calcification or cardiovascular events in a study cohort at high risk of cardiovascular events over 3 years of treatment. These results strongly suggest that the OPG/RANKL system may not be the common pathway linking adverse skeletal and cardiovascular outcomes.

B. L. Clarke, MD

References

1. Wilson PW, Kauppila LI, O'Donnell CJ, et al. Abdominal aortic calcific deposits are an important predictor of vascular morbidity and mortality. *Circulation.* 2001;103:1529-1534.
2. Kiel DP, Kauppila LI, Cupples LA, Hannan MT, O'Donnell CJ, Wilson PW. Bone loss and the progression of abdominal aortic calcification over a 25 year period: the Framingham Heart Study. *Calcif Tissue Int.* 2001;68:271-276.
3. Naves M, Rodríguez-García M, Díaz-López JB, Gómez-Alonso C, Cannata-Andía JB. Progression of vascular calcifications is associated with greater bone loss and increased bone fractures. *Osteoporos Int.* 2008;19:1161-1166.
4. Hak AE, Pols HA, van Hemert AM, Hofman A, Witteman JC. Progression of aortic calcification is associated with metacarpal bone loss during menopause: a population-based longitudinal study. *Arterioscler Thromb Vasc Biol.* 2000;20:1926-1931.
5. Bagger YZ, Tankó LB, Alexandersen P, Qin G, Christiansen C, Prospective Epidemiological Risk Factors Study Group. Radiographic measure of aorta calcification is a site-specific predictor of bone loss and fracture risk at the hip. *J Intern Med.* 2006;259:598-605.
6. Hofbauer LC, Brueck CC, Shanahan CM, Schoppet M, Dobnig H. Vascular calcification and osteoporosis—from clinical observation towards molecular understanding. *Osteoporos Int.* 2007;18:251-259.

Teriparatide for Idiopathic Osteoporosis in Premenopausal Women: A Pilot Study

Cohen A, Stein EM, Recker RR, et al (Columbia Univ Med Ctr, NY; Creighton Univ Med Ctr, Omaha, NE; et al)

J Clin Endocrinol Metab 98:1971-1981, 2013

Context.—Premenopausal women with idiopathic osteoporosis (IOP) have abnormal cortical and trabecular bone microarchitecture.

Objective.—The purpose of this study was to test the hypotheses that teriparatide increases bone mineral density (BMD) and bone formation and improves trabecular microarchitecture and stiffness in women with IOP.

Design.—This was an open-label pilot study.

Setting.—The setting was a tertiary care referral center.

Patients.—Participants were 21 premenopausal women with unexplained fragility fractures or low BMD.

Intervention.—Teriparatide was administered at 20 μg daily for 18 to 24 months.

Main Outcome Measures.—The primary endpoint was within-subject percent change in lumbar spine BMD. Secondary endpoints included percent change in hip and forearm BMD, transiliac biopsy parameters (trabecular bone volume, microarchitecture, stiffness, and adipocytes), serum N-terminal propeptide of procollagen type 1 (P1NP), and C-telopeptide.

Results.—BMD increased at the spine (10.8 ± 8.3% [SD]), total hip (6.2 ± 5.6%), and femoral neck (7.6 ± 3.4%) (all $P < .001$). Serum P1NP doubled by 1 month, peaked at 6 months, and returned to baseline by 18 to 24 months. Transiliac biopsies demonstrated significant increases in cortical width and porosity and trabecular bone volume and number increased, mirrored by a 71% increase in trabecular bone stiffness ($P < .02-.001$). Adipocyte area, perimeter, and volume/marrow volume decreased, with no change in adipocyte number. Four women had no increase in BMD and a blunted, delayed increase in serum P1NP. Nonresponders had markedly lower baseline bone formation rate (0.002 ± 0.001 vs 0.011 ± 0.006 $mm^2/mm/y$; $P < .001$) and higher serum IGF-1 (208 ± 54 vs 157 ± 44 ng/mL; $P = .03$).

Conclusions.—Teriparatide was associated with increased spine and hip BMD and improved trabecular microarchitecture and stiffness at the iliac crest in the majority of women with IOP.

▶ Young, healthy women may be affected by idiopathic osteoporosis with intact gonadal function and no evident secondary cause of bone loss or fragility.[1] Compared with normal premenopausal women, women with idiopathic osteoporosis have abnormal bone microarchitecture, with thinner cortices; fewer, thinner, and more widely separated and heterogeneously distributed trabeculae; more rodlike trabecular structure; lower trabecular stiffness; and higher marrow fat.[2] Bone remodeling as assessed by serum bone turnover markers[1] or transiliac bone biopsies[2] showed normal or increased bone turnover in some and low bone formation and increased serum insulinlike growth factor-1 (IGF-1) levels in others. Because IGF-1 has anabolic effects on osteoblasts, the increased IGF-1 levels in some premenopausal women with idiopathic osteoporosis have been interpreted as suggesting IGF-1 resistance in osteoblasts.[2] This open-label pilot study was done to assess the effects of the anabolic agent teriparatide on bone formation and trabecular microarchitecture and stiffness in 21 premenopausal women with idiopathic osteoporosis. The study showed increased bone mineral density (BMD) at the lumbar spine, total hip, and femoral neck, with an increase in serum P1NP by 1 month, peaking at 6 months, and returning to baseline at 18 to 24 months. Paired bone biopsy data showed increased cortical width and porosity, with trabecular bone volume and number increased, with a 71% increase in trabecular bone stiffness. Marrow adipocyte area, perimeter, and volume/marrow volume decreased, with no change in adipocyte number. Four women had no increase in BMD and a blunted, delayed increase in serum P1NP, with markedly lower baseline bone formation rate and higher serum IGF-1 levels. The study concluded that teriparatide significantly increased lumbar spine and hip BMD, and improved trabecular microarchitecture and stiffness in most women with idiopathic osteoporosis.

This important study suggests that teriparatide is effective treatment for most premenopausal women with idiopathic osteoporosis who experience fractures or who have severe and progressive bone loss. Nonresponders to teriparatide may have a defective osteoblast response to teriparatide, perhaps mediated by osteoblast resistance to IGF-1.

B. L. Clarke, MD

References

1. Cohen A, Recker RR, Lappe J, et al. Premenopausal women with idiopathic low-trauma fractures and/or low bone mineral density. *Osteoporos Int.* 2012;23:171-182.
2. Cohen A, Dempster DW, Recker RR, et al. Abnormal bone microarchitecture and evidence of osteoblast dysfunction in premenopausal women with idiopathic osteoporosis. *J Clin Endocrinol Metab.* 2011;96:3095-3105.

Risk Factors for Treatment Failure With Antiosteoporosis Medication: The Global Longitudinal Study of Osteoporosis in Women (GLOW)

Díez-Pérez A, for the Global Longitudinal Study of Osteoporosis in Women (GLOW) Investigators (Hosp del Mar-IMIM-Autonomous Univ of Barcelona, Spain; et al)

J Bone Miner Res 29:260-267, 2014

Antiosteoporosis medication (AOM) does not abolish fracture risk, and some individuals experience multiple fractures while on treatment. Therefore, criteria for treatment failure have recently been defined. Using data from the Global Longitudinal Study of Osteoporosis in Women (GLOW), we analyzed risk factors for treatment failure, defined as sustaining two or more fractures while on AOM. GLOW is a prospective, observational cohort study of women aged ≥55 years sampled from primary care practices in 10 countries. Self-administered questionnaires collected data on patient characteristics, fracture risk factors, previous fractures, AOM use, and health status. Data were analyzed from women who used the same class of AOM continuously over 3 survey years and had data available on fracture occurrence. Multivariable logistic regression was used to identify independent predictors of treatment failure. Data from 26,918 women were available, of whom 5550 were on AOM. During follow-up, 73 of 5550 women in the AOM group (1.3%) and 123 of 21,368 in the non-AOM group (0.6%) reported occurrence of two or more fractures. The following variables were associated with treatment failure: lower Short Form 36 Health Survey (SF-36) score (physical function and vitality) at baseline, higher Fracture Risk Assessment Tool (FRAX) score, falls in the past 12 months, selected comorbid conditions, prior fracture, current use of glucocorticoids, need of arms to assist to standing, and unexplained weight loss ≥10 lb (≥4.5 kg). Three variables remained predictive of treatment failure after multivariable analysis: worse SF-36 vitality score (odds ratio [OR] per 10-point increase, 0.85; 95% confidence interval [CI], 0.76–0.95; $p = 0.004$); two or more falls in the past year (OR, 2.40; 95% CI, 1.34–4.29; $p = 0.011$), and prior fracture (OR, 2.93; 95% CI, 1.81–4.75; $p < 0.0001$). The C statistic for the model was 0.712. Specific strategies for fracture prevention should therefore be developed for this subgroup of patients.

► A number of antiosteoporosis medications are found to be efficacious in treatment of postmenopausal osteoporosis by reducing fracture risk.[1] A smaller subset of these women do not respond to treatment as expected and continue to have fractures, even in those that are compliant with their medications. These fractures are not unexpected because available osteoporosis medications have been found to reduce fractures by up to 70% at the spine, 20% for nonvertebral sites, and 40% for the hip.[2-8] Treatment failure has been defined by an expert committee of the International Osteoporosis Foundation as having 2 or more fractures occur while on treatment.[9] This study evaluated characteristics of postmenopausal women ≥55 years who sustained 2 or more fractures while on continuous antiosteoporosis therapy in the Global Longitudinal Study of Osteoporosis, a prospective cohort study of postmenopausal women. The study administered self-reported questionnaires regarding patient characteristics, fracture risk factors, previous fractures, antiosteoporosis medications used, and health status. Fracture data were analyzed in women who had taken the same antiosteoporosis medication for 3 years continuously. Treatment failure was associated with lower physical function and vitality SF-36 score at baseline, higher FRAX score, falls in the last 12 months, comorbid conditions, prior fracture, current use of glucocorticoids, need of arms to assist with standing, and unexplained weight loss of ≥10 pounds. After multivariate analysis, worse Short Form 36 Health Survey vitality score, 2 or more falls in the last year, and prior fracture remained significant predictors of treatment failure.

These findings offer insight into which patients may continue to fracture despite use of US Food and Drug Administration—approved osteoporosis medications. Use of efficacious antiosteoporosis therapies may not prevent fractures in weak or frail individuals, or those who fall frequently, or those who have had prior fractures. The study findings suggest that specific strategies beyond currently available antiosteoporosis medications should be developed for fracture prevention in this subgroup of patients.

B. L. Clarke, MD

References

1. MacLean C, Newberry S, Maglione M, et al. Systematic review: comparative effectiveness of treatments to prevent fractures in men and women with low bone density or osteoporosis. *Ann Intern Med.* 2008;148:197-213.
2. Ettinger B, Black DM, Mitlak BH, et al. Reduction of vertebral fracture risk in postmenopausal women with osteoporosis treated with raloxifene: results from a 3-year randomized clinical trial. Multiple Outcomes of Raloxifene Evaluation (MORE) Investigators. *JAMA.* 1999;282:637-645.
3. Levis S, Quandt SA, Thompson D, et al. Alendronate reduces the risk of multiple symptomatic fractures: results from the fracture intervention trial. FIT Research Group. *J Am Geriatr Soc.* 2002;50:409-415.
4. Watts NB, Josse RG, Hamdy RC, et al. Risedronate prevents new vertebral fractures in postmenopausal women at high risk. *J Clin Endocrinol Metab.* 2003; 88:542-549.
5. Mackey DC, Black DM, Bauer DC, et al. Effects of antiresorptive treatment on nonvertebral fracture outcomes. *J Bone Miner Res.* 2011;26:2411-2418.
6. Silverman SL, Christiansen C, Genant HK, Vukicevic S, Zanchetta JR, de Villiers TJ, Constantine GD, Chines AA. Efficacy of bazedoxifene in reducing new vertebral fracture risk in postmenopausal women with osteoporosis: results from a 3-year, randomized, placebo-, and active-controlled clinical trial. *J Bone Miner Res.* 2008;23:1923-1934.

7. Black DM, Delmas PD, Eastell R, et al. HORIZON Pivotal Fracture Trial. Once-yearly zoledronic acid for treatment of postmenopausal osteoporosis. *N Engl J Med.* 2007;356:1809-1822.
8. Cummings SR, San Martin J, McClung MR, et al. FREEDOM Trial. Denosumab for prevention of fractures in postmenopausal women with osteoporosis. *N Engl J Med.* 2009;361:756-765.
9. Díez-Pérez A, González-Macías J. Inadequate responders to osteoporosis treatment: proposal for an operational definition. *Osteoporos Int.* 2008;19:1511-1516.

Novel Osteoporosis Therapies

Effects of Odanacatib on BMD and Safety in the Treatment of Osteoporosis in Postmenopausal Women Previously Treated With Alendronate: A Randomized Placebo-Controlled Trial

Bonnick S, De Villiers T, Odio A, et al (Clinical Res Ctr of North Texas, Denton, TX; Stellenbosch Univ, Cape Town, South Africa; Alta California Med Group and Heritage Med Res Inst, Simi Valley; et al)
J Clin Endocrinol Metab 98:4727-4735, 2013

Context.—Odanacatib (ODN) is a selective cathepsin K inhibitor being developed to treat osteoporosis.

Objective.—The effects of ODN were evaluated on bone mineral density (BMD), biochemical markers of bone turnover, and safety in patients previously treated with alendronate.

Design.—This was a randomized, double-blind, placebo-controlled, 24-month study.

Setting.—The study was conducted at private or institutional practices.

Participants.—Postmenopausal women (n = 243) ≥60 years of age with low BMD at the total hip, femoral neck, or trochanter (T-score ≤−2.5 but >−3.5 without prior fracture or ≤−1.5 but >−3.5 with prior fracture) on alendronate for ≥3 years.

Intervention.—The intervention included ODN 50 mg or placebo weekly.

Main Outcome Measures.—The primary end point was percentage change from baseline of femoral neck BMD at month 24. BMD was assessed by dual-energy x-ray absorptiometry at baseline and 6, 12, and 24 months. Biochemical markers of bone turnover (serum C-telopeptides of type 1 collagen, urinary N-telopeptides of type 1 collagen, serum bone specific alkaline phosphatase, and serum N-terminal propeptide of type 1 collagen) were measured at baseline and 3, 6, 12, 18, and 24 months.

Results.—In the ODN group, BMD changes from baseline at the femoral neck, trochanter, total hip, and lumbar spine at 24 months (1.7%, 1.8%, 0.8%, and 2.3%, respectively) were significantly different from the placebo group. ODN significantly decreased urinary N-telopeptides of type 1 collagen to creatinine ratio and significantly increased serum N-terminal propeptide of type 1 collagen compared with placebo. Serum C-telopeptides of type 1 collagen was unexpectedly increased with ODN treatment. The safety profile appeared similar between groups.

Conclusions.—ODN provided incremental BMD gains in osteoporotic women after alendronate treatment.

▶ Cathepsin K is the primary protease secreted by osteoclasts to digest organic matrix during bone resorption.[1] Preclinical studies in animal models of estrogen deficiency showed that odanacatib, a cathepsin K inhibitor, prevented bone loss and increased bone mass and strength.[2-4] Unlike with bisphosphonate or denosumab treatment, osteoclast number is not reduced with odanacatib treatment.[5] Clinical studies showed that odanacatib reduced serum markers of bone formation less than markers of bone resorption.[6] Bone loss resumes relatively quickly after stopping odanacatib treatment.[7]

This study evaluated the effects of weekly odanacatib versus placebo on bone mineral density (BMD), serum markers of bone turnover, and safety in postmenopausal osteoporotic women previously treated with alendronate for a minimum of 3 years. Odanacatib caused a mild increase in BMD at the lumbar spine and hip sites over 2 years of treatment, and decreased urine and serum N-terminal telopeptides as expected. Unexpectedly, serum C-terminal (CTx) telopeptides increased on treatment. Safety appeared similar between the odanacatib and placebo groups. The study concluded that odanacatib treatment caused further mild increases in BMD after alendronate treatment.

These findings suggest that weekly dosing of the moderately potent cathepsin K inhibitor odanacatib is able to stimulate further increases in BMD after long-term bisphosphonate therapy. The unexpected increase in serum CTx telopeptide was attributed to odanacatib inhibition of new bone resorption with metalloproteinase release of older β-CTx accumulated during previous alendronate therapy. Odanacatib appears to be safe and well tolerated.

B. L. Clarke, MD

References

1. Costa AG, Cusano NE, Silva BC, Cremers S, Bilezikian JP. Cathepsin K: its skeletal actions and role as a therapeutic target in osteoporosis. *Nat Rev Rheumatol.* 2011; 7:447-456.
2. Cusick T, Chen CM, Pennypacker BL, et al. Odanacatib treatment increases hip bone mass and cortical thickness by preserving endocortical bone formation and stimulating periosteal bone formation in the ovariectomized adult rhesus monkey. *J Bone Miner Res.* 2012;27:524-537.
3. Masarachia PJ, Pennypacker BL, Pickarski M, et al. Odanacatib reduces bone turnover and increases bone mass in the lumbar spine of skeletally mature ovariectomized rhesus monkeys. *J Bone Miner Res.* 2012;27:509-523.
4. Pennypacker BL, Duong le T, Cusick TE, et al. Cathepsin K inhibitors prevent bone loss in estrogen-deficient rabbits. *J Bone Miner Res.* 2011;26:252-262.
5. D'Amelio P, Grimaldi A, Di Bella S, et al. Risedronate reduces osteoclast precursors and cytokine production in postmenopausal osteoporotic women. *J Bone Miner Res.* 2008;23:373-379.
6. Bone HG, McClung MR, Roux C, et al. Odanacatib, a cathepsin-K inhibitor for osteoporosis: a two-year study in postmenopausal women with low bone density. *J Bone Miner Res.* 2010;25:937-947.
7. Eisman JA, Bone HG, Hosking DJ, et al. Odanacatib in the treatment of postmenopausal women with low bone mineral density: three-year continued therapy and resolution of effect. *J Bone Miner Res.* 2011;26:242-251.

Romosozumab in Postmenopausal Women with Low Bone Mineral Density
McClung MR, Grauer A, Boonen S, et al (Oregon Osteoporosis Ctr, Portland; Amgen, Thousand Oaks, CA; Leuven Univ, Belgium; et al)
N Engl J Med 370:412-420, 2014

Background.—Sclerostin is an osteocyte-derived inhibitor of osteoblast activity. The monoclonal antibody romosozumab binds to sclerostin and increases bone formation.

Methods.—In a phase 2, multicenter, international, randomized, placebo-controlled, parallelgroup, eight-group study, we evaluated the efficacy and safety of romosozumab over a 12-month period in 419 postmenopausal women, 55 to 85 years of age, who had low bone mineral density (a T score of −2.0 or less at the lumbar spine, total hip, or femoral neck and −3.5 or more at each of the three sites). Participants were randomly assigned to receive subcutaneous romosozumab monthly (at a dose of 70 mg, 140 mg, or 210 mg) or every 3 months (140 mg or 210 mg), subcutaneous placebo, or an open-label active comparator — oral alendronate (70 mg weekly) or subcutaneous teriparatide (20 μg daily). The primary end point was the percentage change from baseline in bone mineral density at the lumbar spine at 12 months. Secondary end points included percentage changes in bone mineral density at other sites and in markers of bone turnover.

Results.—All dose levels of romosozumab were associated with significant increases in bone mineral density at the lumbar spine, including an increase of 11.3% with the 210-mg monthly dose, as compared with a decrease of 0.1% with placebo and increases of 4.1% with alendronate and 7.1% with teriparatide. Romosozumab was also associated with large increases in bone mineral density at the total hip and femoral neck, as well as transitory increases in bone-formation markers and sustained decreases in a bone-resorption marker. Except for mild, generally nonrecurring injection-site reactions with romosozumab, adverse events were similar among groups.

Conclusions.—In postmenopausal women with low bone mass, romosozumab was associated with increased bone mineral density and bone formation and with decreased bone resorption. (Funded by Amgen and UCB Pharma; ClinicalTrials.gov number, NCT00896532.)

▶ Sclerostin is a glycoprotein inhibitor of osteoblast activity produced by osteocytes. This protein is encoded by the gene *SOST*, and has been identified as a pivotal regulator of bone formation. Sclerostin inhibits Wnt and bone morphogenetic protein signaling pathways, both of which stimulate osteoblast proliferation and function, leading to inhibition of bone formation.[1] Sclerostin expression is limited to the skeleton, making it an attractive target for osteoporosis therapies, because its limited expression should limit off-target effects of therapies targeting this molecule.[2] Patients with genetic deficiency of sclerostin have a high bone mass phenotype, with increased bone strength and reduced fracture risk.[3] Mice in which the sclerostin gene was deleted had increased bone formation and bone mass and strength.[4] Estrogen-deficient rat and monkey models of postmenopausal osteoporosis showed improved bone mass and bone strength compared with control animals when treated with sclerostin antibodies.[5] Inhibition of sclerostin leading to Wnt activation has been associated with decreased bone resorption in both humans and animal models.[6] Romosozumab is a humanized monoclonal antisclerostin antibody. This study was a 1-year phase 2 study that showed efficacy and safety in treatment of postmenopausal women with low bone mineral density. The findings suggest that romosozumab, 210 mg given subcutaneously once a month, increased lumbar spine bone mineral density (BMD) by 11.3%, twice as much as the comparator drug teriparatide, the only currently available anabolic agent, and also caused large increases in femoral neck and total hip BMD. These effects were associated with transitory increases in bone formation markers and sustained decreases in resorption markers. Other than mild, generally nonrecurring injection site reactions seen with romosozumab, adverse events were similar to those seen with alendronate and teriparatide.

These findings suggest that this new antisclerostin antibody stimulates increased BMD and bone formation, while simultaneously inhibiting bone resorption. A phase 3 trial is currently underway to determine whether romosozumab might be an effective treatment for osteoporosis.

B. L. Clarke, MD

References

1. Krause C, Korchynskyi O, de Rooij K, et al. Distinct modes of inhibition by sclerostin on bone morphogenetic protein and Wnt signaling pathways. *J Biol Chem.* 2010;285:41614-41626.
2. Baron R, Rawadi G. Targeting the Wnt/beta-catenin pathway to regulate bone formation in the adult skeleton. *Endocrinology.* 2007;148:2635-2643.
3. Balemans W, Ebeling M, Patel N, et al. Increased bone density in sclerosteosis is due to the deficiency of a novel secreted protein (SOST). *Hum Mol Genet.* 2001;10:537-543.
4. Li X, Ominsky MS, Niu QT, et al. Targeted deletion of the sclerostin gene in mice results in increased bone formation and bone strength. *J Bone Miner Res.* 2008;23: 860-869.
5. Li X, Ominsky MS, Warmington KS, et al. Sclerostin antibody treatment increases bone formation, bone mass, and bone strength in a rat model of postmenopausal osteoporosis. *J Bone Miner Res.* 2009;24:578-588.
6. Baron R, Kneissel M. WNT signaling in bone homeostasis and disease: from human mutations to treatments. *Nat Med.* 2013;19:179-192.

Metabolic Bone Disease

Persistent Hyperparathyroidism Is a Major Risk Factor for Fractures in the Five Years After Kidney Transplantation

Perrin P, Caillard S, Javier RM, et al (Univ Hosp, Strasbourg, France)

Am J Transplant 13:2653-2663, 2013

The risk of fractures after kidney transplantation is high. Hyperparathyroidism frequently persists after successful kidney transplantation and contributes to bone loss, but its impact on fracture has not been demonstrated. This longitudinal study was designed to evaluate hyperparathyroidism and its associations with mineral disorders and fractures in the 5 posttransplant years. We retrospectively analyzed 143 consecutive patients who underwent kidney transplantation between August 2004 and April 2006. The biochemical parameters were determined at transplantation and at 3, 12 and 60 months posttransplantation, and fractures were recorded. The median intact parathyroid hormone (PTH) level was 334 ng/L (interquartile 151–642) at the time of transplantation and 123 ng/L (interquartile 75–224) at 3 months. Thirty fractures occurred in 22 patients. The receiver operating characteristic (ROC) curve analysis for PTH at 3 months (area under the ROC curve = 0.711, p = 0.002) showed that a good threshold for predicting fractures was 130 ng/L (sensitivity = 81%, specificity = 57%). In a multivariable analysis, independent risk factors for fracture were PTH > 130 ng/L at 3 months (adjusted hazard ratio [AHR] = 7.5, 95% CI 2.18–25.50), and pretransplant osteopenia (AHR = 2.7, 95% CI 1.07–7.26). In summary, this study demonstrates for the first time that persistent hyperparathyroidism is an independent risk factor for fractures after kidney transplantation.

▶ Kidney transplant recipients have higher fracture risk than dialysis patients or the general population.[1-3] Fractures in this population are associated with increased morbidity and mortality,[1] as in other populations. The increased risk of fractures after transplantation results from glucocorticoid therapy,[4] other immunosuppressive medications, diabetes,[5] female sex, and older age.[2] Preexisting renal osteodystrophy may also play a role, as fracture incidence is associated with duration of dialysis before renal transplantation.[6] After renal transplantation, hyperparathyroidism persists in many patients and contributes to bone loss.[7] The effect of persistent hyperparathyroidism on fractures in renal transplant patients has not yet been found.

This report shows for the first time that persistent hyperparathyroidism is an independent risk factor for fractures after kidney transplantation. The study evaluated fractures in 143 consecutive kidney transplant recipients at an academic medical center over 5 years after transplantation. Measured parathyroid hormone levels were increased at the time of transplantation and gradually decreased over time. Thirty fractures occurred in 22 patients, with fracture risk increased with parathyroid hormone levels greater than 130 pg/mL at 3 months after transplant and with pretransplant osteopenia.

These findings indicate that persistent hyperparathyroidism during the first 5 years after renal transplantation may be associated with increased fracture risk. The study suggests that better control of pre- and posttransplant hyperparathyroidism may help reduce fractures. Randomized studies will be required to show whether cinacalcet reduces fracture risk in renal transplant patients with persistent hyperparathyroidism.

B. L. Clarke, MD

References

1. Abbott KC, Oglesby RJ, Hypolite IO, et al. Hospitalizations for fractures after renal transplantation in the United States. *Ann Epidemiol.* 2001;11:450-457.
2. Ball AM, Gillen DL, Sherrard D, et al. Risk of hip fracture among dialysis and renal transplant recipients. *JAMA*. 2002;288:3014-3018.
3. Grotz WH, Mundinger FA, Gugel B, Exner V, Kirste G, Schollmeyer PJ. Bone fracture and osteodensitometry with dual energy X-ray absorptiometry in kidney transplant recipients. *Transplantation.* 1994;58:912-915.
4. Nikkel LE, Hollenbeak CS, Fox EJ, Uemura T, Ghahramani N. Risk of fractures after renal transplantation in the United States. *Transplantation.* 2009;87:1846-1851.
5. Nisbeth U, Lindh E, Ljunghall S, Backman U, Fellström B. Increased fracture rate in diabetes mellitus and females after renal transplantation. *Transplantation.* 1999;67:1218-1222.
6. O'Shaughnessy EA, Dahl DC, Smith CL, Kasiske BL. Risk factors for fractures in kidney transplantation. *Transplantation.* 2002;74:362-366.
7. Akaberi S, Lindergård B, Simonsen O, Nyberg G. Impact of parathyroid hormone on bone density in long-term renal transplant patients with good graft function. *Transplantation.* 2006;82:749-752.

Normocalcemic Hyperparathyroidism and Hypoparathyroidism in Two Community-Based Nonreferral Populations

Cusano NE, Maalouf NM, Wang PY, et al (Columbia Univ, NY; Univ of Texas Southwestern Med Ctr, Dallas; Oregon Health and Science Univ, Portland; et al)

J Clin Endocrinol Metab 98:2734-2741, 2013

Context.—Normocalcemic primary hyperparathyroidism is typically identified after referral to a specialty clinic. At diagnosis, patients demonstrate features seen in hypercalcemic primary hyperparathyroidism. Normocalcemic hypoparathyroidism has been discovered after hypocalcemia unmasked after bisphosphonate administration.

Objective.—We hypothesized that screening unselected, nonreferral populations, such as The Osteoporotic Fractures in Men (MrOS) study and Dallas Heart Study (DHS), would identify asymptomatic subjects with normocalcemic hyperparathyroidism and hypoparathyroidism.

Methods.—Normocalcemic hyperparathyroidism was defined as serum PTH greater than the upper reference range with normal albumin-adjusted serum calcium, excluding common secondary causes (renal failure [estimated glomerular filtration rate <60 mL/min], 25-hydroxyvitamin D <20 ng/mL, and thiazide use), and normocalcemic hypoparathyroidism as PTH below the reference range with normocalcemia. Cross-sectional data were obtained from MrOS, and longitudinal data (baseline and 8 years) from DHS.

Results.—In 2364 men from MrOS, we identified 9 with normocalcemic hyperparathyroidism (prevalence 0.4%) and 26 with normocalcemic hypoparathyroidism (1.1%). In 3450 men and women from DHS, we identified 108 with normocalcemic hyperparathyroidism (3.1%) and 68 with normocalcemic hypoparathyroidism (1.9%). Of the 108 normocalcemic hyperparathyroid subjects, 64 had follow-up data. Hypercalcemic primary hyperparathyroidism developed in 1 subject whereas 13 (0.6% of the follow-up cohort) showed persistently elevated PTH levels with normocalcemia. Of the 26 normocalcemic hypoparathyroid subjects with follow-up data, none developed overt hypoparathyroidism and 2 (0.09%) had persistent evidence of normocalcemic hypoparathyroidism.

Conclusions.—This study documents normocalcemic primary hyperparathyroidism and hypoparathyroidism identified among community-dwelling individuals. Larger studies are needed to determine the true prevalence and natural history of these parathyroid disorders.

► Normocalcemic primary hyperparathyroidism is a recently recognized form of primary hyperparathyroidism in which serum calcium is normal and parathyroid hormone increased in the absence of vitamin D deficiency or renal disease.[1-3] Normocalcemic hypoparathyroidism has been reported in occasional cases in which hypocalcemia developed after bisphosphonate infusion in patients who were not previously recognized as having hypoparathyroidism.[4-6] The epidemiology and natural history of these uncommon forms of parathyroid disease are not well understood.

This study attempted to clarify the prevalence and natural history of normocalcemic primary hyperparathyroidism and normocalcemic hypoparathyroidism in 2 community-dwelling populations, men in the Osteoporotic Fractures in Men (MrOS) study and men and women in the Dallas Heart Study. In 2364 men in the MrOS study, 9 were identified with normocalcemic hyperparathyroidism, for a prevalence of 0.4%, and 26 were identified with normocalcemic hypoparathyroidism, for a prevalence of 1.1%. In 3450 men and women in the Dallas Heart Study, 108 were identified with normocalcemic hyperparathyroidism, for a prevalence of 3.1%, and 68 were identified with normocalcemic hypoparathyroidism, for a prevalence of 1.9%. Development of hypercalcemic primary hyperparathyroidism occurred in 1 patient during follow-up, whereas 13 showed persistently elevated parathyroid hormone (PTH) levels with normocalcemia. Of the 26 normocalcemic hypoparathyroid subjects with follow-up data, none developed overt hypoparathyroidism, and 2 (0.09%) had persistent evidence of normocalcemic hypoparathyroidism.

This important study clarifies that normocalcemic primary hyperparathyroidism occurs in 0.4% to 3.1% of community-dwelling patients and that normocalcemic hypoparathyroidism occurs in 1.1% to 1.9% of these individuals. Because the MrOS study and Dallas Heart Study are relatively small, short-term cohort studies, larger and longer-term follow-up studies will be required to fully define the prevalence and natural history of these uncommon forms of primary hyperparathyroidism.

B. L. Clarke, MD

References

1. Maruani G, Hertig A, Paillard M, Houillier P. Normocalcemic primary hyperparathyroidism: evidence for a generalized target-tissue resistance to parathyroid hormone. *J Clin Endocrinol Metab.* 2003;88:4641-4648.
2. Silverberg SJ, Bilezikian JP. "Incipient" primary hyperparathyroidism: a "forme fruste" of an old disease. *J Clin Endocrinol Metab.* 2003;88:5348-5352.
3. Rao DS, Wilson RJ, Kleerekoper M, Parfitt AM. Lack of biochemical progression or continuation of accelerated bone loss in mild asymptomatic primary hyperparathyroidism: evidence for biphasic disease course. *J Clin Endocrinol Metab.* 1988; 67:1294-1298.
4. Schussheim DH, Jacobs TP, Silverberg SJ. Hypocalcemia associated with alendronate. *Ann Intern Med.* 1999;130:329.
5. Kashyap AS, Kashyap S. Hypoparathyroidism unmasked by alendronate. *Postgrad Med J.* 2000;76:417-418.
6. Cömlekçi A, Biberoglu S, Hekimsoy Z, et al. Symptomatic hypocalcemia in a patient with latent hypoparathyroidism and breast carcinoma with bone metastasis following administration of pamidronate. *Intern Med.* 1998;37:396-397.

Efficacy and safety of recombinant human parathyroid hormone (1–84) in hypoparathyroidism (REPLACE): a double-blind, placebo-controlled, randomised, phase 3 study

Mannstadt M, Clarke BL, Vokes T, et al (Massachusetts General Hosp and Harvard Med School, Boston; Mayo Clinic, Rochester, MN; Univ of Chicago Medicine, IL; et al)

Lancet Diabetes Endocrinol 1:1-9, 2013

Background.—Hypoparathyroidism results in impaired mineral homoeostasis, including hypocalcaemia and hyperphosphataemia. Treatment with high-dose oral calcium and active vitamin D does not provide adequate or consistent control of biochemical indices and can lead to serious long-term complications. We aimed to test the efficacy, safety, and tolerability of once-daily recombinant human parathyroid hormone 1–84 (rhPTH[1–84]) in adults with hypoparathyroidism.

Methods.—In this double-blind, placebo-controlled, randomised phase 3 study (REPLACE), we recruited patients with hypoparathyroidism (≥18 months duration) aged 18–85 years from 33 sites in eight countries. After an optimisation period, during which calcium and active vitamin D doses were adjusted to achieve consistent albumin-corrected serum calcium, patients were randomly assigned (2:1) via an interactive voice response system to 50 μg per day of rhPTH(1–84) or placebo for 24 weeks. Active vitamin D and calcium were progressively reduced, while rhPTH(1–84) could be titrated up from 50 μg to 75 μg and then 100 μg (weeks 0–5). The primary endpoint was the proportion of patients at week 24 who achieved a 50% or greater reduction from baseline in their daily dose of oral calcium and active vitamin D while maintaining a serum calcium concentration greater than or the same as baseline concentrations and less than or equal to the upper limit of normal, analysed by intention to treat. This trial is registered with ClinicalTrials.gov, number NCT00732615.

Findings.—Between June 23, 2009, and Feb 28, 2011, 134 eligible patients were recruited and randomly assigned to rhPTH(1−84) (n = 90) or placebo (n = 44). Six patients in the rhPTH(1−84) group and seven in the placebo group discontinued before study end. 48 (53%) patients in the rhPTH(1−84) group achieved the primary endpoint compared with one (2%) patient in the placebo group (percentage difference 51·1%, 95% CI 39·9−62·3; $p < 0{\cdot}0001$). The proportions of patients who had at least one adverse event were similar between groups (84 [93%] patients in the rhPTH[1−84] group *vs* 44 [100%] patients in the placebo group), with hypocalcaemia, muscle spasm, paraesthesias, headache, and nausea being the most common adverse events. The proportions of patients with serious adverse events were also similar between the rhPTH(1−84) group (ten [11%] patients) and the placebo group (four [9%] patients).

Interpretation.—50 μg, 75 μg, or 100 μg per day of rhPTH(1−84), administered subcutaneously in the outpatient setting, is efficacious and well tolerated as a PTH replacement therapy for patients with hypoparathyroidism.

▶ Hypoparathyroidism is a rare disorder characterized by low serum calcium and absent or deficient production of parathyroid hormone (PTH). Most cases in adults result from postsurgical hypoparathyroidism. PTH deficiency is responsible for disturbances in mineral homeostasis, including decreased calcium absorption caused by reduced renal conversion of 25-hydroxyvitamin D to active 1,25-dihydroxyvitamin D, and hypercalciuria caused by decreased PTH-dependent renal tubular calcium reabsorption. Bone turnover is also decreased, leading to increased bone mineral density.[1-3] Most hormone deficiency states are treated with the missing hormone, but hypoparathyroidism continues to be treated with large doses of oral calcium and vitamin D because of lack of US Food and Drug Administration (FDA)-approved PTH therapy, an approach that leads to complications, including calcifications in the kidneys, brain, and elsewhere, as well as reduced renal function.[4,5] This study was performed to test the efficacy, safety, and tolerability of human recombinant parathyroid hormone 1-84 (rhPTH[1−84]) given once daily by subcutaneous injection in adult patients with hypoparathyroidism. A total of 134 patients were randomly assigned 2:1 to rhPTH(1−84) or placebo. Of these, 53% of patients in the rhPTH(1−84) group achieved the primary endpoint compared with 2% in the placebo group, defined as the proportion of patients at week 24 who achieved a 50% or greater reduction from baseline in their daily dose of oral calcium and active vitamin D while maintaining a serum calcium concentration greater than or the same as baseline concentrations and less than or equal to the upper limit of normal by intention-to-treat analysis. Adverse events were similar between the treatment groups, with hypocalcaemia, muscle spasm, paraesthesias, headache, and nausea being the most common adverse events. The study concluded that 50 μg, 75 μg, or 100 μg per day of rhPTH(1−84) administered subcutaneously in the outpatient setting was efficacious and well tolerated as a PTH replacement therapy.

This is the first phase III study to show that recombinant human PTH(1–84) may be useful in the treatment of patients with hypoparathyroidism in the outpatient setting. The findings show that rhPTH(1–84) is efficacious as a replacement for endogenous PTH in patients with hypoparathyroidism and show that doses between 50 and 100 μg may be useful in treating individual patients. It is not clear from this short-term trial, however, whether reduction in high-dose calcium and vitamin D supplements will reduce long-term complications from these supplements.

B. L. Clarke, MD

References

1. Bilezikian JP, Khan A, Potts JT Jr, et al. Hypoparathyroidism in the adult: epidemiology, diagnosis, pathophysiology, target-organ involvement, treatment, and challenges for future research. *J Bone Miner Res.* 2011;26:2317-2337.
2. Shoback D. Clinical practice. Hypoparathyroidism. *N Engl J Med.* 2008;359: 391-403.
3. Rejnmark L, Sikjaer T, Underbjerg L, Mosekilde L. PTH replacement therapy of hypoparathyroidism. *Osteoporos Int.* 2013;24:1529-1536.
4. Goswami R, Sharma R, Sreenivas V, Gupta N, Ganapathy A, Das S. Prevalence and progression of basal ganglia calcification and its pathogenic mechanism in patients with idiopathic hypoparathyroidism. *Clin Endocrinol (Oxf).* 2012;77: 200-206.
5. Weber G, Cazzuffi MA, Frisone F, et al. Nephrocalcinosis in children and adolescents: sonographic evaluation during long-term treatment with 1,25-dihydroxycholecalciferol. *Child Nephrol Urol.* 1988;9:273-276.

Incidence and Prevalence of Primary Hyperparathyroidism in a Racially Mixed Population

Yeh MW, Ituarte PHG, Zhou HC, et al (UCLA David Geffen School of Medicine; Kaiser Permanente Southern California, Pasadena, CA; et al)
J Clin Endocrinol Metab 98:1122-1129, 2013

Context.—The epidemiology of primary hyperparathyroidism (PHPT) has generally been studied in Caucasian populations.

Objective.—The aim was to examine the incidence and prevalence of PHPT within a racially mixed population.

Design.—A descriptive epidemiologic study was performed.

Patients/Setting.—The study population included 3.5 million enrollees within Kaiser Permanente Southern California.

Methods.—All patients with at least one elevated serum calcium level (>10.5 mg/dL, 2.6 mmol/L) between 1995 and 2010 were included. Cases of PHPT were identified by electronic query of laboratory values using biochemical criteria, after exclusion of secondary or renal and tertiary hyperparathyroidism cases. The incidence and prevalence rates of PHPT were calculated according to sex, race, age group by decade, and year.

Results.—Initial case finding identified 15,234 patients with chronic hypercalcemia, 13,327 (87%) of which had PHPT as defined by elevated or inappropriately normal parathyroid hormone levels. The incidence of PHPT fluctuated from 34 to 120 per 100 000 person-years (mean 66) among women, and from 13 to 36 (mean 25) among men. With advancing age, incidence increased and sex differences became pronounced (incidence 12–24 per 100 000 for both sexes younger than 50 y; 80 and 36 per 100 000 for women and men aged 50–59 y, respectively; and 196 and 95 for women and men aged 70–79 y, respectively). The incidence of PHPT was highest among blacks (92 women; 46 men, $P < .0001$), followed by whites (81 women; 29 men), with rates for Asians (52 women, 28 men), Hispanics (49 women, 17 men), and other races (25 women, 6 men) being lower than that for whites ($P < .0001$). The prevalence of PHPT tripled during the study period, increasing from 76 to 233 per 100 000 women and from 30 to 85 per 100 000 men. Racial differences in prevalence mirrored those found in incidence.

Conclusions.—PHPT is the predominant cause of hypercalcemia and is increasingly prevalent. Substantial differences are found in the incidence and prevalence of PHPT between races.

► Most epidemiologic studies of the relatively common endocrine disorder, primary hyperparathyroidism, have focused on largely white populations in Scandinavian countries and Rochester, Minnesota. Even though this disorder is commonly cited as the most common cause of outpatient hypercalcemia, with the prevalence estimate in different populations ranging between 1 and 7 cases per 1000 adults,[1-4] the perception has been that this disorder largely affects the white population. Primary hyperparathyroidism affects mainly older adults, and women appear to be affected 2 to 3 times as often as men.[5] Incidence estimates have been harder to obtain, but available estimates range from 0.4 to 21.6 cases per 100 000 person years,[4,6] with the variation in estimates explained by differences in screening methods, case definitions, populations studied, and annual fluctuations in incidence within the same population that are not clearly understood.

This study attempted to determine the incidence and prevalence of primary hyperparathyroidism in the racially mixed enrollee population of Kaiser Permanente Southern California, an integrated health care delivery system serving about 3.5 million patients, by applying a uniform biochemical algorithm. All patients with at least one serum calcium level of 10.5 mg/dL or higher between 1995 and 2010 were included, with confirmation of diagnosis of primary hyperparathyroidism in 87% of cases by review of laboratory values, including parathyroid hormone, after exclusion of secondary and tertiary hyperparathyroidism. The incidence among women ranged between 34 and 120 per 100 000 person-years, with the mean 66 per 100 000 person-years, and among men between 13 and 36 per 100 000 person-years, with the mean 25 per 100 000 person-years. The incidence increased with age across both sexes and among different racial groups. The incidence of primary hyperparathyroidism was greatest in blacks, followed by whites, and then Asians, Hispanics, and other races. The prevalence of the disorder tripled during the study period for unclear reasons.

These significant findings clearly extend previous observations regarding the incidence and prevalence of primary hyperparathyroidism and show for the first time clear racial differences. Primary hyperparathyroidism was the predominant cause of hypercalcemia in this cohort, and the prevalence increased across the study interval for unclear reasons. Further research will be required to clarify the reason(s) for the racial differences and increasing prevalence of the disorder.

B. L. Clarke, MD

References

1. Adami S, Marcocci C, Gatti D. Epidemiology of primary hyperparathyroidism in Europe. *J Bone Miner Res.* 2002;17:N18-N23.
2. Christensson T, Hellström K, Wengle B, Alveryd A, Wikland B. Prevalence of hypercalcaemia in a health screening in Stockholm. *Acta Med Scand.* 1976;200: 131-137.
3. Wermers RA, Khosla S, Atkinson EJ, Hodgson SF, O'Fallon WM, Melton LJ 3rd. The rise and fall of primary hyperparathyroidism: a population-based study in Rochester, Minnesota, 1965–1992. *Ann Intern Med.* 1997;126:433-440.
4. Yu N, Donnan PT, Murphy MJ, Leese GP. Epidemiology of primary hyperparathyroidism in Tayside, Scotland, UK. *Clin Endocrinol.* 2009;71:485-493.
5. Fraser WD. Hyperparathyroidism. *Lancet.* 2009;374:145-158.
6. Wermers RA, Khosla S, Atkinson EJ, et al. Incidence of primary hyperparathyroidism in Rochester, Minnesota, 1993–2001: An update on the changing epidemiology of the disease. *J Bone Miner Res.* 2006;21:171-177.

Primary Hyperparathyroidism Is Associated With Abnormal Cortical and Trabecular Microstructure and Reduced Bone Stiffness in Postmenopausal Women

Stein EM, Silva BC, Boutroy S, et al (Columbia Univ, NY)
J Bone Miner Res 28:1029-1040, 2013

Typically, in the milder form of primary hyperparathyroidism (PHPT), now seen in most countries, bone density by dual-energy X-ray absorptiometry (DXA) and detailed analyses of iliac crest bone biopsies by histomorphometry and micro–computed tomography (μCT) show detrimental effects in cortical bone, whereas the trabecular site (lumbar spine by DXA) and the trabecular compartment (by bone biopsy) appear to be relatively well preserved. Despite these findings, fracture risk at both vertebral and nonvertebral sites is increased in PHPT. Emerging technologies, such as high-resolution peripheral quantitative computed tomography (HRpQCT), may provide additional insight into microstructural features at sites such as the forearm and tibia that have heretofore not been easily accessible. Using HRpQCT, we determined cortical and trabecular microstructure at the radius and tibia in 51 postmenopausal women with PHPT and 120 controls. Individual trabecula segmentation (ITS) and micro–finite element (μFE) analyses of the HRpQCT images were also performed to further understand how the abnormalities seen by HRpQCT might translate into effects on bone strength. Women with PHPT showed, at both sites, decreased volumetric densities at trabecular and cortical compartments, thinner cortices, and more widely spaced and heterogeneously distributed trabeculae. At the radius, trabeculae were thinner and fewer in PHPT. The radius was affected to a greater extent in the trabecular compartment than the tibia. ITS analyses revealed, at both sites, that plate-like trabeculae were depleted, with a resultant reduction in the plate/rod ratio. Microarchitectural abnormalities were evident by decreased plate-rod and plate-plate junctions at the radius and tibia, and rod-rod junctions at the radius. These trabecular and cortical abnormalities resulted in decreased whole-bone stiffness and trabecular stiffness. These results provide evidence that in PHPT, microstructural abnormalities are pervasive and not limited to the cortical compartment, which may help to account for increased global fracture risk in PHPT.

► Since the 1970s, primary hyperparathyroidism has presented most commonly with mild bone disease, which is distinctly different from the classical presentation with severe bone disease commonly seen during the first 7 decades after the disorder was described.[1] This change has occurred because most patients with primary hyperparathyroidism today have a mildly symptomatic or asymptomatic form of the disease.[2-4] Milder forms of primary hyperparathyroidism are characterized by decreased bone mineral density (BMD), particularly at the one-third distal radius site, which is predominantly composed of cortical bone. In contrast, the lumbar spine, which is largely composed of trabecular bone, tends to remain stable.[5]

This study evaluated changes in bone microstructure in 51 postmenopausal women with primary hyperparathyroidism and 120 healthy control subjects using high-resolution peripheral quantitative computed tomography scanning of the distal radius and tibia. The postmenopausal women had decreased volumetric densities in both the trabecular and cortical compartments, thinner cortices, and more widely spaced and heterogeneous trabecular elements. At the radius, trabecular elements were thinner and fewer in the women with primary hyperparathyroidism, and trabecular effects were more pronounced at the radius than the tibia. Platelike trabeculae were decreased at both the radius and tibia, with reduction in the plate:rod ratio. These changes resulted in decreased whole bone and trabecular stiffness and, correspondingly, decreased bone strength.

These findings demonstrate that primary hyperparathyroidism causes microstructural skeletal effects at both the cortical and trabecular compartments. Previous dual-energy x-ray absorptiometry bone mineral density and bone histomorphometry studies have shown cortical bone loss with preservation of trabecular bone. The microstructural changes seen in this important study likely contribute to the increased vertebral and nonvertebral fracture risk seen in patients with primary hyperparathyroidism.

B. L. Clarke, MD

References

1. Cope O. The study of hyperparathyroidism at the Massachusetts General Hospital. *N Engl J Med.* 1966;274:1174-1182.
2. Rubin MR, Bilezikian JP, McMahon DJ, et al. The natural history of primary hyperparathyroidism with or without parathyroid surgery after 15 years. *J Clin Endocrinol Metab.* 2008;93:3462-3470.
3. Silverberg SJ, Shane E, Jacobs TP, Siris E, Bilezikian JP. A 10-year prospective study of primary hyperparathyroidism with or without parathyroid surgery. *N Engl J Med.* 1999;341:1249-1255.
4. Bilezikian JP, Brandi ML, Rubin M, Silverberg SJ. Primary hyperparathyroidism: new concepts in clinical, densitometric and biochemical features. *J Intern Med.* 2005;257:6-17.
5. Silverberg SJ, Shane E, de la Cruz L, et al. Skeletal disease in primary hyperparathyroidism. *J Bone Miner Res.* 1989;4:283-291.

6 Adrenal Cortex

Introduction

The duality of volume expansion and vasopressor function frequently seen in systems that regulate the blood pressure is also visible in the adrenal glands and their typical secretory products (and metabolites), steroid hormones, and catecholamines. These are relatively small molecules and little changes in the structure determine very different functions. For some molecules, the differences between the distinct steroid hormones are too small to be sufficiently recognized by the steroid hormone receptors. This explains why progesterone binds to its progesterone receptor and also has antimineralocorticoid and antiandrogenic activities. Similarly, the development of antibodies, which are relatively large molecules, and the invention of immunoassays helped much in the measurements of steroid hormone or catecholamine concentrations. However, they are limited in their specificity to detect one steroid hormone only. One advantage of mass spectrometry (MS), coupled to chromatographic methods, over immunoassays is the increase in the specificity of assays; the other is that concentrations of multiple "small" hormones can be assessed simultaneously. This allows for steroid profiling or profiling of catecholamines along with their precursors and metabolites.

This year's collection of commentaries on recently published articles in the adrenal field recognizes this development and highlights papers employing LC-MS/MS-based technology to study the physiology of adrenal gland-derived hormones. Rege et al used adrenal venous sampling as a window to the human adrenal cortex, metabolizing dehydroepiandrostenedione to androstenedione and androstenediol and further converting these steroids to testosterone. Steroid profiling of urinary samples is more convenient and was shown to differentiate between true and apparent cortisone reductase deficiency (Laver et al), starting to establish genotype-phenotype relationships. Such efforts were extended in the CaHASE-cohort (Krone et al). However, the results allow the interpretation that genotype-phenotype relationships can get lost during therapy for congenital adrenal hyperplasia. This may be good news in that treatment of severe and mild cases with this disorder may have the same clinical outcome. However, it does not necessarily suggest that affected patients have an outcome comparable to that of normal subjects. Indeed, the treatment of male patients with congenital adrenal hyperplasia did not prevent the appearance of testicular adrenal rest tumors in a substantial number of cases (Reisch et al). In addition,

GC-MS analysis of urinary samples of patients with adrenocortical cancer showed that not only the breakdown of glucocorticoids is forced up but also that the 5α-reductase activity declines in the presence of mitotane (Chortis et al), also leading to hypogonadism.

Another advantage of MS-based methods over conventional assays is the fact that immunologically similar steroids can be well-differentiated by their mass when these steroids are deuterated. Such an approach enabled Boonen et al to show that the cortisol metabolism is reduced during critical illness. Interestingly, it turned out that immune cells within the adrenal gland rather than steroid-producing cells are the major regulators of the immune–adrenal cross talk in experimental sepsis (Kanczkowski et al). The friendly co-existence of the adrenal cortex and the adrenal medulla led Dekkers et al to study metanephrine as a marker of selectivity that performs superior to cortisol during adrenal venous sampling for primary hyperaldosteronism. This approach made more adrenal venous sampling studies informative. However, changes in the microenvironment of the adrenal gland cause a disruption of its morphology and a new example for this relationship was recently found: intraglandular secretion of corticotropin (ACTH) underlies the formation of ACTH-independent macronodular adrenal hyperplasia (Louiset et al).

Other articles were highlighted because of the unique combination of advances in genetics and their translational part showing the mechanistic consequences behind mutations. One such work demonstrated how a mutation in the glucocorticoid receptor causes Chrousos' syndrome (primary generalized glucocorticoid resistance) and one that indentified a mutated factor associated with ACTH-independent macronodular adrenal hyperplasia. Last, but not least, the three groups of M. Reincke (Beuschlein et al), R. Lifton (Scholl et al) and M. Brown (Azizan et al) added significantly to the understanding of the pathophysiology of Conn's syndrome, all showing that aldosterone-producing adenomas may form when membrane channel and pump mutations cause a rise in intracellular calcium and result in calcium-related signaling.

Holger S. Willenberg, MD

Adrenal Hormone Secretion and Pathology

Liquid Chromatography–Tandem Mass Spectrometry Analysis of Human Adrenal Vein 19-Carbon Steroids Before and After ACTH Stimulation

Rege J, Nakamura Y, Satoh F, et al (Georgia Health Sciences Univ, Augusta; Tohoku Univ School of Medicine, Sendai, Japan; et al)

J Clin Endocrinol Metab 98:1182-1188, 2013

Context.—A broad analysis of adrenal gland-derived 19-carbon (C_{19}) steroids has not been reported. This is the first study that uses liquid chromatography–tandem mass spectrometry to quantify 9 C_{19} steroids

TABLE 1.—Effects of ACTH on AV Concentration of C_{19} Steroids and Estrogens in Women

Steroid	Pre-ACTH, nmol/L	Post-ACTH, nmol/L	*P* Value	Fold Change
DHEA	125 ± 56.9	2659 ± 666	<.05	21.2
DHEA-S	3827 ± 1317	18 266 ± 3842	<.05	4.8
Androstenediol	1.15 ± 0.24	20.7 ± 6.46	<.05	18.0
Androstenedione	79.0 ± 46.9	585 ± 199	<.05	7.4
11OHA	157 ± 96.2	811 ± 260	<.05	5.2
11KA	0.99 ± 0.33	3.18 ± 0.63	<.05	3.2
Testosterone	0.78 ± 0.26	5.71 ± 1.42	<.05	7.3
11OHT	0.48 ± 0.17	2.62 ± 0.74	<.05	5.5
11KT	0.39 ± 0.09	0.49 ± 0.11	.35	1.3
DHT	0.10 ± 0.03	0.10 ± 0.03	.40	1.0
Estrone	0.08 ± 0.03	0.29 ± 0.06	<.05	3.5
Estradiol	0.05 ± 0.03	0.05 ± 0.03	.61	1.0

Values are expressed as mean ± SEM (n = 7 women). The fold change increase after ACTH infusion is calculated by dividing the mean post-ACTH concentrations by the mean pre-ACTH concentrations.

[a]LC-MS/MS was used to quantify the above C19 steroids (except DHEA-S which was analyzed by RIA) and estrogens in the adrenal vein before andafter 15 min of iv ACTH administration.

(androgens and their precursors), estrone, and estradiol in the adrenal vein (AV) of women, before and after ACTH stimulation.

Objective.—The objective of this study was to define the adrenal androgen metabolome in women before and after ACTH infusion.

Design.—This was a retrospective study.

Patients.—Seven women, aged 50.4 ± 5.4 years, with suspected diagnosis of an adrenal aldosterone-producing adenoma were included in the study.

Methods.—AV and iliac serum samples were collected before and after administration of ACTH (15 minutes). AV samples were analyzed using for concentrations of 9 unconjugated C_{19} steroids, estrone, and estradiol. Dehydroepiandrosterone sulfate (DHEA-S) was quantified by radioimmunoassay.

Results.—AV levels of DHEA-S were the highest among the steroids measured. The most abundant unconjugated C_{19} steroids in AV were 11β-hydroxyandrostenedione (11OHA), dehydroepiandrosterone (DHEA), and androstenedione (A4). ACTH significantly increased the adrenal output of 9 of the 12 steroids that were measured. ACTH increased the mean AV concentration of DHEA-S by 5-fold, DHEA by 21-fold, A4 by 7-fold, and 11OHA by 5-fold. 11β-Hydroxytestosterone and testosterone were found to be potent androgen receptor agonists when tested with an androgen-responsive cell reporter model.

Conclusion.—The current study indicates that the adrenal gland secretes primarily 3 weak androgens, namely DHEA, 11OHA, and A4. Active androgens, including testosterone and 11β-hydroxytestosterone, are also produced but to a lesser degree (Table 1).

► Several steroid hormones are clearly derived from the adrenal gland, including aldosterone and cortisol. Other steroid hormones, however, including androstenedione and dehydroepiandrostenedione, are also produced in the gonads.

Because adrenal venous sampling (AVS) is the study of choice in the determination of the location of excess aldosterone secretion, such a procedure is done on regular occasions. Now, the authors used AVS studies to better investigate the portion of androgens and androgen precursors secreted by adrenal cortical cells in women. They used a protocol with infusion of corticotropin and analyzed the concentrations of C19 steroid hormones in adrenal venous outflows at basal conditions and 15 minutes after corticotropin infusion by liquid chromatography and mass spectrometry. They found that dehydroepiandrostenedione is metabolized to androstenedione and androstenediol and that both of these steroids can be further converted to testosterone in the adrenal itself. In addition, adrenal 11β-hydroxylase synthesizes 11-hydroxy-androstenedione and 11-hydroxy-testosterone from androstenedione and testosterone, respectively and type 2 11β-hydroxysteroid dehydrogenase makes 11-keto-androstenedione and 11-keto-testosterone from 11-hydroxy-androstenedione and 11-hydroxy-testosterone, respectively. Thus, within the adrenal gland, a number of relevant androgen (precursor) steroids are produced in dependency of corticotropin. This study also showed that although androstenedione and 11-hydroxy-androstenedione are minor activators of the androgen receptor, these steroids can easily become activated by 17β-hydroxysteroid dehydrogenases and play a relevant androgenic role in target tissues.

H. S. Willenberg, MD

Detection of Circulating Tumor Cells in Patients With Adrenocortical Carcinoma: A Monocentric Preliminary Study

Pinzani P, Scatena C, Salvianti F, et al (Univ of Florence, Italy)

J Clin Endocrinol Metab 98:3731-3738, 2013

Context.—Adrenocortical carcinoma (ACC) is a rare malignancy, the prognosis of which is mainly dependent on stage at diagnosis. The identification of disease-associated markers for early diagnosis and drug monitoring is mandatory. Circulating tumor cells (CTCs) are released into the bloodstream from primary tumor/metastasis. CTC detection in blood samples may have enormous potential for assisting in the diagnosis of malignancy, estimating prognosis, and monitoring the disease.

Objective.—The aim of the study was to investigate the presence of CTCs in blood samples of patients with ACC or benign adrenocortical adenoma (ACA).

Setting.—We conducted the study at a university hospital.

Intervention.—CTC analysis was performed in blood samples from 14 ACC patients and 10 ACA patients. CTCs were isolated on the basis of cell size by filtration through ScreenCell devices, followed by identification according to validated morphometric criteria and immunocytochemistry.

Main Outcome Measure.—We measured the difference in CTC detection between ACC and ACA.

Results.—CTCs were detected in all ACC samples, but not in ACA samples. Immunocytochemistry confirmed the adrenocortical origin. When

ACC patients were stratified according to the median value of tumor diameter and metastatic condition, a statistically significant difference was found in the number of CTCs detected after surgery. A significant correlation between the number of CTCs in postsurgical samples and clinical parameters was found for tumor diameter alone.

Conclusions.—Our findings provide the first evidence for adrenocortical tumors that CTCs may represent a useful marker to support differential diagnosis between ACC and ACA. The correlation with some clinical parameters suggests a possible relevance of CTC analysis for prognosis and noninvasive monitoring of disease progression and drug response.

► Sometimes it is difficult to safely distinguish between benign or malignant adrenocortical carcinoma (ACC) lesions preoperatively. Usually, computed tomography and magnetic resonance imaging studies are used for characterization of such adrenal lesions. More recently, these techniques have been combined with the information from positron emission tomography studies or with the results of steroid profiling in 24-hour urine samples. Here, the authors tried a different technique, which seemed to be suitable to distinguish malignant from benign disease. They screened blood samples of patients with ACC or benign adrenocortical tumors for the appearance of supposedly circulating tumor cells (CTC) of adrenocortical origin and malignant behavior. This supports the concept of others who used this technique for other tumor types.

However, before such an approach is put into place or facilities offering such a service are established to aid clinicians in their decision process, it is necessary to show that a blinded analysis of blood samples for the presence of CTCs renders similar results. In addition, it is also important to demonstrate that the cells identified as CTCs behave malignantly. Above all, however, it needs to be shown in prospective trials that patients with ACC do not have CTCs when they remain free of disease over the long term when other patients who have CTCs will relapse.

If this technique works reliably, it may become useful in the care of patients with adrenocortical tumors.

H. S. Willenberg, MD

Hypothalamo-pituitary and immune-dependent adrenal regulation during systemic inflammation

Kanczkowski W, Alexaki V-I, Tran N, et al (Technical Univ Dresden, Germany; Univ Dresden, Germany; Univ Hosp Frankfurt, Germany; et al)

Proc Natl Acad Sci U S A 110:14801-14806, 2013

Inflammation-related dysregulation of the hypothalamic–pituitary–adrenal (HPA) axis is central to the course of systemic inflammatory response syndrome or sepsis. The underlying mechanisms, however, are not well understood. Initial activation of adrenocortical hormone production during early sepsis depends on the stimulation of hypothalamus and pituitary mediated by cytokines; in late sepsis, there is a shift from neuroendocrine to local immune–adrenal regulation of glucocorticoid production. Therefore, the modulation of the local immune–adrenal cross talk, and not of the neuroendocrine circuits involved in adrenocorticotropic hormone production, may be more promising in the prevention of the adrenal insufficiency associated with prolonged sepsis. In the present work, we investigated the function of the crucial Toll-like receptor (TLR) adaptor protein myeloid differentiation factor 88 (MyD88) in systemic and local activation of adrenal gland inflammation and glucocorticoid production mediated by lipopolysachharides (LPSs). To this end, we used mice with a conditional MyD88 allele. These mice either were interbred with Mx1 Cre mice, resulting in systemic MyD88 deletion, predominantly in the liver and hematopoietic system, or were crossed with Akr1b7 Cre transgenic mice, resulting thereby in deletion of MyD88, which was adrenocortical-specific. Although reduced adrenal inflammation and HPA-axis activation mediated by LPS were found in $Mx1^{Cre+}$-$MyD88^{fl/fl}$ mice, adrenocortical-specific MyD88 deletion did not alter the adrenal inflammation or HPA-axis activity under systemic inflammatory response syndrome conditions. Thus, our data suggest an important role of immune cell rather than adrenocortical MyD88 for adrenal inflammation and HPA-axis activation mediated by LPS.

▶ In sepsis, the activation of the hypothalamo-pituitary-adrenal (HPA) axis serves the organism for the concentration of its energy metabolism on absolutely essential functions and to prevent a potentially harmful overactivation of the immune system. The stimulation of HPA axis is believed to be mediated by cytokines to a large extent and seems to happen on several levels, including directly in the adrenal gland. This also seems to be the case in experimental animal models using lipopolysaccharides (LPS) as pathogenic agents. LPS particles are ligands of pattern recognition receptors such as toll-like receptors (TLRs), which are expressed on adrenocortical cells as well as immune and other cells. Absence of TLRs has been found to correlate with increased basal levels of corticotropin (TLR2 knock-down) or corticosterone and an enlargement of the adrenal cortex (TLR4 knock-down). In addition, it is associated with a reduced adrenal response in steroidogenesis to LPS. Myeloid differentiation factor 88 (MyD88) is important for TLR signaling and consequent activation of nuclear factor κB. Based on these thoughts, the contribution of adrenal TLR activation to the overall response of the HPA axis to LPS exposure was studied in genetically modified mice models.

The authors found that inactivation of MyD88 in hematopoietic cells, but not in adrenocortical cells, resulted in a decreased secretion of both corticotropin and corticosterone in response to LPS. In addition, mice without MyD88 in their hematopoietic cells displayed reduced LPS-mediated, inflammation-triggered neutrophil recruitment to the adrenal gland and had decreased concentrations of proinflammatory cytokines and chemokines in the adrenal gland as well as in the circulation. However, such observations were not made when MyD88 was absent in adrenocortical cells. Thus, surprisingly, this study suggests that immune cells likely recruited to the adrenal gland rather than steroid-producing cells are the major regulators of the immune–adrenal cross talk as seen in experimental sepsis.

H. S. Willenberg, MD

Imaging Work-Up for Screening of Paraganglioma and Pheochromocytoma in *SDHx* Mutation Carriers: A Multicenter Prospective Study from the PGL.EVA Investigators

Gimenez-Roqueplo A-P, Caumont-Prim A, Houzard C, et al (Assistance Publique-Hôpitaux de Paris, France; Département de Médecine Vasculaire et d'Hypertension Artérielle, Paris, France; et al)

J Clin Endocrinol Metab 98:E162-E173, 2013

Context.—Recommendations have not been established concerning imaging to screen *SDHx* mutation carriers for paraganglioma and pheochromocytoma.

Objective.—Our objective was to compare the performance of gadolinium-enhanced magnetic resonance angiography, contrast-enhanced computed tomography, and [^{123}I]metaiodo-benzylguanidine and somatostatin receptor scintigraphies for detecting head and neck and thoracic-abdominal-pelvic paragangliomas in *SDHx* mutation carriers.

Design and Setting.—We conducted a prospective, multicenter study from June 2005 to December 2009 at 23 French medical centers.

Patients.—A total of 238 index cases or relatives carrying mutations in *SDHD, SDHB*, or *SDHC* genes were included.

Intervention.—Images obtained by each technique were analyzed blind, without knowledge of results from other tests, first in each local center and then centrally.

Main Outcome Measures.—We evaluated sensitivity, specificity, and likelihood ratios for individual and combinations of tests, the gold standard being the consensus of an expert committee.

Results.—Two hundred two tumors were diagnosed in 96 subjects. At local assessment, the sensitivity of anatomical imaging for detecting all tumors was higher (85.7%) than that of both scintigraphic techniques (42.7% for [^{123}I] metaiodo-benzylguanidine and 69.5% for somatostatin receptor scintigraphy), except for thoracic localizations where somatostatin receptor scintigraphy was more sensitive (61.5 *vs.* 46.2% for anatomical imaging and 30.8% for [^{123}I]metaiodo-benzylguanidine scintigraphy). The best diagnostic performance during local assessment was obtained by combining anatomical imaging tests and somatostatin receptor scintigraphy (sensitivity 91.7%). Central assessment significantly increased the sensitivity (98.6%) of tests in combination.

Conclusions.—In routine practice, the imaging work-up for screening *SDHx* mutation carriers should include thoraco-abdomino-pelvic computed tomography, head and neck magnetic angiography, and

somatostatin receptor scintigraphy. Expert centralized image assessment is recommended.

▶ Pheochromocytomas and paragangliomas are neuroendocrine tumors arising from the adrenal medulla or the sympathetic or parasympathetic paraganglia. They can manifest sporadically or as a consequence of an inherited mutation. Of the latter, aberrations in the genes for succinate dehydrogenase (SDH) subunits A, B, C, and D, or in the SDH assembly factor 2 (SDHAF2) are of special importance because they lead to changes in the energy metabolism of affected cells promoting glycolysis. In addition, carriers of an SDHB mutation have a higher risk for malignant disease. Therefore, imaging studies must be performed on regular occasions. A wide range of imaging studies is currently available, including anatomic tests with high resolution, such as computed tomography (CT) and magnetic resonance imaging (MRI), and functional imaging based on radioactivity, such as 18F-3,4-dihydroxyphenylalanine (DOPA), 18F-fluoro-2-deoxy-D-glucose (18F-FDG), 18F-fluorodopamine, metaiodobenzylguanidine incorporation and somatostatin receptor expression, and the combination of both imaging modalities. Therefore, a guide to rational diagnostic imaging is very important.

This study found that the sensitivity of picking up lesions with CT, MRI, and octreoscan is more than 90% in *SDHx*-positive individuals and that it can be further pushed by providing the interpreting radiologist with clinical information. Thus, the word: "Use your ear and your eye before lab and MRI" is supported by the data and acknowledges the clinician's work and values biochemical testing. Although pheochromocytomas were never missed, the screening for thoracic paragangliomas requires a nuclear examination.

However, it is troublesome to learn that a central analysis of pictures performed much better than local analysis. This finding may indicate that it takes a great deal of experience to understand the clinical problem and that such a level of experience can hardly be achieved with patients from a single center. An alternative explanation to this could also be that central evaluation of imaging studies is done by more dedicated people or people who invest more time for analysis. The latter may become a problem for the future and should, therefore, be prevented at any cost.

A problem is that other studies showed that metastases in SDHB-positive patients may nevertheless better be picked up by 18F-fluorodopamine-PET, 18F-DOPA-PET, or 8F-FDG-PET when the aforementioned methods are not available.[1] Because the study by Gimenez-Roqueplo et al could not compare their algorithm with that of others, the conclusion that somatostatin receptor scintigraphy should be used with CT and MRI can actually not be drawn. However, provided that such imaging is done under the optimal conditions as present during this study, the sensitivities are high enough to justify such an approach in clinical practice.

H. S. Willenberg, MD

Reference

1. Timmers HJ, Chen CC, Carrasquillo JA, et al. Comparison of 18F-fluoro-L-DOPA, 18F-fluoro-deoxyglucose, and 18F-fluorodopamine PET and 123I-MIBG scintigraphy in the localization of pheochromocytoma and paraganglioma. *J Clin Endocrinol Metab*. 2009;94:4757-4767.

Congenital Adrenal Hyperplasia

Novel H6PDH mutations in two girls with premature adrenarche: 'apparent' and 'true' CRD can be differentiated by urinary steroid profiling

Lavery GG, Idkowiak J, Sherlock M, et al (Univ of Birmingham, UK; et al)
Eur J Endocrinol 168:K19-K26, 2013

Context.—Inactivating mutations in the enzyme hexose-6-phosphate dehydrogenase (H6PDH, encoded by *H6PD*) cause apparent cortisone reductase deficiency (ACRD). H6PDH generates cofactor NADPH for 11β-hydroxysteroid dehydrogenase type 1 (11β-HSD1, encoded by *HSD11B1*) oxo-reductase activity, converting cortisone to cortisol. Inactivating mutations in *HSD11B1* cause true cortisone reductase deficiency (CRD). Both ACRD and CRD present with hypothalamic-pituitary-adrenal (HPA) axis activation and adrenal hyperandrogenism.

Objective.—To describe the clinical, biochemical and molecular characteristics of two additional female children with ACRD and to illustrate the diagnostic value of urinary steroid profiling in identifying and differentiating a total of six ACRD and four CRD cases.

Design.—Clinical, biochemical and genetic assessment of two female patients presenting during childhood. In addition, results of urinary steroid profiling in a total of ten ACRD/CRD patients were compared to identify distinguishing characteristics.

Results.—Case 1 was compound heterozygous for R109*AfsX3* and a novel P146L missense mutation in *H6PD*. Case 2 was compound heterozygous for novel nonsense mutations Q325X and Y446X in *H6PD*. Mutant expression studies confirmed loss of H6PDH activity in both cases. Urinary steroid metabolite profiling by gas chromatography/mass spectrometry suggested ACRD in both cases. In addition, we were able to establish a steroid metabolite signature differentiating ACRD and CRD, providing a basis for genetic diagnosis and future individualised management.

Conclusions.—Steroid profile analysis of a 24-h urine collection provides a diagnostic method for discriminating between ACRD and CRD. This will provide a useful tool in stratifying unresolved adrenal hyperandrogenism in children with premature adrenarche and adult females with polycystic ovary syndrome (PCOS).

▶ The conversion of cortisol to cortisone by 11β-hydroxylase type 2 has several effects, one of which is the protection of the mineralocorticoid receptor against the influence of the hypothalamo-pituitary-adrenal (HPA) axis. Another major effect is the conservation and transport of inactive cortisol precursors (eg, cortisone) with reconstitution to an active glucocorticoid (eg, cortisol) at the site of action by 11β-hydroxylase type 1 (HSD11B1). Therefore, diminished HSD11B1 activity results in a shortage of cortisol and is the molecular basis of the syndrome of (true) cortisone reductase deficiency (CRD). Nicotinamide adenine dinucleotide phosphate-oxidase (NADPH) is a necessary cofactor of HSD11B1 action and is provided by the activity of hexose-6-phosphate dehydrogenase (H6PDH). Loss-of-function mutations in this enzyme cause a decreased activity of HSD11B1 and are termed *apparent CRD*. The consequent activation of the HPA axis in both conditions also leads to generation of adrenal androgens and androgen precursors as a sideline of adrenal steroidogenesis not separately regulated by a negative feedback loop. Clinically, affected girls may present with premature adrenarche or hyperandrogenemia with a phenotype seen in polycystic ovary syndrome. Biochemically, the ratio of cortisol (metabolites) to cortisone (metabolites) is changed in favor of cortisone (metabolites), and androgen precursors are elevated.

Besides the elegant expression and functional studies of mutated genes and proteins, the authors showed that a thorough characterization of a clinical phenotype helps in predicting genetic aberrations, and, in the presented cases, new H6PDH mutations were found. Above all, the authors were able to distinguish true CRD from apparent CRD by analysis of urine samples collected over 24 hours using gas chromatography/mass spectrometry. Apparent CRD seems to be more severe but phenotypically also slightly different from true CRD as shown by indices reflecting 5α-reductase and 5β-reductase activities. This may open the door to the discovery of new pathophysiologic relationships between enzymes and co-enzymes in steroid hormone metabolism.

H. S. Willenberg, MD

Genotype-Phenotype Correlation in 153 Adult Patients With Congenital Adrenal Hyperplasia due to 21-Hydroxylase Deficiency: Analysis of the United Kingdom Congenital Adrenal Hyperplasia Adult Study Executive (CaHASE) Cohort

Krone N, Wiebke Arlt for the United Kingdom Congenital adrenal Hyperplasia Adult Study Executive (CaHASE) (Univ of Birmingham, UK; et al)
J Clin Endocrinol Metab 98:E346-E354, 2013

Context.—In congenital adrenal hyperplasia (CAH) due to 21-hydroxylase deficiency, a strong genotype-phenotype correlation exists in childhood. However, similar data in adults are lacking.

Objective.—The objective of the study was to test whether the severity of disease-causing CYP21A2 mutations influences the treatment and health status in adults with CAH.

Research Design and Methods.—We analyzed the genotype in correlation with treatment and health status in 153 adults with CAH from the United Kingdom Congenital adrenal Hyperplasia Adult Study Executive cohort.

Results.—CYP21A2 mutations were distributed similarly to previously reported case series. In 7 patients a mutation was identified on only 1 allele. Novel mutations were detected on 1.7% of alleles (5 of 306). Rare mutations were found on 2.3% of alleles (7 of 306). For further analysis, patients were categorized into CYP21A2 mutation groups according to predicted residual enzyme function: null (n = 34), A (n = 42), B (n = 36), C (n = 34), and D (n = 7). Daily glucocorticoid dose was highest in group null and lowest in group C. Fludrocortisone was used more frequently in patients with more severe genotypes. Except for lower female height in group B, no statistically significant associations between genotype and clinical parameters were found. Androgens, blood pressure, lipids, blood glucose, and homeostasis model assessment of insulin resistance were not different between groups. Subjective health status was similarly impaired across groups.

Conclusions.—In adults with classic CAH and women with nonclassic CAH, there was a weak association between genotype and treatment, but health outcomes were not associated with genotype. The underrepresentation of males with nonclassic CAH may reflect that milder genotypes result in a milder condition that is neither diagnosed nor followed up in adulthood. Overall, our results suggest that the impaired health status of adults with CAH coming to medical attention is acquired rather than genetically determined and therefore could potentially be improved through modification of treatment.

▶ Impairment of 21-hydroxylation of progesterone, 17α-hydroxyprogesterone, and 21-deoxycortisol causes diminished generation of glucocorticoids and sometimes mineralocorticoids with increases in the secretion of corticotropin and, consequently, cortisol precursor steroids. These intermediate steroidogenesis products have partly progestogenic and antimineralocorticoid activities and can be metabolized to active androgens. This and other consortia observed that adult patients with congenital adrenal hyperplasia have a suboptimal health status with a poor metabolic profile as well as impairment in fertility and quality of life. Therefore, the authors wanted to know whether such problems are associated with the severity of the genotype causing congenital adrenal hyperplasia. The major findings deserve attention because there was no statistical difference regarding blood pressure, glucose metabolism, and lipid profiles between the groups with different enzyme activities. This finding suggests that the genetic phenotype does not directly translate into clinical outcome, which may be because there were differences between the amounts of glucocorticoids (and mineralocorticoids) given to the patients with different mutational statuses. Finally, this may also lead to a more or less equal biochemical disease control despite different genotypes in the patient groups. An alternative interpretation would be that the prediction of the phenotype from the genotype does not really function. However, the fact that male patients with congenital adrenal hyperplasia seem to be underrepresented in the groups with a rather mild impairment of the 21-hydroxylase function may constitute an argument in favor of a correct genotype-phenotype association. Nevertheless, the absence of men in the study cohort may point to a comparably better quality of life but does not necessarily mean that these affected subjects perform normally in all of the above-mentioned tests. A side effect of this study was the discovery of 5 new mutations in the *CYP21A2* gene, and a genotype-phenotype relation actually needs to be established for these defects.

H. S. Willenberg, MD

Testicular Adrenal Rest Tumors Develop Independently of Long-Term Disease Control: A Longitudinal Analysis of 50 Adult Men With Congenital Adrenal Hyperplasia due to Classic 21-Hydroxylase Deficiency

Reisch N, Rottenkolber M, Greifenstein A, et al (Univ Hosp Munich, Germany; Ludwig-Maximilians-Universität, Munich, Germany; et al)

J Clin Endocrinol Metab 98:E1820-E1826, 2013

Context.—Testicular adrenal rest tumors (TARTs) and hypogonadotropic hypogonadism are the two most common causes for male infertility in classic 21-hydroxylase deficiency. Current hypotheses suggest the quality of disease control to be one of the main pathogenic factors for TART development.

Objective.—The aim was to study long-term predictors for TART development in a retrospective longitudinal study.

Design.—Fifty men with classic 21-hydroxylase deficiency (31 salt wasting, 19 simple virilizing) were investigated. Testicular ultrasound at a median age at investigation of 27 years detected TARTs in 28 of 50 subjects (19 salt wasting, 9 simple virilizing). TART presence was correlated with long-term parameters of disease control during childhood and adolescence obtained from patients' charts: 24-hour urine pregnanetriol, serum 17-hydroxyprogesterone, onset and stage of pubic hair development, testicular growth, and bone age in relation to chronological age.

Results.—There was no difference in pregnanetriol excretion over lifetime between patients with and without TARTs. Similarly, neither development of pubic hair and testicular volume (Tanner) nor bone age in relation to chronological age differed between the two groups. Furthermore, the two groups had the same body mass index and the same impairment of final height in relation to midparental target height.

Conclusion.—Our longitudinal analysis demonstrates no association between TART presence and parameters of disease control. These data, therefore, argue for other mechanisms more relevant for TART induction including those occurring during fetal development.

▶ As in other metabolic diseases, patients with congenital adrenal hyperplasia (CAH) may face short-term complications and consequences that arise from long-term maltreatment. Among the latter, chronic hypercortisolism or impairment in fertility would seem typical. In men, another such problem may contribute to the development of testicular adrenal rest tumors (TARTs). Because gonads and adrenal cortex share the same primordial tissue, it is hypothesized that during embryogenesis, the Leydig cell and adrenocortical cell precursors do not separate entirely. Thus, Leydig cells and other testicular cells may stay intermingled with adrenocortical cells that would develop into hyperplastic tissue after chronic stimulation of adrenocortical cells by corticotropin. This view is supported by the observation that TARTs seem to respond to suppressive treatment with glucocorticoids in a substantial number of cases. Consequently, it is believed that chronic maltreatment may promote genesis of TARTs. The authors found that the total amount of urinary pregnanetriol, a metabolite of the unconverted cortisol precursor 17-hydroxyprogesterone, did not differ between patients with TARTs and those without. Other measures of glucocorticoid treatment, such as the amount of glucocorticoid, also did not differ. Therefore, the authors concluded that TARTs seem to develop irrespective of patient treatment. It was speculated that rather, the amount of adrenocortical cells and the exposure to corticotropin are factors to influence TART growth. The latter hypothesis is supported by the finding that CAH patients of this cohort came to diagnosis rather late during childhood and not by screening. In addition, patients with TARTs had been more frequently on hydrocortisone treatment. It can be added that in a murine CAH model, even relatively high doses of glucocorticoids are not able to fully suppress corticotropin secretion.[1] In humans, it was observed that corticotropin (and generation of adrenal androgen precursors) is only suppressed by glucocorticoids when the dose is high enough to induce hypercortisolism.[2] Haase and colleagues[3] once discussed that before birth and sometime thereafter, the feedback to corticotropin secretion may be adjusted to a less-sensitive level or that even some corticotroph cells develop autonomy and form the basis for a tertiary hypercorticotropinism.

H. S. Willenberg, MD

References

1. Tajima T, Ma XM, Bornstein SR, Aguilera G. Prenatal dexamethasone treatment does not prevent alterations of the hypothalamic pituitary adrenal axis in steroid 21-hydroxylase deficient mice. *Endocrinology.* 1999;140:3354-3362.
2. Merke DP. Approach to the adult with congenital adrenal hyperplasia due to 21-hydroxylase deficiency. *J Clin Endocrinol Metab.* 2008;93:653-660.
3. Haase M, Schott M, Kaminsky E, et al. Cushing's disease in a patient with steroid 21-hydroxylase deficiency. *Endocr J.* 2011;58:699-706.

Glucocorticoid Receptors/Glucocorticoid Sensitivity

A Novel Point Mutation in the DNA-Binding Domain (DBD) of the Human Glucocorticoid Receptor Causes Primary Generalized Glucocorticoid Resistance by Disrupting the Hydrophobic Structure of its DBD

Roberts ML, Kino T, Nicolaides NC, et al (Univ of Athens Med School, Greece; Eunice Kennedy Shriver Natl Inst of Child Health and Human Development, Bethesda, MD; et al)

J Clin Endocrinol Metab 98:E790-E795, 2013

Context.—Primary generalized glucocorticoid resistance is a rare genetic condition characterized by partial end-organ insensitivity to glucocorticoids. Most affected subjects present with clinical manifestations of mineralocorticoid and androgen excess. The condition has been associated with inactivating mutations in the human glucocorticoid receptor (hGR) gene, which impair the molecular mechanisms of hGRα action, thereby reducing tissue sensitivity to glucocorticoids.

Objective.—The aim of our study was to investigate the molecular mechanisms through which one previously described natural heterozygous V423A mutation, the second mutation detected in the DNA-binding domain (DBD) of the hGRα, affects glucocorticoid signal transduction.

Design and Results.—Compared with the wild-type receptor, hGRαV423A demonstrated a 72% reduction in its ability to transactivate the glucocorticoid-inducible mouse mammary tumor virus promoter in response to dexamethasone. The hGRαV423A receptor showed a significant reduction in its ability to bind to glucocorticoid-response elements of glucocorticoid-responsive genes, owing to structural alterations of the DBD confirmed by computer-based structural analysis. In addition, hGRαV423A demonstrated a 2.6-fold delay in nuclear translocation following exposure to the ligand, although it did not exert a dominant negative effect on the wild-type hGRα, had a similar affinity to the ligand with the wild-type receptor, and displayed a normal interaction with the GRIP1 coactivator in vitro.

Conclusions.—The natural mutant receptor hGRαV423A causes primary generalized glucocorticoid resistance by affecting multiple steps in the cascade of glucocorticoid receptor action, which primarily involve decreased ability to bind to target glucocorticoid response elements and delayed translocation into the nucleus.

▶ Primary generalized resistance to glucocorticoids, also termed *Chrousos syndrome*, leads to high levels corticotropin because of the interruption of glucocorticoid feedback. Therefore, this condition provokes symptoms seen in adrenal insufficiency together with excess secretion (and action) of androgens and mineralocorticoids. To date, several cases have been described. The authors cornered the hGRαV423A variant and present data on the mechanism for how the glucocorticoid receptor is prevented from physiologic action. This study derives its elegance from the systematic investigation into ligand affinity, translocation, interaction with a coactivator, binding to glucocorticoid-response elements, transactivation of a promoter, structure, and interaction with a wild-type glucocorticoid receptor.

The authors found that the hydrophobic valin at position 423 shields 4 zinc-binding cysteines from water. The replacement of valin by arginine in the DNA-binding domain permits water to diffuse into the ion-binding region of the glucocorticoid receptor, where it is captured by hydrogen bonds. This reduces the affinity of this domain for zinc and for the phosphate backbone of the DNA and results in a greater energy penalty with decreased binding of the mutant receptor to DNA. Whether the description of such mechanisms helps develop drugs with differential glucocorticoid actions remains open.

H. S. Willenberg, MD

11β-Hydroxysteroid dehydrogenase blockade prevents age-induced skin structure and function defects

Tiganescu A, Tahrani AA, Morgan SA, et al (Univ of Birmingham, Edgbaston, UK; et al)

J Clin Invest 123:3051-3060, 2013

Glucocorticoid (GC) excess adversely affects skin integrity, inducing thinning and impaired wound healing. Aged skin, particularly that which has been photo-exposed, shares a similar phenotype. Previously, we demonstrated age-induced expression of the GC-activating enzyme 11β-hydroxysteroid dehydrogenase type 1 (11β-HSD1) in cultured human dermal fibroblasts (HDFs). Here, we determined 11β-HSD1 levels in human skin biopsies from young and older volunteers and examined the aged 11β-HSD1 KO mouse skin phenotype. 11β-HSD1 activity was elevated in aged human and mouse skin and in PE compared with donor-matched photo-protected human biopsies. Age-induced dermal atrophy with deranged collagen structural organization was prevented in 11β-HSD1 KO mice, which also exhibited increased collagen density. We found that treatment of HDFs with physiological concentrations of cortisol inhibited rate-limiting steps in collagen biosynthesis and processing. Furthermore, topical 11β-HSD1 inhibitor treatment accelerated healing of full-thickness mouse dorsal wounds, with improved healing also observed in aged 11β-HSD1 KO mice. These findings suggest that elevated 11β-HSD1 activity in aging skin leads to increased local GC generation, which may account for adverse changes occurring in the elderly, and 11β-HSD1 inhibitors may be useful in the treatment of age-associated impairments in dermal integrity and wound healing.

► Clinically, it sometimes becomes very difficult to distinguish the skin from elderly people from that of patients with glucocorticoid excess. Both conditions promote flattening of the normally undulating rete ridges at the dermal-epidermal junction, decrease in dermal cellularity and collagen content, and shrinkage of subcutaneous fat. As a consequence, such atrophic skin is characterized by easy bruising and increased fragility with poor wound healing. The skin similarities found in both conditions led the authors to assume that the common basis is an enhancement in glucocorticoid action. Because endogenous glucocorticoids are not elevated to a degree that explains the above-mentioned observations, it was hypothesized that the availability of active glucocorticoid as provided by 11β-HSD1 activity is upregulated in aging. The 11β-HSD1 inhibitor, RO151, reversed age-induced skin atrophy and improved wound healing. Such a specific therapy would especially help patients on chronic glucocorticoid medication, patients in intensive care units, and patients with infections. However, the experiments may be extended to models of chronic exposure to environmental ultraviolet radiation or artificial photoaging in the future. Because the data were partly obtained in human samples and from in vivo experiments while previous studies were limited to in vitro models, a specific therapy seems realistic and within reach.

H. S. Willenberg, MD

Mitotane Therapy in Adrenocortical Cancer Induces CYP3A4 and Inhibits 5α-Reductase, Explaining the Need for Personalized Glucocorticoid and Androgen Replacement

Chortis V, Taylor AE, Schneider P, et al (Univ of Birmingham, UK; et al)
J Clin Endocrinol Metab 98:161-171, 2013

Context.—Mitotane [1-(2-chlorophenyl)-1-(4-chlorophenyl)-2,2-dichloroethane] is the first-line treatment for metastatic adrenocortical carcinoma (ACC) and is also regularly used in the adjuvant setting after presumed complete removal of the primary tumor. Mitotane is considered an adrenolytic substance, but there is limited information on distinct effects on steroidogenesis. However, adrenal insufficiency and male hypogonadism are widely recognized side effects of mitotane treatment.

Objective.—Our objective was to define the impact of mitotane treatment on *in vivo* steroidogenesis in patients with ACC.

Setting and Design.—At seven European specialist referral centers for adrenal tumors, we analyzed 24-h urine samples ($n = 127$) collected from patients with ACC before and during mitotane therapy in the adjuvant setting ($n = 23$) or for metastatic ACC ($n = 104$). Urinary steroid metabolite excretion was profiled by gas chromatography/mass spectrometry in comparison with healthy controls ($n = 88$).

Results.—We found a sharp increase in the excretion of 6β-hydroxycortisol over cortisol ($P < 0.001$), indicative of a strong induction of the major drug-metabolizing enzyme cytochrome P450 3A4. The contribution of 6β-hydroxycortisol to total glucocorticoid metabolites increased from 2% (median, interquartile range 1–4%) to 56% (39–71%) during mitotane treatment. Furthermore, we documented strong inhibition of systemic 5α-reductase activity, indicated by a significant decrease in 5α-reduced steroids, including 5α-tetrahydrocortisol, 5α-tetrahydrocorticosterone, and androsterone (all $P < 0.001$). The degree of inhibition was similar to that in patients with inactivating 5α-reductase type 2 mutations ($n = 23$) and patients receiving finasteride ($n = 5$), but cluster analysis of steroid data revealed a pattern of inhibition distinct from these two groups. Longitudinal data showed rapid onset and long-lasting duration of the observed effects.

Conclusions.—Cytochrome P4503A4 induction by mitotane results in rapid inactivation of more than 50% of administered hydrocortisone, explaining the need for doubling hydrocortisone replacement in mitotane-treated patients. Strong inhibition of 5α-reductase activity is in line with the clinical observation of relative inefficiency of testosterone replacement in mitotane-treated men, calling for replacement by 5α-reduced androgens.

▶ Adrenocortical cancer (ACC) is a tumor with high mortality. It harms patients through its malignant behavior and tumor complications but also through other mechanisms, one of which is excess hormone secretion in a substantial number of cases. Treatment of ACC may help patients to prevent tumor-related problems but may also put the patient at risk for medication side effects. The latter includes reversal of hormone excess, increased binding of glucocorticoids, a higher inactivation rate of glucocorticoids, and the formation of intermediate steroids that may interfere with cortisol immunoassays. All these properties of mitotane may facilitate manifestation of adrenal insufficiency. Therefore, every study that better characterizes the action of this compound and the mechanism through which side effects develop is most welcome. The study by Chortis et al yields an explanation for why male patients on mitotane come down with hypogonadism and why testosterone treatment is less effective in such patients than others. This is because 5α-reductase activity declines in the presence of mitotane. Of note, overall steroidogenesis seems to be inhibited by mitotane without affecting 11β-hydroxylase activity, as seen by the decrease in the sum of total androgen and mineralocorticoid metabolites excreted into the urine.

In addition, this study elegantly confirms the incremental inactivation of glucocorticoids and androstenedione through CYP3A4 when mitotane is administered.

H. S. Willenberg, MD

Essential role of stress hormone signaling in cardiomyocytes for the prevention of heart disease

Oakley RH, Ren R, Cruz-Topete D, et al (Natl Inst of Environmental Health Sciences, Research Triangle Park, NC; et al)

Proc Natl Acad Sci U S A 110:17035-17040, 2013

Heart failure is a leading cause of death in humans, and stress is increasingly associated with adverse cardiac outcomes. Glucocorticoids are primary stress hormones, but their direct role in cardiovascular health and disease is poorly understood. To determine the in vivo function of glucocorticoid signaling in the heart, we generated mice with cardiomyocyte-specific deletion of the glucocorticoid receptor (GR). These mice are born at the expected Mendelian ratio, but die prematurely from spontaneous cardiovascular disease. By 3 mo of age, mice deficient in cardiomyocyte GR display a marked reduction in left ventricular systolic function, as evidenced by decreases in ejection fraction and fractional shortening. Heart weight and left ventricular mass are elevated, and histology revealed cardiac hypertrophy without fibrosis. Removal of endogenous glucocorticoids and mineralocorticoids neither augmented nor lessened the hypertrophic response. Global gene expression analysis of knockout hearts before pathology onset revealed aberrant regulation of a large cohort of genes associated with cardiovascular disease as well as unique disease genes associated with inflammatory processes. Genes important for maintaining cardiac contractility, repressing cardiac hypertrophy, promoting cardiomyocyte survival, and inhibiting inflammation had decreased expression in the GR-deficient hearts. These findings demonstrate that a deficiency in cardiomyocyte glucocorticoid signaling leads to spontaneous cardiac hypertrophy, heart failure, and death, revealing an obligate role for GR in maintaining normal cardiovascular function. Moreover, our findings suggest that selective activation of cardiomyocyte GR may represent an approach for the prevention of heart disease.

▶ When it comes down to hormones and heart, the issues of thyroid hormone and epinephrine are usually discussed first. In the last decade, however, a possible direct action of mineralocorticoids in the heart is increasingly discussed. In addition, there are studies focusing on the influence of insulin (-like growth factor) on heart failure in murine models. The authors open with a statement saying that there is a lot of information on glucocorticoid function, and glucocorticoids are widely used. They are correct when they say that the direct biological actions of glucocorticoids in the heart remain poorly understood. Therefore, the authors created a cardiomyocyte-specific knock down of the glucocorticoid receptor (GR) and found that the GR plays an obligate role for the regulation of a large cohort of genes involved in cardiovascular (~150) and inflammatory (~1000) disease processes. To control for glucocorticoid signaling, the adrenal glands were removed. But this experiment did not change the results, suggesting that the consequences of GR knock down only result from a deficiency in GR action. These findings also explain why patients with adrenal insufficiency may develop heart failure, although they only rarely become hypertensive. Oakley and colleagues also discuss the influence of stress in heart physiology.

H. S. Willenberg, MD

Cushing's Disease: Diagnosis and Treatment

Mitotane levels predict the outcome of patients with adrenocortical carcinoma treated adjuvantly following radical resection

Terzolo M, Baudin AE, Ardito A, et al (Univ of Turin, Orbassano, Italy; IGR, Villejuif, France, Univ Hosp of Würzburg, Germany; et al)

Eur J Endocrinol 169:263-270, 2013

Context.—Mitotane plasma concentrations ≥14 mg/l have been shown to predict tumor response and better survival in patients with advanced adrenocortical carcinoma (ACC). A correlation between mitotane concentrations and patient outcome has not been demonstrated in an adjuvant setting.

Objective.—To compare recurrence-free survival (RFS) in patients who reached and maintained mitotane concentrations ≥14 mg/l vs patients who did not.

Design and Setting.—Retrospective analysis at six referral European centers.

Patients.—Patients with ACC who were radically resected between 1995 and 2009 and were treated adjuvantly with mitotane targeting concentrations of 14–20 mg/l.

Main Outcome Measures.—RFS (primary) and overall survival (secondary).

Results.—Of the 122 patients included, 63 patients (52%) reached and maintained during a median follow-up of 36 months the target mitotane concentrations (group 1) and 59 patients (48%) did not (group 2). ACC recurrence was observed in 22 patients of group 1 (35%) and 36 patients in group 2 (61%). In multivariable analysis, the maintenance of target mitotane concentrations was associated with a significantly prolonged RFS (hazard ratio (HR) of recurrence: 0.418, 0.22–0.79; $P = 0.007$), while the risk of death was not significantly altered (HR: 0.59, 0.26–1.34; $P = 0.20$). Grades 3–4 toxicity was observed in 11 patients (9%) and was managed with temporary mitotane discontinuation. None of the patients discontinued mitotane definitively for toxicity.

Conclusions.—Mitotane concentrations ≥14 mg/l predict response to adjuvant treatment being associated with a prolonged RFS. A monitored adjuvant mitotane treatment may benefit patients after radical removal of ACC.

▶ Adrenocortical carcinoma (ACC) is a rare disease with malignant behavior. More than 50% of patients experience relapse of the disease. Although the mainstay of therapy is surgery, resection of tumor material remains often noncurative. Therefore, adjuvant therapy is necessary. In the past, it was shown that mitotane therapy might be advantageous for patients with ACC. However, there is debate if it is at all and, if so, how long and at what dosages mitotane therapy is useful. Terzolo et al now showed that patients who were able to consistently maintain mitotane levels of more than 14 mg/L had a significantly reduced risk of recurrence compared with patients who failed to do so. So far, this target concentration has been ascertained only in patients with local or metastatic tumor burden. Therefore, this study contributes to the debate of whether mitotane should be used in patients who are supposedly free of adrenal carcinoma remnant tissue.

However, this study is also to be interpreted with caution because it was retrospective and nonrandomized, as are almost all other studies focusing on the issue of mitotane treatment. The basis is formed to justify treatment with mitotane when tumor is still present or in an adjuvant setting. However, because mitotane interferes with other antitumor medication and is washed out rather slowly, future studies on the value of mitotane in ACC should be done in a prospective design.

H. S. Willenberg, MD

ARMC5 Mutations in Macronodular Adrenal Hyperplasia with Cushing's Syndrome

Assié G, Libé R, Espiard S, et al (Université Paris Descartes, France; et al)
N Engl J Med 369:2105-2114, 2013

Background.—Corticotropin-independent macronodular adrenal hyperplasia may be an incidental finding or it may be identified during evaluation for Cushing's syndrome. Reports of familial cases and the involvement of both adrenal glands suggest a genetic origin of this condition.

Methods.—We genotyped blood and tumor DNA obtained from 33 patients with corticotropin-independent macronodular adrenal hyperplasia (12 men and 21 women who were 30 to 73 years of age), using single-nucleotide polymorphism arrays, microsatellite markers, and whole-genome and Sanger sequencing. The effects of armadillo repeat containing 5 (*ARMC5*) inactivation and overexpression were tested in cell-culture models.

Results.—The most frequent somatic chromosome alteration was loss of heterozygosity at 16p (in 8 of 33 patients for whom data were available [24%]). The most frequent mutation identified by means of whole-genome sequencing was in *ARMC5*, located at 16p11.2. *ARMC5* mutations were detected in tumors obtained from 18 of 33 patients (55%). In all cases, both alleles of *ARMC5* carried mutations: one germline and the other somatic. In 4 patients with a germline *ARMC5* mutation, different nodules from the affected adrenals harbored different secondary *ARMC5* alterations. Transcriptome-based classification of corticotropin-independent macronodular adrenal hyperplasia indicated that *ARMC5* mutations influenced gene expression, since all cases with mutations clustered together. *ARMC5* inactivation decreased steroidogenesis in vitro, and its overexpression altered cell survival.

Conclusions.—Some cases of corticotropin-independent macronodular adrenal hyperplasia appear to be genetic, most often with inactivating mutations of *ARMC5*, a putative tumor-suppressor gene. Genetic testing for this condition, which often has a long and insidious prediagnostic course, might result in earlier identification and better management. (Funded by Agence Nationale de la Recherche and others.)

▶ Corticotropin (ACTH)-independent macronodular adrenal hyperplasia (AIMAH) is a clinical condition with several unresolved aspects. It comes with well-defined clinical syndromes, such as the McCune-Albright syndrome, or may present as a sporadic condition. It was observed that AIMAH tissue responds to stimuli different from ACTH with an increase in glucocorticoid synthesis. The ectopic expression or eutopic overexpression of predominantly G-protein—coupled receptors connected the intracellular steroidogenic apparatus of affected adrenocortical cells with hormonal signals that are usually not suppressed by glucocorticoid feedback.[1] However, the phenomenon of unphysiologic receptor expression may explain the phenotype, but it remains unclear why such illicit receptors are expressed.

Following the hypothesis of a genetic origin, Assié et al were able to identify mutations in the armadillo repeat containing 5 (*ARMC5*) gene. It is noteworthy that affected patients had a germline mutation on one allele and a genetic aberration affecting the other. The somatic hit on the second allele, however, could be different between the nodules even in the same hyperplastic gland (Fig 3 in the original article). Interestingly, after silencing the ARMC5 message, the expression of 17α-hydroxylase and 21α-hydroxylase as well as the generation of cortisol increased, although the ACTH receptor and steroidogenic factor-1 were down regulated.

The function of *ARMC5* is unknown. It encodes a protein that contains an armadillo repeat domain, suggesting interactions with other proteins, possibly including β-catenin, which also contains armadillo repeats and is mutated in adrenocortical tumors in a substantial number of cases. Loss of function, however, seems to prevent apoptosis. Whether mutation in the *ARMC5* gene led to aberrant hormone receptor expression remains open. This is also because 3 patients with food-dependent Cushing's syndrome from this cohort were negative for mutated *ARMC5*.

H. S. Willenberg, MD

Reference

1. Lacroix A, Bourdeau I, Lampron A, Mazzuco TL, Tremblay J, Hamet P. Aberrant G-protein coupled receptor expression in relation to adrenocortical overfunction. *Clin Endocrinol (Oxf)*. 2010;73:1-15.

Intraadrenal Corticotropin in Bilateral Macronodular Adrenal Hyperplasia

Louiset E, Duparc C, Young J, et al (Rouen Univ, Mont-Saint-Aignan, France; Univ Paris Sud, France; et al)

N Engl J Med 369:2115-2125, 2013

Background.—Bilateral macronodular adrenal hyperplasia is a rare cause of primary adrenal Cushing's syndrome. In this form of hyperplasia, hypersecretion of cortisol suppresses the release of corticotropin by pituitary corticotrophs, which results in low plasma corticotropin levels. Thus, the disease has been termed corticotropin-independent macronodular adrenal hyperplasia. We examined the abnormal production of corticotropin in these hyperplastic adrenal glands.

Methods.—We obtained specimens of hyperplastic macronodular adrenal tissue from 30 patients with primary adrenal disease. The corticotropin precursor proopiomelanocortin and corticotropin expression were assessed by means of a polymerase-chain-reaction assay and immunohistochemical analysis. The production of corticotropin and cortisol was assessed in 11 specimens with the use of incubated explants and cell cultures coupled with hormone assays. Corticotropin levels were measured in adrenal and peripheral venous blood samples from 2 patients.

Results.—The expression of proopiomelanocortin messenger RNA (mRNA) was detected in all samples of hyperplastic adrenal tissue. Corticotropin was detected in steroidogenic cells arranged in clusters that were disseminated throughout the adrenal specimens. Adrenal corticotropin levels were higher in adrenal venous blood samples than in peripheral venous samples, a finding that was consistent with local production of the peptide within the hyperplastic adrenals. The release of adrenal corticotropin was stimulated by ligands of aberrant membrane receptors but not by corticotropin-releasing hormone or dexamethasone. A semiquantitative score for corticotropin immunostaining in the samples correlated with basal plasma cortisol levels. Corticotropin-receptor antagonists significantly inhibited in vitro cortisol secretion.

Conclusions.—Cortisol secretion by the adrenals in patients with macronodular hyperplasia and Cushing's syndrome appears to be regulated by corticotropin, which is produced by a subpopulation of steroidogenic cells in the hyperplastic adrenals. Thus, the hypercortisolism associated with bilateral macronodular adrenal hyperplasia appears to be corticotropin-dependent. (Funded by the Agence Nationale de la Recherche and others.)

▶ The results of this study suggest that the name *corticotropin (ACTH)-independent macronodular adrenal hyperplasia* (AIMAH) is actually wrong because in this condition, ACTH seems to be generated within the hyperplastic nodules causing excess cortisol secretion by diseased cells. This fact adds to the myths that accompany this syndrome. The condition of AIMAH is known for the responsiveness of the adrenal tissue to stimuli other than ACTH. This phenomenon is believed to be conferred by aberrant expression of mainly G protein–coupled receptors, for example, glucose-dependent insulinotropic peptide (GIP).[1]

The authors found that venous outflows of AIMAH adrenals contain concentrations of ACTH high enough to prove the pituitary origin if taken from the inferior petrosal sinuses in ACTH-dependent Cushing's syndrome. In addition, the basal cortisol concentrations seem to correlate with AIMAH tissue content of ACTH. In cell cultures, affected adrenal cells secreted ACTH along with cortisol, which could be lowered by corticostatin, an ACTH receptor antagonist. Interestingly, exposure of cultured hyperplastic adrenal cells to GIP led to an increase in ACTH and cortisol concentrations.

H. S. Willenberg, MD

Reference

1. Lacroix A, Bourdeau I, Lampron A, Mazzuco TL, Tremblay J, Hamet P. Aberrant G-protein coupled receptor expression in relation to adrenocortical overfunction. *Clin Endocrinol (Oxf)*. 2010;73:1-15.

Adrenal Function

Reduced Cortisol Metabolism during Critical Illness

Boonen E, Vervenne H, Meersseman P, et al (KU Leuven, Belgium; et al)

N Engl J Med 368:1477-1488, 2013

Background.—Critical illness is often accompanied by hypercortisolemia, which has been attributed to stress-induced activation of the hypothalamic–pituitary–adrenal axis. However, low corticotropin levels have also been reported in critically ill patients, which may be due to reduced cortisol metabolism.

Methods.—In a total of 158 patients in the intensive care unit and 64 matched controls, we tested five aspects of cortisol metabolism: daily levels of corticotropin and cortisol; plasma cortisol clearance, metabolism, and production during infusion of deuterium-labeled steroid hormones as tracers; plasma clearance of 100 mg of hydrocortisone; levels of urinary cortisol metabolites; and levels of messenger RNA and protein in liver and adipose tissue, to assess major cortisol-metabolizing enzymes.

Results.—Total and free circulating cortisol levels were consistently higher in the patients than in controls, whereas corticotropin levels were lower ($P < 0.001$ for both comparisons). Cortisol production was 83% higher in the patients ($P = 0.02$). There was a reduction of more than 50% in cortisol clearance during tracer infusion and after the administration of 100 mg of hydrocortisone in the patients ($P \leq 0.03$ for both comparisons). All these factors accounted for an increase by a factor of 3.5 in plasma cortisol levels in the patients, as compared with controls ($P < 0.001$). Impaired cortisol clearance also correlated with a lower cortisol response to corticotropin stimulation. Reduced cortisol metabolism was associated with reduced inactivation of cortisol in the liver and kidney, as suggested by urinary steroid ratios, tracer kinetics, and assessment of liver-biopsy samples ($P \leq 0.004$ for all comparisons).

Conclusions.—During critical illness, reduced cortisol breakdown, related to suppressed expression and activity of cortisol-metabolizing enzymes, contributed to hypercortisolemia and hence corticotropin suppression. The diagnostic and therapeutic implications for critically ill patients are unknown. (Funded by the Belgian Fund for Scientific Research and others; ClinicalTrials.gov numbers, NCT00512122 and NCT00115479; and Current Controlled Trials numbers, ISRCTN49433936, ISRCTN49306926, and ISRCTN08083905.)

▶ This study is noteworthy because it adds significant information to our knowledge of generation and metabolization of cortisol in critically ill patients. With its part on cortisol metabolism, it extends other investigations into the diagnosis of adrenal reserve or glucocorticoid application in intensive care unit (ICU) patients.

The starting point was that patients had very low adrenocorticotropic hormone (ACTH) plasma levels. This is also true for other studies.[1] On the other hand, normal subjects had rather high basal ACTH levels that made the difference between patients and controls unbelievable. Nonetheless, the elevated cortisol levels in ICU patients did not seem to be explained by plasma ACTH values, although ACTH concentrations were inadequately high for plasma cortisol concentrations. This observation stimulated metabolic studies using labeled D4-cortisol (deuterated) showing that the clearance of cortisol is reduced. Although this has been known since the 1950s, the authors elegantly determined the amount or activities of cortisol metabolizing enzymes, including 11β-hydroxysteroid dehydrogenases and 5α and 5β-reductases, which was not possible at that time, and they showed that the activities of these enzymes were reduced indeed. Thus, urinary excretion of glucocorticoids was rather high, but diuresis of inactivated glucocorticoids remained rather low. This result is in support of the initial finding of relatively low ACTH levels as a relative minor causative agent for increased cortisol concentrations in ICU patients. This view is supported by findings of others showing low androgen precursor levels in patients with sepsis.[2] As an alternative explanation, the authors offer that cytokines, including interleukin-6, have a direct influence on adrenal steroidogenesis in critically ill patients. Thus, the results are in concordance with those of an earlier study on the influence of interleukin-6 on corticotropin and its dissociation from cortisol secretion in ill subjects.

H. S. Willenberg, MD

References

1. Marx C, Petros S, Bornstein SR, et al. Adrenocortical hormones in survivors and nonsurvivors of severe sepsis: diverse time course of dehydroepiandrosterone, dehydroepiandrosterone-sulfate, and cortisol. *Crit Care Med.* 2003;31:1382-1388.
2. Mastorakos G, Chrousos GP, Weber JS. Recombinant interleukin-6 activates the hypothalamic-pituitary-adrenal axis in humans. *J Clin Endocrinol Metab.* 1993; 77:1690-1694.

Primary Aldosteronism

Somatic mutations in *ATP1A1* and *ATP2B3* lead to aldosterone-producing adenomas and secondary hypertension

Beuschlein F, Boulkroun S, Osswald A, et al (Ludwig-Maximilians-Universität München, Germany; Paris Cardiovascular Res Ctr, France; et al)
Nat Genet 45:440-444, 2013

Primary aldosteronism is the most prevalent form of secondary hypertension. To explore molecular mechanisms of autonomous aldosterone secretion, we performed exome sequencing of aldosterone-producing adenomas (APAs). We identified somatic hotspot mutations in the *ATP1A1* (encoding an Na^+/K^+ ATPase α subunit) and *ATP2B3* (encoding a Ca^{2+} ATPase) genes in three and two of the nine APAs, respectively. These ATPases are expressed in adrenal cells and control sodium, potassium and calcium ion homeostasis. Functional *in vitro* studies of ATP1A1 mutants showed loss of pump activity and strongly reduced affinity for potassium. Electrophysiological *ex vivo* studies on primary adrenal adenoma cells provided further evidence for inappropriate depolarization of cells with ATPase alterations. In a collection of 308 APAs, we found 16 (5.2%) somatic mutations in *ATP1A1* and 5 (1.6%) in *ATP2B3*. Mutation-positive cases showed male dominance, increased plasma aldosterone concentrations and lower potassium concentrations compared with mutation-negative cases. In summary, dominant somatic alterations in two members of the ATPase gene family result in autonomous aldosterone secretion.

► The application of whole exome sequencing in adrenal disease helped clarify the pathophysiology of the third form of familial aldosteronism[1] and the discovery of somatic KCNJ5 mutations in a substantial number of cases with Conn syndrome (please see the 2013 edition of this Year Book). Using this modern methodologic approach in well-defined patients with primary aldosteronism, it was possible to identify somatic mutations in the α subunit of a Na^+/K^+ ATPase and in a Ca^{2+} ATPase. An interesting part of the report, however, is the presentation of functional studies. Using patch clamp, it was shown that the affected proteins cause inappropriate depolarization of adrenocortical cells (Fig 3d in the original article). This directly (in the case of *ATP2B3* mutations) or indirectly (in the case of *ATP1A1* mutations) results in activation of the calcium-calmodulin signaling pathway, to the expression of the aldosterone synthase gene and generation of aldosterone. In contrast to the mutations in the *KCNJ5* gene, the ATPase variants were predominantly found in male subjects.

H. S. Willenberg, MD

Reference

1. Choi M, Scholl UI, Yue P, et al. K+ channel mutations in adrenal aldosterone-producing adenomas and hereditary hypertension. *Science*. 2011;331:768-772.

Somatic and germline *CACNA1D* calcium channel mutations in aldosterone-producing adenomas and primary aldosteronism

Scholl UI, Goh G, Stölting G, et al (Yale Univ School of Medicine, New Haven, CT; Inst of Complex Systems, Jülich, Germany; et al)

Nat Genet 45:1050-1054, 2013

Adrenal aldosterone-producing adenomas (APAs) constitutively produce the salt-retaining hormone aldosterone and are a common cause of severe hypertension. Recurrent mutations in the potassium channel gene *KCNJ5* that result in cell depolarization and Ca^{2+} influx cause ~40% of these tumors. We identified 5 somatic mutations (4 altering Gly403 and 1 altering Ile770) in *CACNA1D*, encoding a voltage-gated calcium channel, among 43 APAs without mutated *KCNJ5*. The altered residues lie in the S6 segments that line the channel pore. Both alterations result in channel activation at less depolarized potentials; Gly403 alterations also impair channel inactivation. These effects are inferred to cause increased Ca^{2+} influx, which is a sufficient stimulus for aldosterone production and cell proliferation in adrenal glomerulosa. We also identified *de novo* germline mutations at identical positions in two children with a previously undescribed syndrome featuring primary aldosteronism and neuromuscular abnormalities. These findings implicate gain-of-function Ca^{2+} channel mutations in APAs and primary aldosteronism.

▶ The group that described *KCNJ5* mutations to occur in sporadic and hereditary forms of primary aldosteronism[1] followed up on their own investigations into this matter and found somatic mutations in the pore-forming α1-subunit calcium channel CaV1.3 (CACNA1D) in about 11% of aldosterone-producing adenomas; similar frequencies were reported by Azizan et al.[2] In addition, 2 subjects with early-onset primary aldosteronism were identified who harbored germline variants at the same positions mutated in tumors, p.Gly403Asp and p.Ile770Met, respectively. These variants were not present in the unaffected parents (de novo mutations). The rarity of such mutations, together with their location at positions identical to those in tumors, led the authors to conclude that they are implicated in the patient's disease process.

Functional studies of somatic and germline variants showed activation of mutated CaV1.3 calcium channels at less depolarizing membrane potentials. Immunohistochemical analysis showed the CaV1.3 calcium channel to be present on zona glomerulosa cells.

In addition, the 2 subjects with the germline *CACNA1D* mutations were notable for their neurologic features, including cerebral palsy and seizures among other symptoms, representing a novel channelopathy with cardiac and neurologic symptoms. Interestingly, homologous mutations in the *CACNA1F* and *CACNA1A* genes had been implicated in autosomal dominant congenital stationary night blindness and familial hemiplegic migraine.

H. S. Willenberg, MD

References

1. Choi M, Scholl UI, Yue P, et al. K+ channel mutations in adrenal aldosterone-producing adenomas and hereditary hypertension. *Science*. 2011;331:768-772.
2. Azizan EA, Poulsen H, Tuluc P, et al. Somatic mutations in ATP1A1 and CACNA1D underlie a common subtype of adrenal hypertension. *Nat Genet*. 2013; 45:1055-1060.

Somatic mutations in *ATP1A1* and *CACNA1D* underlie a common subtype of adrenal hypertension

Azizan EAB, Poulsen H, Tuluc P, et al (Addenbrooke's Hosp, Univ of Cambridge, UK; Aarhus Univ, Denmark; Univ of Innsbruck, Austria; et al)

Nat Genet 45:1055-1060, 2013

At least 5% of individuals with hypertension have adrenal aldosterone-producing adenomas (APAs). Gain-of-function mutations in *KCNJ5* and apparent loss-of-function mutations in *ATP1A1* and *ATP2A3* were reported to occur in APAs. We find that *KCNJ5* mutations are common in APAs resembling cortisol-secreting cells of the adrenal zona fasciculata but are absent in a subset of APAs resembling the aldosterone-secreting cells of the adrenal zona glomerulosa. We performed exome sequencing of ten zona glomerulosa–like APAs and identified nine with somatic mutations in either *ATP1A1*, encoding the Na^+/K^+ ATPase α1 subunit, or *CACNA1D*, encoding $Ca_v1.3$. The *ATP1A1* mutations all caused inward leak currents under physiological conditions, and the *CACNA1D* mutations induced a shift of voltage-dependent gating to more negative voltages, suppressed inactivation or increased currents. Many APAs with these mutations were <1 cm in diameter and had been overlooked on conventional adrenal imaging. Recognition of the distinct genotype and phenotype for this subset of APAs could facilitate diagnosis.

► The report by Beuschlein et al[1] was followed by another report that used whole exome sequencing in search for new genes to be involved in the pathophysiology of primary aldosteronism. More specifically, because the *KCNJ5* mutations may come with cosecretion of cortisol and are thought to cause a zona fasciculata-like phenotype of the adenomatous cells, the authors applied this technique to tissue of aldosterone-producing adenomas (APAs) that had a zona glomerulosa-like appearance. Light microscopy impressions were reflected by the results of the immunostaining to aldosterone synthase (CYP11B2) and 11β-hydroxylase type 1 as well as by cluster analysis of the sequencing data. Thus, all 10 zona glomerulosa-like APAs expressed the aldosterone synthase and were negative for *KCNJ5* mutations. Nine of them, however, were positive for mutations in the Na^+/K^+ ATPase or in the α1 subunit of the L-type voltage-gated calcium channel $Ca_v1.3$. Functional analyses were carried through in depth and showed that the mutations interfere with pumping of potassium, protons, sodium, and calcium as well as the membrane potentials in a differential way. However, as a common consequence, the expression of aldosterone synthase and the production of aldosterone are increased. This is true for basal conditions in culture and stimulation with angiotensin II.

H. S. Willenberg, MD

Reference

1. Beuschlein F, Boulkroun S, Osswald A, et al. Somatic mutations in ATP1A1 and ATP2B3 lead to aldosterone-producing adenomas and secondary hypertension. *Nat Genet*. 2013;45:440-444.

Plasma Metanephrine for Assessing the Selectivity of Adrenal Venous Sampling

Dekkers T, Deinum J, Schultzekool LJ, et al (Radboud Univ Nijmegen Med Ctr, The Netherlands; et al)

Hypertension 62:1152-1157, 2013

Adrenal vein sampling is used to establish the origins of excess production of adrenal hormones in primary aldosteronism. Correct catheter positioning is confirmed using adrenal vein measurements of cortisol, but this parameter is not always reliable. Plasma metanephrine represents an alternative parameter. The objective of our study was to determine the use of plasma metanephrine concentrations to establish correct catheter positioning during adrenal vein sampling with and without cosyntropin stimulation. We included 52 cosyntropin-stimulated and 34 nonstimulated sequential procedures. Plasma cortisol and metanephrine concentrations were measured in adrenal and peripheral venous samples. Success rates of sampling, using an adrenal to peripheral cortisol selectivity index of 3.0, were compared with success rates of metanephrine using a selectivity index determined by receiver operating characteristic curve analysis. Among procedures assessed as selective using cortisol, the adrenal to peripheral vein ratio of metanephrine was 6-fold higher than that of cortisol (94.0 versus 15.5; $P < 0.0001$). There were significant positive relationships between adrenal to peripheral vein ratios of cortisol and metanephrine for cosyntropin-stimulated samplings but not for nonstimulated samplings. Receiver operating characteristic curve analysis indicated a plasma metanephrine selectivity index cutoff of 12. Using this cutoff, concordance in sampling success rates determined by cortisol and metanephrine was substantially higher in cosyntropin-stimulated than in nonstimulated samplings (98% versus 59%). For the latter procedures, sampling success rates determined by metanephrine were higher ($P < 0.01$) than those determined by cortisol (91% versus 56%). In conclusion, metanephrine provides a superior analyte compared with cortisol in assessing the selectivity of adrenal vein sampling during procedures without cosyntropin stimulation.

▶ Adrenal venous sampling (AVS) is the gold standard for classifying patients with primary aldosteronism as having unilateral or bilateral disease. However, this technique requires experience in cannulating the right adrenal vein. So far, cautiously performed venographies are performed to distinguish the right adrenal vein from hepatic veins but rupture of the small adrenal vessel is a possible complication. In the past, it was shown that aldosterone concentrations are lower in hepatic veins[1] compared with peripheral values and that rapid assessment of cortisol helps verify a correct catheter position.[2,3]

However, aldosterone measurements have not been available as fast tests so far, and the determination of cortisol has certain disadvantages. Fast cortisol assays last 20 minutes at a minimum, and it is buffered as inactive cortisone or bound to transcortin. Therefore, the half-life of cortisol is relatively long, a fact that lowers the step-up in cortisol concentrations between adrenal and peripheral veins. On the other hand, metanephrine is an unbound metabolite of the adrenal medulla and has a short half-life, which leads to a huge concentration gradient.

Using this phenomenon, Dekkers et al show that the measurement of plasma metanephrine is superior to the measurement of cortisol in determining success of adrenal vein sampling. Interestingly, most AVS studies that were thought to have failed following the cortisol data had been successful on the basis of metanephrine analysis. Whether determination of plasma metanephrine also leads to a more sensitive recognition of asymmetric aldosterone secretion, however, needs to be studied.

H. S. Willenberg, MD

References

1. Solar M, Ceral J, Krajina A, et al. Adrenal venous sampling: where is the aldosterone disappearing to? *Cardiovasc Intervent Radiol.* 2010;33:760-765.
2. Mengozzi G, Rossato D, Bertello C, et al. Rapid cortisol assay during adrenal vein sampling in patients with primary aldosteronism. *Clin Chem.* 2007;53:1968-1971.
3. Betz MJ, Degenhart C, Fischer E, et al. Adrenal vein sampling using rapid cortisol assays in primary aldosteronism is useful in centers with low success rates. *Eur J Endocrinol.* 2011;165:301-306.

Pheochromocytomas: Diagnosis and Treatment

Genotype-Specific Abnormalities in Mitochondrial Function Associate with Distinct Profiles of Energy Metabolism and Catecholamine Content in Pheochromocytoma and Paraganglioma

Rao JU, Engelke UFH, Rodenburg RJT, et al (Radboud Univ Nijmegen Med Centre, the Netherlands; et al)

Clin Cancer Res 19:3787-3795, 2013

Purpose.—Pheochromocytomas and paragangliomas (PGL) are neuroendocrine tumors of sympathetic and parasympathetic paraganglia. This study investigated the relationships between genotype-specific differences in mitochondrial function and catecholamine content in PGL tumors.

Experimental Design.—Respiratory chain enzyme assays and ^{1}H-nuclear magnetic resonance (NMR) spectroscopy at 500 MHz were conducted on homogenates of 35 sporadic PGLs and 59 PGLs from patients with hereditary mutations in succinate dehydrogenase subunits B and D (*SDHB, SDHD*), succinate dehydrogenase assembly factor 2, von Hippel-Lindau (*VHL*), rearranged during transfection (*RET*), neurofibromatosis type 1 (*NF1*), and myc-associated factor X.

Results.—In SDHx-related PGLs, a significant decrease in complex II activity ($P < 0.0001$) and a significant increase in complex I, III, and IV enzyme activities were observed when compared to sporadic, RET, and NF1 tumors. Also, a significant increase in citrate synthase ($P < 0.0001$) enzyme activity was observed in SDHx related PGLs when compared to sporadic-, VHL-, RET-, and NF1-related tumors. An increase in succinate accumulation ($P < 0.001$) and decrease in ATP/ADP/AMP accumulation ($P < 0.001$) was observed when compared to sporadic PGLs and PGLs of other genotypes. Positive correlations ($P < 0.01$) were observed between respiratory chain complex II activity and total catecholamine content and ATP/ADP/AMP and total catecholamine contents in tumor tissues.

Conclusions.—This study for the first time establishes a relationship between determinants of energy metabolism, like activity of respiratory chain enzyme complex II, ATP/ADP/AMP content, and catecholamine content in PGL tumors. Also, this study for the first time successfully uses NMR spectroscopy to detect catecholamines in PGL tumors and provides *ex vivo* evidence for the accumulation of succinate in PGL tumors with an SDHx mutation.

▶ The biochemist Otto Warburg suggested that cancer cells develop when respiration, the cellular process of oxidative phosphorylation, is mildly impaired. He suggested that defective mitochondrial activity forces cells to meet their energy needs by switching to fermentation, glycolysis, despite aerobic conditions. During oxidative phosphorylation, mitochondrial complexes transfer electrons via a transport chain from donors to acceptors and generate ATP. The respiration chain is functionally completed by the Krebs (citrate) cycle. Malfunction of succinate dehydrogenases (SDH) results in ineffective metabolization of succinate, which puts the cell under oxidative stress. The SDH enzyme complex consists of different subgroups, including A, B, C, and D, and operates with the SDH assembly factor 2. Such defects were identified as a cause for hereditary paraganglioma syndromes.

This study shows that tumors with a defect in the SDH enzyme complex have a very low respiratory chain enzyme activity of complex II, leading to an increase in succinate content. As a result, generation of ATP, ADP, or AMP is significantly decreased and leads to an interrupted synthesis of (nor-) epinephrine. In the tissue of SDHx-associated PGL, the activities of respiratory chain complexes I, III, and IV and the function of citrate synthase are increased but cannot compensate for loss of SDH performance. This study is important because it closes the gap between Warburg's observations in ascites cancer cells and the suggestions derived by the molecular studies in SDHx-linked PGL disease. It links genotype to phenotype and shows differences in respiration and the metabolite contents of such tumors. The functional data can now be used to develop novel tools for differential diagnosis, localization, and treatment of SDHx-associated PGL.

H. S. Willenberg, MD

7 Reproductive Endocrinology

Introduction

I have selected a variety of studies for this year, including pediatric endocrinology, hormonal action of estrogen and androgens, menopause, the influence of hormones on bone metabolism, polycystic ovary syndrome, aging, hypogonadism in men, and male and female hormone action.

Each year there are many studies of polycystic ovary disease that extend our understanding of the pathophysiology. In "Clinical Review: Lifecycle of Polycystic Ovary Syndrome (PCOS): From In Utero to Menopause" Welt and Carmina proposed a model from in utero to adolescence where factors affected the development of PCOS. The model includes both genetic and early environmental factors, to which fetal androgen exposure and low birth weight contribute. Daughters of women with PCOS have a larger follicular ovarian component. Hyperandrogenism in women with PCOS persists in menopause. The details of the model require further study.

A topic that is currently controversial is whether testosterone replacement therapy is beneficial and the criteria used to identify men in whom therapy is safe and prolongs quality of life. The factors known to affect serum testosterone concentration include age, obesity, cardiovascular disease, type 2 diabetes, hypertension, depression, smoking, and insulin resistance. Shi and associates investigated these factors and serum testosterone levels ("Longitudinal Changes in Testosterone over Five Years in Community-Dwelling Men"). The testosterone decline was significantly affected by lifestyle factors and chronic conditions. They concluded that testosterone decline with age was not inevitable and is particularly affected by smoking, changes in health status, obesity, and depression.

Testosterone replacement therapy is reported in many studies each year, but the study of Finkelstein and colleagues ("Gonadal Steroids and Body Composition, Strength, and Sexual Function in Men") merits recognition. The criteria used by some for replacement therapy might not justify the therapy. The study took into consideration testosterone and its potent metabolites, dihydrotestosterone and estradiol 17-beta. The effects of sex steroids on body composition, strength, and sexual function under suppression of endogenous testosterone and estradiol were studied. The authors were able to confirm that lean body mass and muscle size were, as expected, androgen dependent. Body fat increases were estrogen dependent. The somewhat unexpected finding was that both androgen and estrogen influenced sexual function.

Another study that merits focus is "Effects of Estrogen on Bone mRNA Levels of Sclerostin and Other Genes Relevant to Bone Metabolism in Postmenopausal Women" by Fujita et al. Estrogen protects bone from development of bone loss and estrogen deficiency enhances bone loss. Fujita et al observed that estrogen inhibited sclerostin, which is known to cause bone loss through molecular means. It is known to inhibit osteoblasts. The development of an antibody to sclerostin has been used to treat osteoporosis successfully.

A. Wayne Meikle, MD

Pediatrics

Delayed Puberty and Estrogen Resistance in a Woman With Estrogen Receptor α Variant

Quaynor SD, Stradtman EW Jr, Kim H-G, et al (Georgia Regents Univ, Augusta; et al)
N Engl J Med 369:164-171, 2013

Although androgen resistance has been characterized in men with a normal chromosome complement and mutations in the androgen-receptor gene, a mutation in the gene encoding estrogen receptor α (*ESR1*) was previously described only in one man and not, to our knowledge, in a woman. We now describe an 18-year-old woman without breast development and with markedly elevated serum levels of estrogens and bilateral multicystic ovaries. She was found to have a homozygous loss-of-function *ESR1* mutation in a completely conserved residue that interferes with estrogen signaling. Her clinical presentation was similar to that in the mouse orthologue knockout. This case shows that disruption of *ESR1* causes profound estrogen resistance in women.

▶ Androgen resistance in humans with 46 XY karyotypes with mutations of the androgen receptor has been well characterized. An estrogen receptor mutation has also been observed in a man previously. Estrogen receptors α and β have been cloned and studied in knockout mice with these genes. Mice with knockout of both forms of estrogen receptor have hypoplastic uteri, poor breast development, and multicystic hemorrhagic ovaries without corpus lutea. Quaynor et al studied the consequences of estrogen receptor α variant in a young woman who had poor breast development, elevated serum estrogens, and bilateral multicystic ovaries. Administration of a progestin reduced the size of her ovaries, gonadotropins, and serum estradiol, suggesting that the pituitary gonadotropin feedback in response to progesterone was intact. She had acne but did not have elevated serum testosterone level. Estrogen resistance would be expected to be associated with reduced bone mass, and she did have lower-than-normal bone mass for her age and elevated bone turnover markers.[1-5]

A. W. Meikle, MD

References

1. Boada M, Antunez C, Lòpez-Arrieta J, et al. Estrogen receptor alpha gene variants are associated with Alzheimer's disease. *Neurobiol Aging*. 2012;33:198.e15-198.e24.
2. Grundberg E, Akesson K, Kindmark A, et al. The impact of estradiol on bone mineral density is modulated by the specific estrogen receptor-alpha cofactor retinoblastoma-interacting zinc finger protein-1 insertion/deletion polymorphism. *J Clin Endocrinol Metab*. 2007;92:2300-2306.
3. Itoh Y, Hayashi H, Miyazawa K, Kojima S, Akahoshi T, Onozaki K. 17beta-estradiol induces IL-1alpha gene expression in rheumatoid fibroblast-like synovial cells through estrogen receptor alpha (ERalpha) and augmentation of transcriptional activity of Sp1 by dissociating histone deacetylase 2 from ERalpha. *J Immunol*. 2007;178:3059-3066.
4. Quigley CA, Friedman KJ, Johnson A, et al. Complete deletion of the androgen receptor gene: definition of the null phenotype of the androgen insensitivity syndrome and determination of carrier status. *J Clin Endocrinol Metab*. 1992;74: 927-933.
5. Brown TR, Lubahn DB, Wilson EM, Joseph DR, French FS, Migeon CJ. Deletion of the steroid-binding domain of the human androgen receptor gene in one family with complete androgen insensitivity syndrome: evidence for further genetic heterogeneity in this syndrome. *Proc Natl Acad Sci U S A*. 1988;85:8151-8155.

Lifecycle of Polycystic Ovary Syndrome (PCOS): From In Utero to Menopause

Welt CK, Carmina E (Massachusetts General Hosp, Boston; Univ of Palermo, Italy)

J Clin Endocrinol Metab 98:4629-4638, 2013

Context.—Polycystic ovary syndrome (PCOS) is diagnosed during the reproductive years when women present with 2 of 3 of the following criteria: 1) irregular menstrual cycles or anovulation, 2) hyperandrogenism, and 3) PCO morphology. However, there is evidence that PCOS can be identified from early infancy to puberty based on predisposing environmental influences. There is also increasing information about the PCOS phenotype after menopause. The goal of this review is to summarize current knowledge about the appearance of PCOS at different life stages and the influence of reproductive maturation and senescence on the PCOS phenotype.

Evidence.—PubMed, the bibliography from the Evidence-Based PCOS Workshop, and the reference lists from identified manuscripts were reviewed.

Evidence Synthesis.—The current data suggest that daughters of women with PCOS have a greater follicle complement and mild metabolic abnormalities from infancy. PCOS is often diagnosed in puberty with the onset of hyperandrogenism and may be preceded by premature pubarche.

During the reproductive years, there is a gradual decrease in the severity of the cardinal features of PCOS. Menopausal data suggest that the majority of women who had PCOS during their reproductive years continue to manifest cardiovascular risk factors. However, the majority do not present an increased risk for cardiovascular morbidity and mortality, perhaps because women with no history of PCOS may catch up after menopause.

Conclusion.—The current data provide a comprehensive starting point to understand the phenotype of PCOS across the lifespan. However, limitations such as a bias of ascertainment in childhood, age-based changes during reproductive life, and the small numbers studied during menopause point to the need for additional longitudinal studies to expand the current knowledge.

▶ Polycystic ovary syndrome (PCOS) is commonly diagnosed during adolescence in association with menstrual irregularities and signs of androgen excess. Welt and Carmina postulated that earlier environmental and genetic factors contribute to the adolescent emergence, even those occurring in utero. The authors reviewed animal models of PCOS that showed that fetal androgen exposure results in a PCOS-like syndrome. Low birth weight is another factor associated with PCOS. The authors found evidence that daughters of women with PCOS had a larger follicle component and some metabolic abnormalities from early life. Metabolic alterations in PCOS lead to cardiovascular risk factors. Hyperandrogenism in women with PCOS persists into menopause compared with that in women without PCOS. The criteria for diagnosis of PCOS in young girls have not been clarified in this study, but it raises hope for continued research that might allow early normalization of the endocrine and metabolic abnormalities. This represents a start to unravel the clinical factors that contribute to PCOS in some women.[1-7]

A. W. Meikle, MD

References

1. Hoeger KM, Legro RS, Welt CK. A patient's guide: polycystic ovary syndrome (PCOS). *J Clin Endocrinol Metab.* 2014;99:35A-36A.
2. Pau C, Saxena R, Welt CK. Evaluating reported candidate gene associations with polycystic ovary syndrome. *Fertil Steril.* 2013;99:1774-1778.
3. Carroll J, Saxena R, Welt CK. Environmental and genetic factors influence age at menarche in women with polycystic ovary syndrome. *J Pediatr Endocrinol Metab.* 2012;25:459-466.
4. Welt CK, Styrkarsdottir U, Ehrmann DA, et al. Variants in DENND1A are associated with polycystic ovary syndrome in women of European ancestry. *J Clin Endocrinol Metab.* 2012;97:E1342-E1347.
5. Abbott DH, Nicol LE, Levine JE, Xu N, Goodarzi MO, Dumesic DA. Nonhuman primate models of polycystic ovary syndrome. *Mol Cell Endocrinol.* 2013;373:21-28.
6. Abbott DH, Barnett DK, Bruns CM, Dumesic DA. Androgen excess fetal programming of female reproduction: a developmental aetiology for polycystic ovary syndrome? *Hum Reprod Update.* 2005;11:357-374.
7. Dumesic DA, Schramm RD, Abbott DH. Early origins of polycystic ovary syndrome. *Reprod Fertil Dev.* 2005;17:349-360.

Androgen Excess in Adolescence

Prevalence of Hyperandrogenic States in Late Adolescent and Young Women: Epidemiological Survey on Italian High-School Students

Gambineri A, Fanelli F, Prontera O, et al (St Orsola-Malpighi Hosp, Bologna, Italy; et al)

J Clin Endocrinol Metab 98:1641-1650, 2013

Context.—Most of the estimates of the prevalence of hyperandrogenic states refer to the general adult population.

Objective.—The objective of the study was to estimate the prevalence of hyperandrogenic states in late adolescence and youth and to evaluate potential independent predictors.

Design.—This was a cross-sectional study.

Setting.—The study was conducted in high schools.

Patients.—Patients included female students, aged 16–19 years.

Main Outcome Measures.—The study protocol was designed with 3 possible levels of participation: the first level consisted of a self-compiled questionnaire; the second level added a medical examination; and the third level added a blood sample for laboratory testing. Liquid chromatography-tandem mass spectrometry was used to measure total testosterone, and a reference interval was established in-house.

Results.—We offered participation to 2052 students, and 1469 of those compiled the questionnaire. Of these, 1038 were examined, and 519 also provided blood samples. Two hundred three of the 1038 examined students and 125 of the 519 students who provided blood samples were subsequently excluded because of treatment with oral contraceptives or because of endocrine disorders. In the sample of women with a questionnaire + a medical examination, 13% were affected by isolated menstrual irregularity, 16.1% by isolated clinical hyperandrogenism, and 3.8% by both states. A similar prevalence of isolated menstrual irregularity (10.2%) and isolated clinical hyperandrogenism (16.7%) was found in the subsample of women with laboratory tests; in addition, 6.6% showed isolated hyperandrogenemia, and 4.3% proved to be affected by polycystic ovary syndrome.

Conclusions.—This study provides for the first time a reliable assessment of the prevalence of hyperandrogenic states in late adolescent and young females and confirms that hyperandrogenic disorders originate at a young age (Table 5).

► Hyperandrogenic conditions often become apparent during adolescence and youth. Polycystic ovary syndrome is the most common. Studies on the prevalence of hyperandrogenism in young females are limited. The diagnostic criteria for adults might be different than for youth, as irregular menses, oligoanovulation, or enlarged ovaries might be associated with normal adolescence. Hirsutism might underestimate the prevalence of hyperandrogenism. Serum concentrations of testosterone should be the best index, but specific reference intervals with specific, sensitive assays are needed. In the study of Gambineri et al,

TABLE 5.—Multivariate Analyses Predicting Hyperandrogenic State (Defined on the Basis of Medical Examination and Blood Sampling)

Variables	Isolated Menstrual Irregularity OR (95% CI)	*P* Value	Isolated Hyperandrogenemia OR (95% CI)[a]	*P* Value	Isolated Clinical Hyperandrogenism OR (95% CI)[b]	*P* Value	PCOS OR (95% CI)[a]	*P* Value
Gynecological age, 1-y increase	0.88 (0.70–1.11)	.3	0.93 (0.71–1.23)	.6	1.37 (1.14–1.64)	.001	1.04 (0.75–1.46)	.8
Mean BMI (SD)	1.00 (0.83–1.22)	.9	1.26 (1.01–1.59)	.033	1.12 (0.97–1.29)	.13	1.42 (1.09–1.84)	.009
Waist circumference, 1-cm increase	0.97 (0.91–1.04)	.3	1.00 (0.93–1.08)	.9	0.95 (0.90–0.99)	.039	0.91 (0.83–1.00)	.060
Acanthosis, yes vs no	2.70 (0.46–15.3)	.3	0.36 (0.03–4.04)	.4	4.03 (1.30–12.6)	.016	1.65 (0.19–14.5)	.6
HDL cholesterol, 1-U increase	1.02 (0.99–1.06)	.12	1.06 (1.03–1.10)	.001	1.00 (0.98–1.03)	.6	1.03 (0.99–1.08)	.2
Glucose levels, 1-mg/dL increase	1.00 (0.97–1.02)	.7	0.98 (0.95–1.01)	.3	1.00 (0.99–1.02)	.4	0.97 (0.92–1.00)	.052

Abbreviations: CI, confidence interval; HDL, high-density lipoprotein. Polytomous logistic regression model included all subjects who compiled the questionnaire were examined and provided blood samples and excluded those who were on active treatment with oral contraceptives and were diagnosed with thyroid dysfunction or hyperprolactinemia (n = 394; see Table 1). For all ORs and relative 95% CIs, the reference category was normality. The following covariates were also tested for significance: age at menarche, weight, waist to hip ratio, percentage of fatty mass, diastolic blood pressure, total cholesterol, triglycerides, fasting insulin, HOMA, and QUICKI. None of them was significant, and they were not included in the final model because of multicollinearity with 1 or more of the covariates reported in the table. Age (nonsignificant in all models) was also excluded because of the relatively scarce sample size to reduce the likelihood of overfitting.

[a]The number of subjects (successes) in this group was very small (fewer than 30): the lack of significance for some covariates could be due to an insufficient statistical power, and the results should be interpreted with caution (see text for more details).

[b]Five subjects had clinical hyperandrogenism combined with hyperandrogenemia.

reference intervals were established, and testosterone was measured by liquid chromatography-tandem mass spectrometry. The criteria used for hyperandrogenic states were menstrual irregularities with more than 6 cycles with a length more than 35 days per year. Clinical hyperandrogenism was defined as the presence of hirsutism. Acne was not considered a clinical sign. Hyperandrogenism was defined by the 97.5th percentile of the reference interval related to the menstrual cycle. The prevalence of hyperandrogenism was determined.[1-5]

A. W. Meikle, MD

References

1. Pinola P, Lashen H, Bloigu A, et al. Menstrual disorders in adolescence: a marker for hyperandrogenaemia and increased metabolic risks in later life? Finnish general population-based birth cohort study. *Hum Reprod.* 2012;27:3279-3286.
2. Alemzadeh R, Kichler J, Calhoun M. Spectrum of metabolic dysfunction in relationship with hyperandrogenemia in obese adolescent girls with polycystic ovary syndrome. *Eur J Endocrinol.* 2010;162:1093-1099.
3. Fruzzetti F, Perini D, Lazzarini V, Parrini D, Genazzani AR. Hyperandrogenemia influences the prevalence of the metabolic syndrome abnormalities in adolescents with the polycystic ovary syndrome. *Gynecol Endocrinol.* 2009;25:335-343.
4. Kushnir MM, Blamires T, Rockwood AL, et al. Liquid chromatography-tandem mass spectrometry assay for androstenedione, dehydroepiandrosterone, and testosterone with pediatric and adult reference intervals. *Clin Chem.* 2010;56: 1138-1147.
5. Meikle AW, Kushnir MM, Rockwood AL, et al. Adrenal steroid concentrations in children seven to seventeen years of age. *J Pediatr Endocrinol Metab.* 2007;20: 1281-1291.

Polycystic Ovary Syndrome

Evidence for Masculinization of Adipokine Gene Expression in Visceral and Subcutaneous Adipose Tissue of Obese Women With Polycystic Ovary Syndrome (PCOS)

Martínez-García MÁ, Montes-Nieto R, Fernández-Durán E, et al (Universidad de Alcalá and Hospital Universitario Ramón y Cajal, Madrid, Spain; Centro de Investigación Biomédica en Red Diabetes y Enfermedades Metabó licas Asociadas, Madrid, Spain)

J Clin Endocrinol Metab 98:E388-E396, 2013

Context.—Sex hormones, particularly androgens, may influence not only adipose tissue distribution but also its functions.

Objective.—We explored the possibility of sexual dimorphism in adipose tissue and skeletal muscle function.

Design.—This was a case-control study.

Setting.—The setting was an academic hospital.

Participants.—Participants were severely obese men (n = 7), control women (n = 7), and hyperandrogenic women presenting with polycystic ovary syndrome (PCOS) (n = 7) submitting to bariatric surgery and an independent series of 40 patients with PCOS and 40 control women matched for age and body mass index.

Interventions.—Samples of subcutaneous (SAT) and visceral adipose tissue (VAT) and skeletal muscle were obtained during bariatric surgery in severely obese subjects.

Main Outcome Measures.—Gene expression of chemerin, lipocalin-2, and omentin-1 in tissue samples was measured. We analyzed the effects of PCOS and obesity on serum concentrations of these adipokines in the larger series of women with PCOS and in control women.

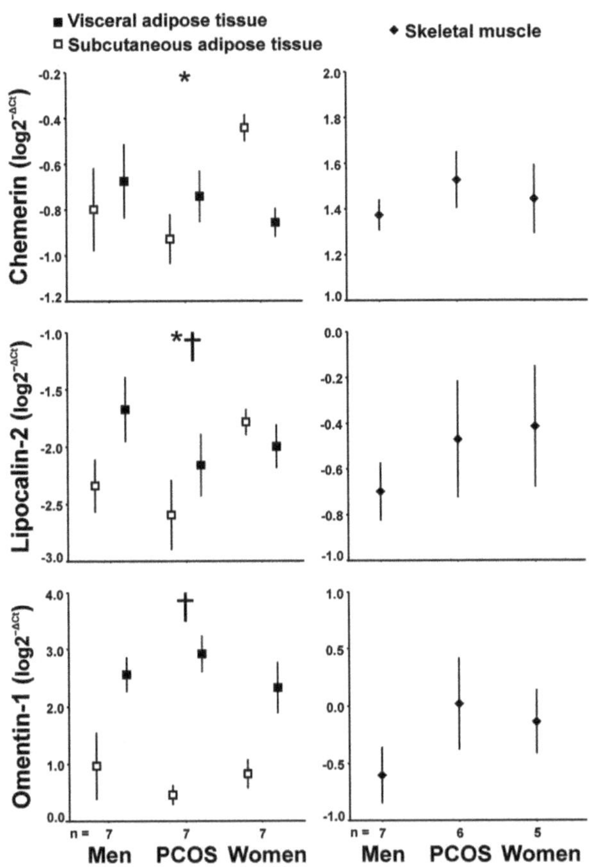

FIGURE 1.—Differences between obese men, obese patients with PCOS, and obese control women in the gene expression of chemerin, lipocalin-2, and omentin-1 in SAT and VAT and in skeletal muscle. Data are means ± SEM. *$P < .05$ or less for the interaction between adipose tissue depot and group of subjects, meaning that the differences in gene expression were not the same in men, patients with PCOS, and control women. †$P < .05$ or less for differences between SAT and VAT considering men, patients with PCOS, and control women as a whole. There were no differences in the global adipose tissue gene expression of chemerin ($P = .540$), lipocalin-2 ($P = .423$), and omentin-1 ($P = .913$) between men, patients with PCOS, and control women. (Reprinted from Martínez-García MÁ, Montes-Nieto R, Fernández-Durán E, et al. Evidence for masculinization of adipokine gene expression in visceral and subcutaneous adipose tissue of obese women with polycystic ovary syndrome (PCOS). *J Clin Endocrinol Metab*. 2013;98:E388-E396, Copyright 2013, with permission from The Endocrine Society.)

Results.—Expression of chemerin and lipocalin-2 was higher in VAT than in SAT in men and women with PCOS; the opposite was observed in control women. Omentin-1 expression was higher in VAT than in SAT in the three groups. No differences were observed in the skeletal muscle expression of these adipokines. Obesity increased serum chemerin and lipocalin-2 levels and tended to decrease omentin-1, irrespective of PCOS.

Conclusions.—The present results suggest that there is sexual dimorphism in some adipose tissue functions and that this dimorphism may be related to differences in androgen concentrations because women with PCOS show a masculinized pattern of expression of some adipokines (Fig 1).

► Diabetes dependent on obesity is common and is associated with considerable morbidity and mortality. Adipose tissue is an endocrine organ with interplay on the genesis of diabetes. In addition to fat cells, adipose tissue also has stromal preadipocytes, immune cells, and endothelium. Adipokines are similar to cytokines. Adipose tissue includes subcutaneous and visceral adipose tissue. Of these fat cells, visceral adipose tissue is associated with more metabolic disorders. Sexual dimorphism of body adipose tissue influences the distribution of adipose tissue and is affected by both estrogens and androgens. Women with polycystic ovary syndrome have higher androgens and have a tendency toward central distribution of fat, particularly visceral fat.[1,2] However, this study suggested that the sexual dimorphism of adipose tissue is not restricted to the distribution of body fat but also influences several adipokines in different adipose deposits. They also suggested that androgen excess might influence adipose tissue function in addition to its distribution.

A. W. Meikle, MD

References

1. Glintborg D, Andersen M. An update on the pathogenesis, inflammation, and metabolism in hirsutism and polycystic ovary syndrome. *Gynecol Endocrinol.* 2010;26:281-296.
2. Spritzer PM, Comim FV, Capp E, D'Avila A. Influence of leptin, androgens and insulin sensitivity on increased GH response to clonidine in lean patients with polycystic ovary syndrome. *Horm Metab Res.* 2005;37:94-98.

Menopause

Changes in Estradiol and Testosterone Levels in Postmenopausal Women After Changes in Body Mass Index

Jones ME, Schoemaker M, Rae M, et al (Univ of London, Sutton, UK)
J Clin Endocrinol Metab 98:2967-2974, 2013

Context.—Endogenous sex hormones are risk factors for postmenopausal breast cancer. A potential route for favorable hormonal modification is weight loss.

Objective.—The objective of the study was to measure change in plasma estradiol and testosterone levels in postmenopausal women in relation to change in body mass index (BMI) and plasma leptin.

Setting.—The setting was a cohort study of over 100 000 female volunteers from the general population, United Kingdom.

Participants.—The participants were a sample of 177 postmenopausal women aged over 45 years who provided blood samples during 2004–2005 and again during 2010–2011.

Main Outcome Measure.—Outcomes were percentage change in plasma estradiol and testosterone levels per 1 kg/m^{2}change in BMI and per 1 ng/mL change in plasma leptin.

Results.—Among women with reduction in BMI, estradiol decreased 12.7% (95% confidence interval: [6.4%, 19.5%]; $P < .0001$) per kg/m^2 and among women with increased BMI estradiol increased 6.4% [0.2%, 12.9%] ($P = .042$). The corresponding figures for testosterone were 10.7% [3.0%, 19.0%] ($P = .006$) and 1.9% [−5.4%, 9.7%] ($P = .61$) per kg/m^2. For women with decreases and increases in leptin, estradiol decreased by 3.6% [1.3%, 6.0%] ($P = .003$) per ng/mL and increased by 1.7% [−0.3%, 3.6%] ($P = .094$), respectively. The corresponding figures for testosterone were 4.8% [2.0%, 7.8%] ($P = .009$) and 0.3% [−2.0%, 2.6%] ($P = .82$) per ng/mL.

Conclusions.—In postmenopausal women, changes in BMI and plasma leptin occurring over several years are associated with changes in estradiol and testosterone levels. The results suggest that fat loss by an individual can result in substantial decreases in postmenopausal estradiol and testosterone levels and provides support for weight management to lessen breast cancer risk (Table 2).

▶ Breast cancer risk in postmenopausal women is associated with body mass index (BMI) and endogenous estrogen concentrations. High BMI is linked to elevated endogenous estrogen concentrations. Serum testosterone concentrations in women are associated with BMI and postmenopausal breast cancer risk. In postmenopausal women, the ovary is less of a contributor to serum estrogen concentrations, and the fat cells become an important source. In short-term studies, exercise or fat cell loss might be important in lowering both serum estrogen and testosterone concentrations. In the 5- to 6-year study by Jones et al, they assessed changes in BMI, estradiol, testosterone, and leptin, which they felt was a more direct measure of body fat than BMI. They observed that both serum estrogen and testosterone concentrations declined over time in association with the changes in BMI and leptin. Although their study does not establish that fat cell loss decreases breast cancer risk in postmenopausal women, it would support the hypothesis, and future studies will be required to establish the link.[1-5]

A. W. Meikle, MD

TABLE 2.—Percentage Change in Total and Free Estradiol and Testosterone, and Sex Hormone Binding Globulin, for a 1 kg/m^2 Change in BMI, for 177[a] Postmenopausal Women from the Breakthrough Generations Study, United Kingdom

	Average Change in Analyte for a 1 kg/m^2 Change in BMI (within the same individual)										
	Women with Decrease in BMI			Women with Increase in BMI[b]				All BMI			
	N	Percent Change in Analyte per 1 kg/m^2	95% Confidence Interval	N	Percent Change in Analyte per 1 kg/m^2	95% Confidence Interval	Difference in Slope (P value)	N	Percent Change in Analyte per 1 kg/m^2	95% Confidence Interval	R^{2c}
Total estradiol	84	12.7	6.4, 19.5	92	6.4	0.2, 12.9	0.27	176	9.6	6.1, 13.1	15.7
Estimated free estradiol	84	15.2	8.7, 21.9	92	8.5	2.2, 15.1	0.24	176	11.8	8.3, 15.5	21.8
Total testosterone	85	10.7	3.0, 19.0	92	1.9	−5.4, 9.7	0.19	177	6.3	2.2, 10.6	5.1
Estimated free testosterone	85	14.7	6.7, 23.3	92	5.9	−1.7, 14.0	0.20	177	10.3	6.0, 14.7	11.9
Sex hormone binding globulin	85	−5.1	−7.3, −3.0	92	−6.2	−8.4, −4.0	0.58	177	−5.7	−6.8, −4.5	33.2

[a]The estradiol assay was unquantifiable for one sample.
[b]BMI was unchanged for 5 women, and these women are counted in this group. (Counting them in either group does not affect the results of the linear regression, which used indicator variables to estimate simultaneously separate slopes for decreases and increases in BMI.)
[c]R^2, coefficient of determination from linear regression.

References

1. Petekkaya I, Sahin U, Gezgen G, et al. Association of breast cancer subtypes and body mass index. *Tumori.* 2013;99:129-133.
2. Dallal CM, Brinton LA, Bauer DC, et al. Obesity-related hormones and endometrial cancer among postmenopausal women: a nested case-control study within the B~FIT cohort. *Endocr Relat Cancer.* 2013;20:151-160.
3. Biglia N, Peano E, Sgandurra P, et al. Body mass index (BMI) and breast cancer: impact on tumor histopathologic features, cancer subtypes and recurrence rate in pre and postmenopausal women. *Gynecol Endocrinol.* 2013;29:263-267.
4. Folkerd EJ, Dixon JM, Renshaw L, A'Hern RP, Dowsett M. Suppression of plasma estrogen levels by letrozole and anastrozole is related to body mass index in patients with breast cancer. *J Clin Oncol.* 2012;30:2977-2980.
5. Liedtke S, Schmidt ME, Vrieling A, et al. Postmenopausal sex hormones in relation to body fat distribution. *Obesity (Silver Spring).* 2012;20:1088-1095.

Contraception

Effect of a new oral contraceptive with estradiol valerate/dienogest on carbohydrate metabolism

De Leo V, Fruzzetti F, Musacchio MC, et al (Univ of Siena, Italy; Univ of Pisa, Italy)

Contraception 88:364-368, 2013

Background.—Insulin resistance may be induced by both the estrogen and progestin component in hormonal contraception. When estrogen dose is reduced from 50 to 20 mcg, the extent of hyperinsulinemia decreases. Recently, the oral combination contraceptive (COC) containing estradiol valerate (E2V) in combination with dienogest (DNG) was developed in a new estrogen step-down, progesterone step-up dosing strategy (Qlaira, Bayer Healthcare Pharmaceuticals). This study was conducted to evaluate of the effect of a 3-month treatment with E2V/DNG on carbohydrate metabolism in women with polycystic ovarian syndrome (PCOS) and insulin resistance.

Study Design.—Study consisted of subjects attending the gynecological clinic of Siena or Pisa, with PCOS and insulin resistance, and without contraindications for the use of COCs. PCOS females ($n = 20$) aged 18 to 33 years were treated with a contraceptive formulation containing E2V/DNG for 3 months. Before treatment and during the third month of therapy, body mass index (BMI) measurement and an oral glucose tolerance test (OGTT) were performed.

Results.—Median values of insulin after treatment were lower than median values before treatment. In particular, the median value of insulin at T_0 was reduced by 54.6% ($p<.001$), and the mean difference between time 0 and 30 min was significantly reduced [42.96 (9.99) mU/mL vs 38.00 (15.10) mU/mL; $p<.05$]. Homeostasis model assessment of insulin resistance levels were significantly decreased following treatment. OGTT after treatment revealed median fasting glucose levels to be stable ($p=.895$) at T_0. At T_{30}, T_{60}, T_{120} and T_{180} min, glucose median values were moderately reduced in comparison to median values before treatment. No significant difference was observed between median BMI values before [26 (4.8) kg/m^2] and after treatment [26 (3.7) kg/m^2].

Conclusions.—Median insulin levels at T_0 and the mean difference between time 0 and 30 of insulin following OGTT were significantly reduced than values before treatment with E2V/DNG for 3 months. Median BMI and glucose levels were not significantly modified. Natural estradiol and nonandrogenic progestogen in the Qlaira formulation could be recommended as an oral contraceptive in women with PCOS who are insulin resistant or who are overweight (Fig 3).

▶ Synthetic steroid contraceptives (SSC) have been implicated in adverse changes in lipoproteins, insulin sensitivity, coagulation and cardiovascular events, and venous stasis with clotting. Some combinations of estrogen and progestin have more adverse effects on these parameters than others. High doses of estrogen and progestin are known to have a more profound effect on modulation of glucose tolerance than preparations with lower doses. Shifting the balance toward a lower dose of estrogen compared with progestin favors reduced hyperinsulinemia. Thus, the combination of birth control preparations has required careful assessment. De Leo et al investigated the effect of a new oral contraceptive formulated with estradiol valerate/dienogest on carbohydrate metabolism. In short-term experiments, insulin requirement improved in participants compared to baseline, and they had improved homeostasis model assessment of insulin resistance after 3 months of therapy. The authors suggest that this SSC might be of benefit, particularly to women with polycystic ovary syndrome, because most of them have insulin resistance. Further study is

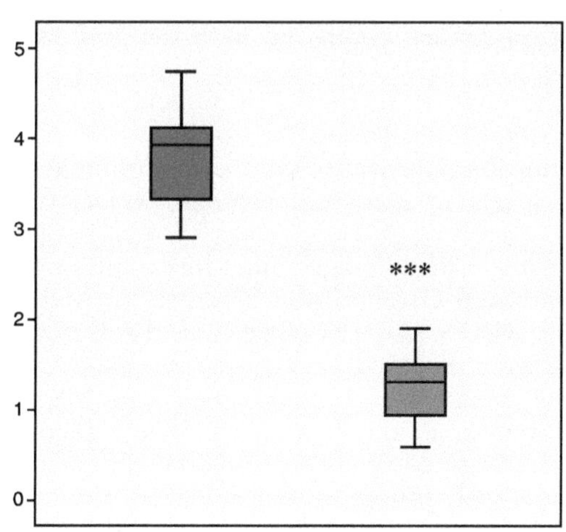

FIGURE 3.—Change in HOMA-IR values at baseline and 3 months after E2V/DNG treatment. Boxes represent value distribution; vertical lines represent on the bottom the minimum value and on the top the maximum value. Data are presented as medians and IOR. ***p<.001. (Reprinted from De Leo V, Fruzzetti F, Musacchio MC, et al. Effect of a new oral contraceptive with estradiol valerate/dienogest on carbohydrate metabolism. *Contraception* 2013;88:364-368, Copyright 2013, with permission from Elsevier.)

required to test the hypothesis that women with polycystic ovarian syndrome and normal women will have beneficial outcomes with long-term use.[1-4]

A. W. Meikle, MD

References

1. Lopez LM, Grimes DA, Schulz KF. Steroidal contraceptives: effect on carbohydrate metabolism in women without diabetes mellitus. *Cochrane Database Syst Rev.* 2012;(4):CD006133.
2. Sitruk-Ware R, Nath A. Metabolic effects of contraceptive steroids. *Rev Endocr Metab Disord.* 2011;12:63-75.
3. Wiegratz I, Stahlberg S, Manthey T, et al. Effects of combined oral contraceptive ethinylestradiol (30 microg) and dienogest (2 mg) on carbohydrate metabolism during 1 year of conventional or extended-cycle use. *Horm Metab Res.* 2010; 42:358-363.
4. Demir B, Ozturkoglu E, Solaroglu A, et al. The effects of estrogen therapy and estrogen combined with different androgenic progestins on carbohydrate and lipid metabolism in overweight-obese younger postmenopausal women. *Gynecol Endocrinol.* 2008;24:347-353.

Estrogen Assays

Comparisons of Immunoassay and Mass Spectrometry Measurements of Serum Estradiol Levels and Their Influence on Clinical Association Studies in Men

Ohlsson C, Nilsson ME, Tivesten Å, et al (Univ of Gothenburg, Sweden; et al)
J Clin Endocrinol Metab 98:E1097-E1102, 2013

Context.—Immunoassay-based techniques, routinely used to measure serum estradiol (E2), are known to have reduced specificity, especially at lower concentrations, when compared with the gold standard technique of mass spectrometry (MS). Different measurement techniques may be responsible for the conflicting results of associations between serum E2 and clinical phenotypes in men.

Objective.—Our objective was to compare immunoassay and MS measurements of E2 levels in men and evaluate associations with clinical phenotypes.

Design and Setting.—Middle-aged and older male subjects participating in the population-based Osteoporotic Fractures in Men (MrOS) Sweden study ($n = 2599$), MrOS US ($n = 688$), and the European Male Aging Study ($n = 2908$) were included.

Main Outcome Measures.—Immunoassay and MS measurements of serum E2 were compared and related to bone mineral density (BMD; measured by dual energy x-ray absorptiometry) and ankle-brachial index.

Results.—Within each cohort, serum E2 levels obtained by immunoassay and MS correlated moderately (Spearman rank correlation coefficient r_S 0.53–0.76). Serum C-reactive protein (CRP) levels associated significantly (albeit to a low extent, $r_S = 0.29$) with immunoassay E2 but not with MS E2 levels. Similar associations of immunoassay E2 and MS E2 were seen with lumbar spine and total hip BMD, independent of serum

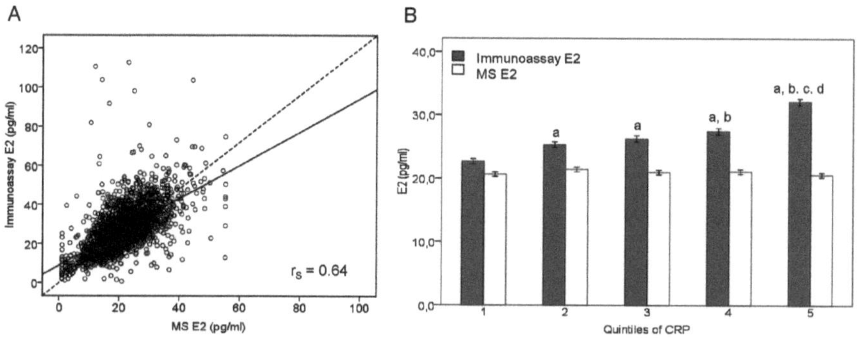

FIGURE 1.—Correlation between immunoassay and MS E2 and relation with CRP levels. A, Scatter plot of the correlation between E2 measured by immunoassay and MS in MrOS Sweden (n = 2599). The Spearman rank correlation coefficient (rS) as well as the linear regression line (solid line) and the line of full agreement (dashed line) is indicated. B, Mean serum E2 levels (± SE), measured either by immunoassay or MS, according to quintiles of serum CRP in MrOS Sweden. Limits of CRP levels were 1.56 or less for quintile 1, greater than 1.56 and 1.92 or less for quintile 2, greater than 1.92 and 2.44 or less for quintile 3, greater than 2.44 and 3.64 or less for quintile 4, and greater than 3.64 mg/L for quintile 5. a, $P < .05$ vs quintile 1; b, $P < .05$ vs quintile 2; c, $P < .05$ vs quintile 3; d, $P < .05$ vs quintile 4. (Reprinted from Ohlsson C, Nilsson ME, Tivesten Å, et al. Comparisons of immunoassay and mass spectrometry measurements of serum estradiol levels and their influence on clinical association studies in men. *J Clin Endocrinol Metab*. 2013;98:E1097-E1102, Copyright 2013, with permission from the Author[s] and The Endocrine Society.)

CRP. However, immunoassay E2, but not MS E2, associated inversely with ankle-brachial index, and this correlation was lost after adjustment for CRP.

Conclusions.—Our findings suggest interference in the immunoassay E2 analyses, possibly by CRP or a CRP-associated factor. Although associations with BMD remain unaffected, this might imply for a reevaluation of previous association studies between immunoassay E2 levels and inflammation-related outcomes (Fig 1).

▶ Estradiol is commonly measured by immunoassays in both clinical and research assessments. With sensitive and specific mass spectrometry (MS)-based estradiol assays, the sensitivity, specificity, and accuracy of immunoassays have been questioned.[1,2] These issues are critical in conducting studies for determining outcomes related to mortality, cardiovascular disease, and bone health. They observed potential interference with the immunoassay with a C-reactive protein (CRP)-associated factor, but it was not associated with hormonal measurement by MS. The nature of the interference with the immunoassay was not ascertained. However, the associations between immunoassay results and bone mineral density (BMD) of the lumbar spine and total hip were still valid, regardless of CRP concentrations. Khosla et al also observed that serum estradiol quantitated by MS showed similar correlations with BMD parameters as found with immunoassays.[3,4] There are limitations of the study. Single measurements of serum estradiol were made, and more specific indirection extraction-based immunoassay methods with MS could not be made.

A. W. Meikle, MD

References

1. Kushnir MM, Rockwood AL, Yue B, Meikle AW. High sensitivity measurement of estrone and estradiol in serum and plasma using LC-MS/MS. *Methods Mole Biol.* 2010;603:219-228.
2. Kushnir MM, Rockwood AL, Bergquist J, et al. High-sensitivity tandem mass spectrometry assay for serum estrone and estradiol. *Am J Clin Pathol.* 2008; 129:530-539.
3. Khosla S, Amin S, Singh RJ, Atkinson EJ, Melton LJ 3rd, Riggs BL. Comparison of sex steroid measurements in men by immunoassay versus mass spectroscopy and relationships with cortical and trabecular volumetric bone mineral density. *Osteoporos Int.* 2008;19:1465-1471.
4. Syed FA, Oursler MJ, Hefferanm TE, Peterson JM, Riggs BL, Khosla S. Effects of estrogen therapy on bone marrow adipocytes in postmenopausal osteoporotic women. *Osteoporos Int.* 2008;19:1323-1330.

Bone Health

Effects of Estrogen on Bone mRNA Levels of Sclerostin and Other Genes Relevant to Bone Metabolism in Postmenopausal Women

Fujita K, Roforth MM, Demaray S, et al (Mayo Clinic College of Medicine, Rochester, MN)

J Clin Endocrinol Metab 99:E81-E88, 2014

Context.—Studies in postmenopausal women have shown that estrogen reduces circulating sclerostin levels, but effects of estrogen on skeletal sclerostin mRNA levels are unknown.

Objective.—The objective of the study was to evaluate the effects of short-term estrogen treatment on bone mRNA levels of sclerostin and other genes relevant to bone metabolism.

Design, Setting, and Patients.—Needle bone biopsies were obtained from 20 postmenopausal women treated with transdermal estrogen for 3 weeks and 20 untreated controls. Quantitative PCR analyses were used to examine the expression of sclerostin and other genes related to bone metabolism, including 71 additional genes linked to bone density/fracture from genome-wide association studies.

Results.—Estrogen treatment was associated with lower bone sclerostin mRNA levels (by 48%, $P < .05$) and with lower (by 54%, $P < .01$) mRNA levels of the sclerostin-related protein, sclerostin domain-containing protein 1 (*SOSTDC1*), which is also a Wnt/bone morphogenetic protein inhibitor. Consistent with studies in mice showing that ovariectomy increased nuclear factor-κB (NF-κB) activation, we found that estrogen treatment was associated with a significant reduction in inflammatory genes as a group ($P = .028$), with bone mRNA levels of *NFKB2* and *RELB* (both encoding proteins in the NF-κB transcription factor complex) being significantly reduced individual genes. Eight of the 71 genome-wide association study-related genes examined were modulated by estrogen ($P < .05$, false discovery rate < 0.10).

Conclusion.—In humans, estrogen-induced decreases in two key inhibitors of Wnt/bone morphogenetic protein signaling, sclerostin and *SOSTDC1*, along with reductions in NF-κB signaling, may be responsible for at least part of the protective effects of estrogen on bone.

► Estrogens are known to protect from increased bone turnover, bone loss, and fracture risk. These effects are attributed to inhibition of osteoclast. Deficiency results in increased remodeling of bone, which is associated with bone resorption. However, it leaves a gap between bone resorption and formation, with resorption keeping ahead of formation. Abrupt withdrawal of estrogen results in a marked increase and decrease in bone turnover as reflected by increase in bone turnover markers. Chronic estrogen therapy in postmenopausal women reverses bone resorption markers. Fujita et al report on the estrogen effects on bone mRNA levels of sclerostin and other genes in bone metabolism. They confirm previous studies that estrogen treatment is associated with reduction in circulating sclerostin serum concentrations and sclerostin, which is known to inhibit osteoblasts. Fujita and associates observed that estrogen inhibited sclerostin bone mRNA as well. Estrogen also inhibited *SOSTDCi*, which Wnt (known to inhibit osteoclastogenesis) and bone morphogenetic protein signal.[1]

A. W. Meikle, MD

Reference

1. Roforth MM, Fujita K, McGregor UI, et al. Effects of age on bone mRNA levels of sclerostin and other genes relevant to bone metabolism in humans. *Bone*. 2014;59:1-6.

Bone Marrow Fat Composition as a Novel Imaging Biomarker in Postmenopausal Women With Prevalent Fragility Fractures

Patsch JM, Li X, Baum T, et al (Univ of California San Francisco)

J Bone Miner Res 28:1721-1728, 2013

The goal of this magnetic resonance (MR) imaging study was to quantify vertebral bone marrow fat content and composition in diabetic and nondiabetic postmenopausal women with fragility fractures and to compare them with nonfracture controls with and without type 2 diabetes mellitus. Sixty-nine postmenopausal women (mean age 63 ± 5 years) were recruited. Thirty-six patients (47.8%) had spinal and/or peripheral fragility fractures. Seventeen fracture patients were diabetic. Thirty-three women (52.2%) were nonfracture controls. Sixteen women were diabetic nonfracture controls. To quantify vertebral bone marrow fat content and composition, patients underwent MR spectroscopy (MRS) of the lumbar spine at 3 Tesla. Bone mineral density (BMD) was determined by dual-energy X-ray absorptiometry (DXA) of the hip and lumbar spine (LS) and quantitative computed tomography (QCT) of the LS. To evaluate associations of vertebral marrow fat content and composition with spinal and/or peripheral fragility fractures and diabetes, we used linear regression models adjusted for age, race, and spine volumetric bone mineral density (vBMD) by QCT. At the LS, nondiabetic and diabetic fracture patients had lower vBMD than controls and diabetics without fractures ($p = 0.018$; $p = 0.005$). However, areal bone mineral density (aBMD) by DXA did not differ between fracture and nonfracture patients. After adjustment for age, race, and spinal vBMD, the prevalence of fragility fractures was associated with −1.7% lower unsaturation levels (confidence interval [CI] −2.8% to −0.5%, $p = 0.005$) and +2.9% higher saturation levels (CI 0.5% to 5.3%, $p = 0.017$). Diabetes was associated with −1.3% (CI −2.3% to −0.2%, $p = 0.018$) lower unsaturation and +3.3% (CI 1.1% to 5.4%, $p = 0.004$) higher saturation levels. Diabetics with fractures had the lowest marrow unsaturation and highest saturation. There were no associations of marrow fat content with diabetes or fracture. Our results suggest that altered bone marrow fat composition is linked with fragility fractures and diabetes. MRS of spinal bone marrow fat may therefore serve as a novel tool for BMD-independent fracture risk assessment (Fig 2).

▶ Links between bone and adipose tissue have been investigated. One link is that mesenchymal stem cells and osteoblasts and adipocytes have a common origin. Another link is that aging and estrogen deficiency, which are associated with osteoporosis, are associated with lower osteogenic and more fat cell linage derived from mesenchymal stem cells. Disorders associated with alteration in fat or fat distribution are observed to have lower bone density. With an interest in bone marrow fat and osteoporosis, noninvasive imaging techniques, such as magnetic resonance spectroscopy, are being used to assess bone quality. Patsch et al investigated the bone marrow fat composition with new imaging

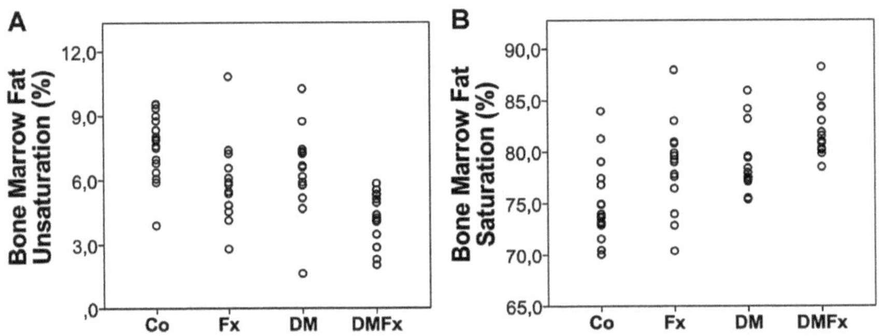

FIGURE 2.—Bone marrow fat composition in controls (Co), postmenopausal women with fragility fractures (Fx), diabetic postmenopausal women without fractures (DM), and diabetic postmenopausal women with fragility fractures (DMFx). (*A*) Unsaturation levels. (*B*) Saturation levels. (Reproduced from Journal of Bone and Mineral Research. Patsch JM, Li X, Baum T, et al. Bone marrow fat composition as a novel imaging biomarker in postmenopausal women with prevalent fragility fractures. *J Bone Miner Res.* 2013;28:1721-1728, with permission from the American Society for Bone and Mineral Research.)

techniques with the goal of evaluating fragility fractures. They found that altered bone marrow fat was associated with fragility fractures and diabetes. How lower unsaturated fat and higher saturation concentrations of bone marrow predispose to fragility fractures requires additional investigation. Total marrow fat content did not differ between those with fractures and those without, irrespective of diabetes. Another surprising finding was that lower unsaturated fat and higher saturated fat components predisposed to a higher fracture risk.

A. W. Meikle, MD

Role of Metabolic Factors in the Association Between Osteocalcin and Testosterone in Chinese Men

Liao M, Guo X, Yu X, et al (First Affiliated Hosp of Guangxi Med Univ, Nanning, Guangxi, People's Republic of China; et al)
J Clin Endocrinol Metab 98:3463-3469, 2013

Objective.—Osteocalcin can regulate energy metabolism and increase testosterone production. Although previous studies have shown the positive association between osteocalcin and testosterone, the effect of metabolic factors in the association is unclear.

Design and Setting.—Osteocalcin, testosterone, and metabolic factors were accessed in 2400 men aged 20 to 69 years, who participated in the population-based Fangchenggang Area Male Health and Examination Survey in Guangxi province of China from September 2009 to December 2009.

Main Outcome Measures.—Metabolic syndrome was defined based on the updated report of National Cholesterol Education Program Adult Treatment Panel III criteria. Serum total osteocalcin, total testosterone (TT), and sex hormone binding globulin (SHBG) were measured, whereas free testosterone (FT) and bioavailable testosterone (BT) were calculated based on Vermeulen's formula. The multivariable linear regression analysis was used.

Results.—Osteocalcin was positively associated with TT, FT, and BT in the unadjusted model (all $P < .001$). After adjusting for age, the positive association between osteocalcin and TT remained statistically significant ($\beta = .17$,95% confidence interval = 0.14–0.20) and was not attenuated in each MetS subgroup including hypertriglyceridemia, hyperglycemia, elevated blood pressure, and low high-density lipoprotein cholesterol, while in the group of central obesity (waist circumstance ≥90 cm), the association appeared significantly stronger ($\beta = 0.21$, 95% confidence interval = 0.12–0.30). After further adjusting for SHBG, osteocalcin was positively associated with TT, FT, and BT in men with central obesity or men with any two MetS components (all $P < .05$).

TABLE 3.—Association Between Osteocalcin and Testosterone in the Linear Regression Analysis

		β-Coefficient[b] (95% CI)	
	Unadjusted	Age-adjusted	Age- and SHBG-adjusted
TT	0.18 (0.15, 0.21); $P<.001$	0.17 (0.14, 0.20); $P<.001$	0.01 (−0.01, 0.04); $P=.217$
FT	0.08 (0.47, 0.78); $P<.001$	0.08 (−0.09, 0.20); $P=.484$	0.08 (−0.01, 0.29); $P=.069$
BT	0.05 (0.04, 0.07); $P<.001$	0.01 (−0.01, 0.02); $P=.485$	0.01 (−0.01, 0.03); $P=.069$

Conclusions.—Serum total osteocalcin is positively associated with testosterone, which is probably modified by SHBG and central obesity (Table 3).

▶ Osteocalcin can be produced in human adipose tissue and has been related to abdominal obesity in men.[1] In a recent cross-sectional study in men with type 2 diabetes mellitus, undercarboxylated osteocalcin (unOC) was positively associated with free testosterone independent of body mass index (BMI).[2] UnOC administration has been shown to regulate gene expression in both adipose and pancreatic β cells, which are involved in the development of the metabolic syndrome and type 2 diabetes mellitus.[3,4] Liao and associates conducted a cross-sectional study to assess the association between osteocalcin and testosterone. They observed a significant positive correction between total testosterone and osteocalcin but not between osteocalcin, free testosterone, bioavailable testosterone, and sex hormone–binding globulin (SHBG). However, osteocalcin, free and total testosterone, bioavailable testosterone, and SHBG were inversely associated with metabolic factors to include BMI, waste circumference, glucose, triglycerides, HOMA, and insulin. The weakness of the study was that it was a cross-sectional design, but it had a large population for the investigation. Additional study is needed to ascertain the long-term clinical impact of the association between unOC and testosterone.

A. W. Meikle, MD

References

1. Buday B, Pach FP, Literati-Nagy B, Vitai M, Vecsei Z, Koranyi L. Serum osteocalcin is associated with improved metabolic state via adiponectin in females versus testosterone in males. Gender specific nature of the bone-energy homeostasis axis. *Bone.* 2013;57:98-104.
2. Varsavsky M, Reyes-García R, García-Martín A, Rozas-Moreno P, Rocio GR, Muñoz-Torres M. Bone turnover markers in patients with prostate carcinoma: influence of sex steroids levels. *J Bone Miner Metab.* 2013 [Epub ahead of print].
3. Strapazzon G, Garolla A, Carraro U, Foresta C. Osteocalcin and its association with testosterone in patients with metabolic diseases. *Osteoporos Int.* 2013;24: 2539-2540.
4. Guntur AR, Rosen CJ. Bone as an endocrine organ. *Endocr Pract.* 2012;18: 758-762.

Hypogonadism in Men

Abrupt decrease in serum testosterone levels after an oral glucose load in men: implications for screening for hypogonadism

Caronia LM, Dwyer AA, Hayden D, et al (Massachusetts General Hosp, Boston; Centre Hospitalier Universitaire Vaudois, Lausanne, Switzerland; et al)

Clin Endocrinol 78:291-296, 2013

Objective.—This study examines the physiological impact of a glucose load on serum testosterone (T) levels in men with varying glucose tolerance (GT).

Design.—Cross-sectional study.

Patients and Methods.—74 men (19–74 years, mean 51·4 ± 1·4 years) underwent a standard 75-g oral glucose tolerance test with blood sampling at 0, 30, 60, 90 and 120 min. Fasting serum glucose, insulin, total T (and calculated free T), LH, SHBG, leptin and cortisol were measured.

Results.—57% of the men had normal GT, 30% had impaired GT and 13% had newly diagnosed type 2 diabetes. Glucose ingestion was associated with a 25% decrease in mean T levels (delta = −4·2 ± 0·3 nm, *P* < 0·0001). T levels remained suppressed at 120 min compared with baseline (13·7 ± 0·6 vs 16·5 ± 0·7 nm, *P* < 0·0001) and did not differ across GT or BMI. Of the 66 men with normal T levels at baseline, 10 (15%) had levels that decreased to the hypogonadal range (<9·7 nm) at one or more time points. SHBG, LH and cortisol levels were unchanged. Leptin levels decreased from baseline at all time points (*P* < 0·0001).

Conclusions.—Glucose ingestion induces a significant reduction in total and free T levels in men, which is similar across the spectrum of glucose tolerance. This decrease in T appears to be because of a direct testicular

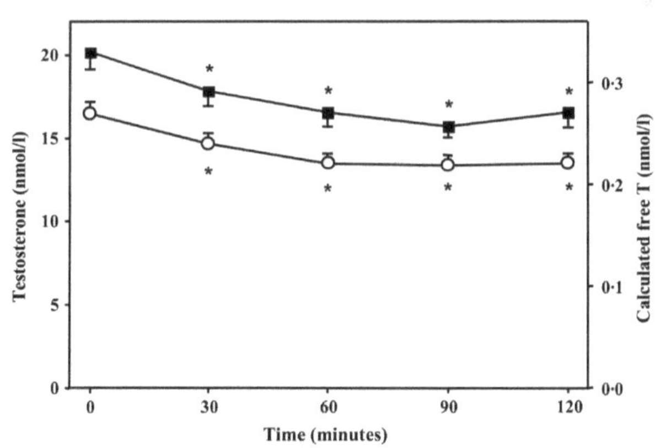

FIGURE 1.—Changes in total testosterone (○) and calculated free testosterone (■) in response to a 75-g oral glucose load (*n* = 74). Each time point represents mean ± SEM, asterisks (*) denote change from baseline (*P* < 0·0001). (Reprinted from Caronia LM, Dwyer AA, Hayden D, et al. Abrupt decrease in serum testosterone levels after an oral glucose load in men: implications for screening for hypogonadism. *Clin Endocrinol.* 2013;78:291-296, with acknowledgement of Wiley-Blackwell.)

defect, but the absence of compensatory changes in LH suggests an additional central component. Men found to have low nonfasting T levels should be re-evaluated in the fasting state (Fig 1).

▶ Several factors affect serum testosterone concentrations in men. Dysfunction of the hypothalamus, pituitary, and Leydig cells are well-characterized abnormalities. Others are less likely to be fully characterized for a mechanism. The associations with testosterone deficiency include obesity, the metabolic syndrome, type 2 diabetes associated with insulin resistance, aging, circadian variation, and nutrient ingestion, which was associated with a 15% to 40% postprandial decline in testosterone or no change.[1-4] The study by Caronia et al observed a decrease in serum testosterone concentration after oral ingestion of glucose. They invoked a direct glucose effect on the testes, but also a possible central effect because there was no apparent change in serum luteinizing hormone. The authors suggest that dietary intake should be taken into consideration when measuring serum testosterone concentrations in men being evaluated for deficiency. A morning blood collection should be taken before breakfast in men suspected of testosterone deficiency. This would control for dietary as well as circadian variation in testosterone secretion.

A. W. Meikle, MD

References

1. Bhasin S, Cunningham GR, Hayes FJ, et al. Testosterone therapy in men with androgen deficiency syndromes: an Endocrine Society clinical practice guideline. *J Clin Endocrinol Metab.* 2010;95:2536-2559.
2. Meikle AW, Stringham JD, Woodward MG, et al. Effects of a fat-containing meal on sex hormones in men. *Metabolism.* 1990;39:943-946.
3. Habito RC, Ball MJ. Postprandial changes in sex hormones after meals of different composition. *Metabolism.* 2001;50:505-511.
4. Volek JS, Gómez AL, Love DM, Avery NG, Sharman MJ, Kraemer WJ. Effects of a high-fat diet on postabsorptive and postprandial testosterone responses to a fat-rich meal. *Metabolism.* 2001;50:1351-1355.

Determinants of testosterone recovery after bariatric surgery: is it only a matter of reduction of body mass index?

Luconi M, Samavat J, Seghieri G, et al (Univ of Florence, Italy; General Hosp, Pistoia, Italy; et al)

Fertil Steril 99:1872-1879.e1, 2013

Objective.—To explore the correlation models between body mass index (BMI) and sex hormones constructed from a male cross-sectional survey and evaluate the effects of surgery-induced weight loss on sex hormones in morbidly obese subjects that are not predicted by the constructed BMI correlation models.

Design.—Cross-sectional population and longitudinal studies.

Setting.—Bariatric surgery center in a university hospital.

Patient(s).—A cross-sectional survey of a male general population of 161 patients (BMI median [interquartile range] = 29.2 [24.8–41.9] kg/m^2) in addition to 24 morbidly obese subjects (BMI = 43.9 [40.8–53.8] kg/m^2) who were undergoing bariatric surgery were prospectively studied for 6 and 12 months.

Intervention(s).—Bariatric surgery on 24 morbidly obese men.

Main Outcome Measure(s).—Cross-sectional population: construction of the best-fitting models describing the relationship between baseline BMI with total (TT) and calculated free (cFT) testosterone, E_2, sex hormone–binding globulin (SHBG), FSH, and LH levels. Longitudinal study deviation between the observed sex hormone levels at 6- and 12-month follow-up and those expected on BMI bases.

Result(s).—The correlation of BMI with sex hormones was not univocally linear (E_2), but the best-fitting model was exponential for TT, cFT, FSH, LH, and TT/E_2 and power for SHBG. In addition to the significant improvement of all parameters observed after surgery in the longitudinal cohort, the increase in TT and SHBG, but not in cFT, was significantly higher than expected from the corresponding weight loss at 6 months from surgery (14.80 [12.30–19.00] nM vs. 12.77 [10.92–13.64] nM

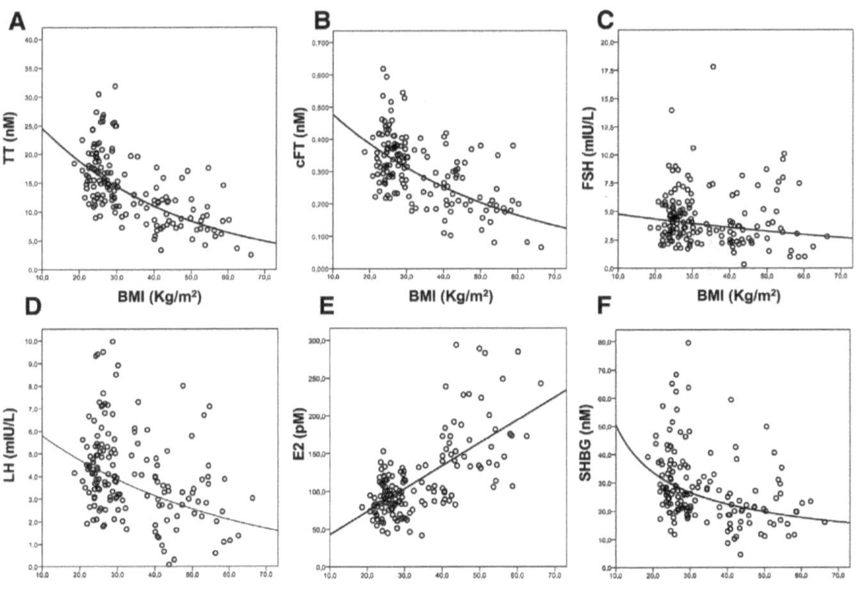

FIGURE 1.—Relationship of BMI with sex steroid hormones in the cross-sectional study. The best-fitting regression curves are shown for the relationship between BMI and TT (A, exponential model), cFT (B, exponential model), FSH (C, exponential model), LH (D, exponential model), E_2 (E, linear model), and SHBG (F, power model) in the cross-sectional cohort of subjects composed of population- and clinic-based samples. Relative equations and parameters are reported in Table 2. (Reprinted from Fertility and Sterility. Luconi M, Samavat J, Seghieri G, et al. Determinants of testosterone recovery after bariatric surgery: is it only a matter of reduction of body mass index? *Fertil Steril.* 2013;99:1872-1879.e1, Copyright 2013, with permission from American Society for Reproductive Medicine.)

and 40.0 [28.9–54.5] nM vs. 24.7 [22.5–25.8] nM for TT and SHBG, respectively), remaining rather stable at 12 months.

Conclusion(s).—The increase in TT and SHBG, but not the increase in cFT, after bariatric surgery is greater than expected based on weight loss (Fig 1).

▶ Obesity in men is associated with several alterations in endocrine and reproductive abnormalities. Total testosterone and sex hormone binding globulin (SHBG) are reduced and estrogen is increased. There is failure of a compensatory increase in gonadotropins. Other factors affecting the gonads in obese men are leptin, kisspeptin, and adipokines. The mechanism for this alteration requires additional study. Few studies have investigated men with morbid obesity before and after weight loss from bariatric surgery.[1-5] Luconi et al extended prior studies by using mathematical models correlating body mass index with different sex hormones or assessing determinates of changes in sex hormone with losing weight. Surgery did not produce a significantly higher recovery of gonadotropins as observed for SHGB and total testosterone. They postulated that the recovery of the hypothalamic-pituitary-gonadal axis after weight loss has a longer latency requiring a longer follow-up. The study has several limitations, including surgery-induced weight loss, total testosterone, and SHBG in morbid obesity. Confirmation of the results requires a larger study and a longer follow-up.

A. W. Meikle, MD

References

1. Corona G, Rastrelli G, Monami M, et al. Body weight loss reverts obesity-associated hypogonadotropic hypogonadism: a systematic review and meta-analysis. *Eur J Endocrinol.* 2013;168:829-843.
2. Hammoud AO, Meikle AW, Reis LO, Gibson M, Peterson CM, Carrell DT. Obesity and male infertility: a practical approach. *Semin Reprod Med.* 2012;30:486-495.
3. Hammoud A, Gibson M, Hunt SC, et al. Effect of Roux-en-Y gastric bypass surgery on the sex steroids and quality of life in obese men. *J Clin Endocrinol Metab.* 2009;94:1329-1332.
4. Hammoud AO, Gibson M, Peterson CM, Meikle AW, Carrell DT. Impact of male obesity on infertility: a critical review of the current literature. *Fertil Steril.* 2008;90:897-904.
5. Hammoud AO, Wilde N, Gibson M, Parks A, Carrell DT, Meikle AW. Male obesity and alteration in sperm parameters. *Fertil Steril.* 2008;90:2222-2225.

Symptomatic Reduction in Free Testosterone Levels Secondary to Crizotinib Use in Male Cancer Patients

Weickhardt AJ, Doebele RC, Purcell WT, et al (Univ of Colorado Anschutz Med Campus, Aurora; et al)

Cancer 119:2383-2390, 2013

Background.—Crizotinib is a tyrosine kinase inhibitor active against *ALK, MET,* and *ROS1.* We previously reported that crizotinib decreases

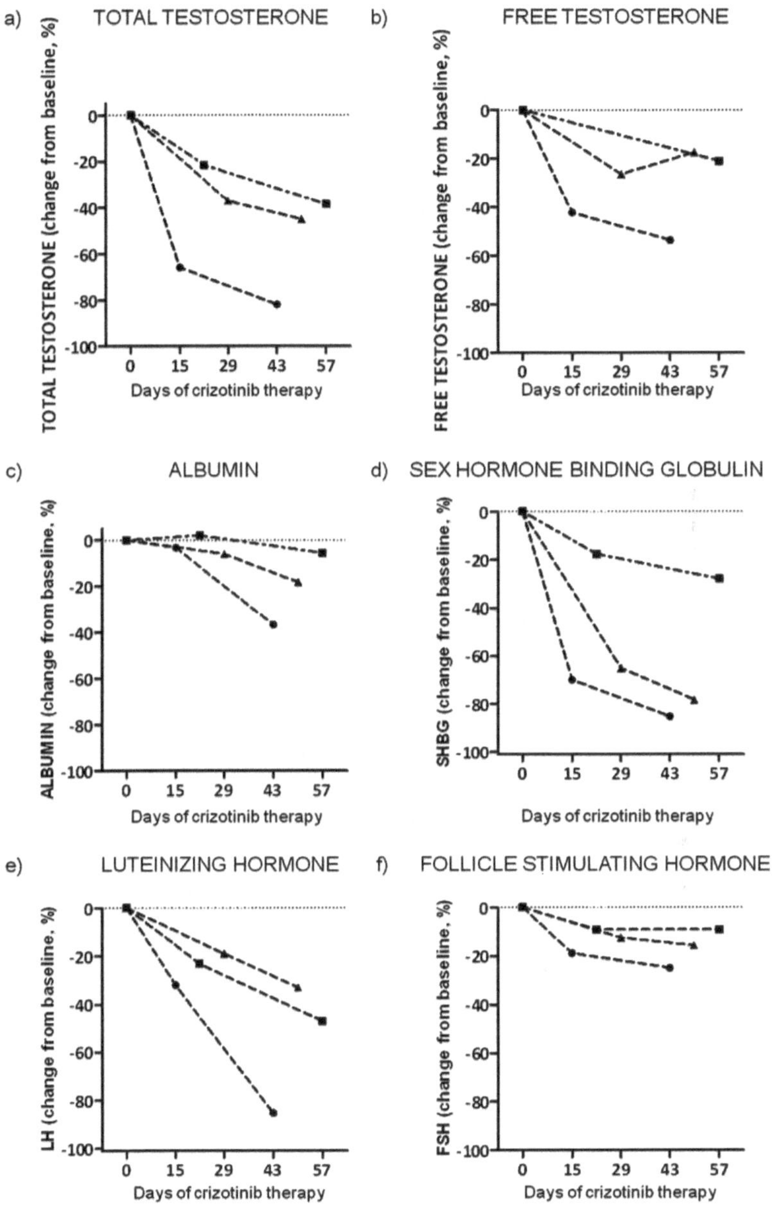

FIGURE 4.—Dynamic assessment of sex hormones and testosterone-binding proteins in 3 patients commenced on crizotinib, showing decrease in total and free testosterone relative to baseline measurement, as well as rapid decreases in LH and FSH, albumin, and sex hormone-binding globulin. (Reprinted from Cancer. Weickhardt AJ, Doebele RC, Purcell WT, et al. Symptomatic reduction in free testosterone levels secondary to crizotinib use in male cancer patients. *Cancer.* 2013;119:2383-2390, Copyright 2013, American Cancer Society. This material is reproduced with permission of Wiley-Liss, Inc., a subsidiary of John Wiley & Sons, Inc., www.interscience.wiley.com.)

testosterone in male patients. The detailed etiology of the effect, its symptomatic significance, and the effectiveness of subsequent testosterone replacement have not been previously reported.

Methods.—Male cancer patients treated with crizotinib had total testosterone levels measured and results compared with non-crizotinib-treated patients. Albumin, sex hormone-binding globulin (SHBG), follicle-stimulating hormone (FSH), and/or luteinizing hormone (LH) were tracked longitudinally. A subset of patients had free testosterone levels measured and a hypogonadal screening questionnaire administered. Patients receiving subsequent testosterone supplementation were assessed for symptomatic improvement.

Results.—Mean total testosterone levels were −25% below the lower limit of normal (LLN) in 32 crizotinib-treated patients (27 of 32 patients below LLN, 84%) compared with +29% above LLN in 19 non-crizotinib-treated patients (6 of 19 below LLN, 32%), $P = .0012$. Levels of albumin and SHBG (which both bind testosterone) declined rapidly with crizotinib, but so did FSH, LH, and free testosterone, suggesting a centrally mediated, true hypogonadal effect. Mean free testosterone levels were −17% below LLN (19 of 25 patients below LLN, 76%). Eighty-four percent (16 of 19) with low free levels, and 79% (19/24) with low total levels had symptoms of androgen deficiency. Five of 9 patients (55%) with low testosterone given testosterone supplementation had improvement in symptoms, coincident with increases in testosterone above LLN.

Conclusions.—Symptoms of androgen deficiency and free or total/free testosterone levels should be tracked in male patients on crizotinib with consideration of testosterone replacement as appropriate (Fig 4).

▶ Crizotinib is an inhibitor of tyrosine kinases and is used to treat various tumors, including anaplastic lymphoma and non–small cell lung cancer.[1] The drug was also observed to decrease serum testosterone concentrations to less than normal in men. The effect on testosterone was reversible and appeared to be suppressed by a central mechanism. It is uncertain whether some of the side effects of crizotinib are drug related or from testosterone deficiency. The study by Weickhardt et al investigated the mechanism for the reduction in testosterone after treatment with crizotinib.[2] They observed that the main binding proteins for testosterone (sex hormone-binding globulin and albumin) declined rapidly, but so did follicle-stimulating hormone, luteinizing hormone, and free testosterone, suggesting that the effect of crizotinib was central. It is unresolved if the effect of crizotinib is at the pituitary or hypothalamic level.[3] Additional studies are needed to determine the mechanism of crizotinib on inhibiting testosterone secretion, and it will likely involve the hypothalamus.

A. W. Meikle, MD

References

1. Timm A, Kolesar JM. Crizotinib for the treatment of non-small-cell lung cancer. *Am J Health Syst Pharm.* 2013;70:943-947.

2. Weickhardt AJ, Rothman MS, Salian-Mehta S, et al. Rapid-onset hypogonadism secondary to crizotinib use in men with metastatic nonsmall cell lung cancer. *Cancer.* 2012;118:5302-5309.
3. Ramalingam SS, Shaw AT. Hypogonadism related to crizotinib therapy: implications for patient care. *Cancer.* 2012;118:E1-E2.

Effects of three different medications on metabolic parameters and testicular volume in patients with hypogonadotropic hypogonadism: 3-year experience

Aydogdu A, Bolu E, Sonmez A, et al (Gulhane School of Medicine, Ankara, Turkey)

Clin Endocrinol 79:243-251, 2013

Introduction.—The aim of this study was to demonstrate the influences of three different treatment strategies on biochemical parameters and testicular volume (TV) in patients with idiopathic hypogonadotropic hypogonadism (IHH).

Subjects Design and Methods.—Seventy-seven never-treated patients with IHH and age and body mass index (BMI)-matched 42 healthy controls were analysed in a retrospective design. Twenty-eight patients were treated with testosterone esters (TE), 25 patients were treated with human chorionic gonadotropin (hCG) and 24 patients were treated with testosterone gel (TG). Biochemical parameters, tanner stages (TS) and TV were evaluated before and after 6 months of treatment.

Results.—Pretreatment TV, TS and biochemical test results were similar among the three treatment subgroup. In the TE-treated group, BMI, haemoglobin, haematocrit, creatinine, triglyceride, total testosterone (TT), TS and TV increased, but HDL-cholesterol (C) and urea level decreased significantly. In the hCG-treated group, triglyceride level decreased, and luteinizing hormone level, TS and TV increased significantly. BMI, TT, TS and TV increased, and leucocyte count, total-C, HDL-C levels decreased significantly in the TG-treated patients. No treatment type resulted in any changes in insulin resistance markers.

Conclusion.—hCG treatment resulted in favourable effects particularly on TV and lipid parameters. When TV improvement is considered less important, TG treatment may be a better option for older patients with IHH because of its easy use, neutral effects on triglyceride, haemoglobin and haematocrit, and its beneficial effects on total cholesterol level (Fig 1).

► Male testosterone deficiency, defined as a morning serum testosterone level of less than 300 ng/dL, is common. The diagnosis is based on symptoms plus laboratory determinations to ascertain the cause. Elevated luteinizing hormone and follicle-stimulating hormone levels suggest primary hypogonadism, whereas inappropriately low gonadotropins suggest pituitary or hypothalamic cause. Although many men are treated with androgen replacement therapy,

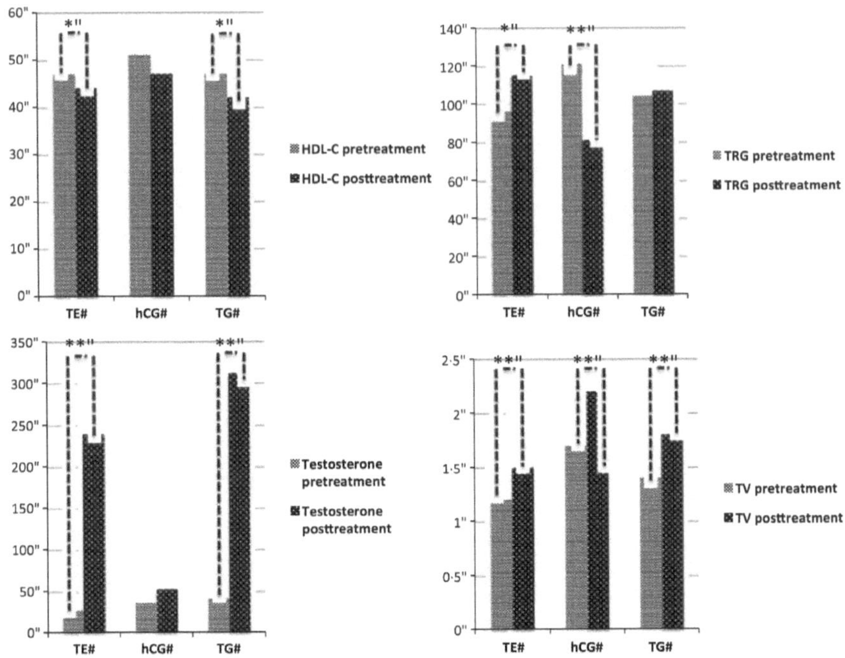

FIGURE 1.—Biochemical parameters and testicular volume before and after treatment with TE, hCG and TG. C, cholesterol; HDL, high density lipoprotein; TRG, Triglyceride; TV, testicular volume; TE, esterized testosterone; hCG, human chorionic gonadotropin; TG, testosterone gel ($*P < 0{\cdot}05$, $**P < 0{\cdot}005$). (Reprinted from Aydogdu A, Bolu E, Sonmez A, et al. Effects of three different medications on metabolic parameters and testicular volume in patients with hypogonadotropic hypogonadism: 3-year experience. *Clin Endocrinol.* 2013;79:243-251, with acknowledgement of Wiley-Blackwell.)

others might desire fertility options. Risk factors for hypogonadism include infertility, grump mood, central obesity, insulin resistance, metabolic syndrome, type 2 diabetes mellitus, coronary artery disease, and death. Aydogdu et al used 3 different treatment plans to assess effects on biochemical parameters and testicular volume in patients with idiopathic hypogonadotropic hypogonadism. The therapies used were testosterone ester injections, testosterone gel, and human chorionic gonadotropin (hCG). Treatment with hCG was most effective for testicular volume. Testosterone gel was better accepted by older men and was not associated with adverse metabolic alteration. The presumption is that larger testicular volume would be associated with fertility potential.[1-6]

A. W. Meikle, MD

References

1. Bolu E, Sonmez A, Tapan S, et al. HDL cholesterol subfractions and the effect of testosterone replacement in hypogonadism. *Horm Metab Res.* 2013;45:443-448.
2. Sonmez A, Haymana C, Bolu E, et al. Metabolic syndrome and the effect of testosterone treatment in young men with congenital hypogonadotropic hypogonadism. *Eur J Endocrinol.* 2011;164:759-764.

3. Bhasin S, Pencina M, Jasuja GK, et al. Reference ranges for testosterone in men generated using liquid chromatography tandem mass spectrometry in a community-based sample of healthy nonobese young men in the Framingham Heart Study and applied to three geographically distinct cohorts. *J Clin Endocrinol Metab.* 2011;96:2430-2439.
4. Bhasin S, Basaria S. Diagnosis and treatment of hypogonadism in men. *Best Pract Res Clin Endocrinol Metab.* 2011;25:251-270.
5. Bhasin S, Cunningham GR, Hayes FJ, et al. Testosterone therapy in men with androgen deficiency syndromes: an Endocrine Society clinical practice guideline. *J Clin Endocrinol Metab.* 2010;95:2536-2559.
6. Matsumoto AM, Snyder PJ, Bhasin S, et al. Stimulation of spermatogenesis with recombinant human follicle-stimulating hormone (follitropin alfa; GONAL-f): long-term treatment in azoospermic men with hypogonadotropic hypogonadism. *Fertil Steril.* 2009;92:979-990.

Effects of Testosterone

Anabolic androgenic steroid use is associated with ventricular dysfunction on cardiac MRI in strength trained athletes

Luijkx T, Velthuis BK, Backx FJG, et al (Univ Med Ctr Utrecht, The Netherlands; et al)

Int J Cardiol 167:664-668, 2013

Background.—Uncertainty remains about possible cardiac adaptation to resistance training. Androgenic anabolic steroids (AAS) use plays a potential role and may have adverse cardiovascular effects.

Objective.—To elucidate the effect of resistance training and of AAS-use on cardiac dimensions and function.

Participants.—Cardiac magnetic resonance (CMR) were performed in 156 male subjects aged 18–40 years: 52 non-athletes (maximum of 3 exercise hours/week), 52 strength-endurance (high dynamic–high static, HD–HS) athletes and 52 strength (low dynamic–high static, LD–HS) trained athletes (athletes ≥6 exercise hours/week). 28 LD–HS athletes denied and 24 admitted to AAS use for an average duration of 5 years (range 3 months–20 years).

Results.—No significant differences were found between non-athletes and non-AAS-using LD–HS athletes. AAS-using LD–HS athletes had significantly larger LV and RV volumes and LV wall mass than non-AAS-using LD–HS athletes, but lower than HD–HS athletes. In comparison to all other groups AAS-using LD–HS athletes showed lower ejection fractions of both ventricles (LV/RV EF 51/48% versus 55–57/51–52%) and lower E/A ratios (LV/RV 1.5/1.2 versus 1.9–2.0/1.4–1.5) as an indirect measure of diastolic function. Linear regression models demonstrated a significant effect of AAS-use on LV EDV, LV EDM, systolic function and mitral valve E/A ratio (all ANOVA-tests $p < 0.05$).

Conclusions.—Strength athletes who use AAS show significantly different cardiac dimensions and biventricular systolic dysfunction and impaired ventricular inflow as compared to non-athletes and non-AAS-using strength athletes. Increased ventricular volume and mass did not

TABLE 2.—Quantitative Ventricular Parameters Adjusted for Body Surface Area

	Non-Athletes	Non-Using LD–HS Athletes	AAS-Using LD–HS Athletes	HD–HS Athletes
n	52	28	24	52
LV				
EDV index (ml/m2)	100 ± 15 (127)‡§	104 ± 19 (138)§	113 ± 17 (154)†§	126 ± 15 (154)†¶‡
ESV index (ml/m2)	43 ± 9.6 (61)‡§	47 ± 12 (73)‡§	56 ± 13 (86)†¶	55 ± 10 (79)†¶
EDM index (ml/m2)	47 ± 8.2 (63)‡§	47 ± 8.5 (64)‡§	59 ± 15 (88)†¶	65 ± 12 (89)†¶
EDD SA (mm)	56 ± 3.8 (63)‡§	58 ± 4.4 (66)‡	61 ± 3.8 (68)†¶	60 ± 4.1 (67)†
EF (%)	57 ± 5.9 (47)‡	55 ± 4.7 (44)‡	51 ± 6.9 (37)†¶§	56 ± 4.8 (45)‡
MV E/A ratio	1.9 ± 0.45 (1.2)‡	1.9 ± 0.48 (1.0)‡	1.5 ± 0.31 (0.9)†¶§	2.0 ± 0.50 (1.3)‡
RV				
EDV index (ml/m2)	110 ± 17 (139)§	110 ± 17 (136)§	119 ± 19 (164)§	141 ± 20 (184)†¶‡
ESV index (ml/m2)	53 ± 11 (72)‡§	54 ± 9.9 (69)‡§	62 ± 13 (91)†¶§	70 ± 13 (97)†¶‡
EDM index (ml/m2)	12 ± 2.3 (15)§	12 ± 1.9 (15)§	11 ± 1.4 (15)§	14 ± 2.4 (21)†¶‡
EDD SA (mm)	45 ± 5.9 (56)§	47 ± 5.8 (57)	48 ± 7.2 (60)	48 ± 5.8 (59)†
EF (%)	52 ± 5.0 (43)‡	51 ± 4.1 (45)‡	48 ± 5.5 (39)†¶§	51 ± 4.1 (44)‡
TV E/A ratio	1.5 ± 0.31 (1.0)‡	1.4 ± 0.30 (1.0)‡	1.2 ± 0.27 (0.9)†¶§	1.5 ± 0.30 (1.0)‡
IVS-WT SA (mm)	9.5 ± 1.3 (12)‡§	9.4 ± 1.5 (13)‡§	12 ± 1.8 (15)†¶	11 ± 1.3 (13)†¶

Data are expressed as mean ± SD (95th percentile or 5th percentile where appropriate), EDV = end-diastolic volume, ESV = end-systolic volume, EDM = end-diastolic mass, EDD = end-diastolic diameter, SA = short axis view, EF = ejection fraction, IVS-WT = interventricular septal wall thickness.

†Significant differences ($p < 0.05$) from non-athletes.

¶Nonusing LD–HS athletes.

‡AAS-using LD–HS athletes.

§HD–HS athletes are indicated.

exceed that of strength–endurance athletes. These findings may help raise awareness of the consequences of AAS use (Table 2).

▶ The effect of androgenic anabolic steroids (AAS) on cardiac changes associated with strength resistance training is unresolved. AAS use has been reported to adversely affect the left ventricle and the cardiovascular system in general. There are various sporting activities that might have different stresses on cardiac function and adaptation. Causes of sudden cardiac death attributed to AAS use have been cardiotoxicity, autonomic deregulation, and thrombosis from polycythemia, homocysteine elevations, and arrhythmias. Luijkx et al evaluated ventricular dysfunction in strength-trained athletes. They compared cardiac function in nonathletes, non-using, low-dynamic-high-static (LD-HS) athletes, AAS-using, LD-HS athletes, and high-dynamic-high-static athletes. They observed that AAS use caused significant dysfunction of the heart ventricles. A limitation of the study is that it could not assess longitudinal changes in cardiac parameters in men using AAS. The participants were not tested for AAS concentrations in the circulation. Their observations have considerable clinical importance in athletes who use AAS.[1-5]

A. W. Meikle, MD

References

1. Luijkx T, Cramer MJ, Prakken NH, et al. Sport category is an important determinant of cardiac adaptation: an MRI study. *Br J Sports Med.* 2012;46:1119-1124.

2. Chaves EA, Fortunato RS, Carvalho DP, Nascimento JH, Oliveira MF. Exercise-induced cardioprotection is impaired by anabolic steroid treatment through a redox-dependent mechanism. *J Steroid Biochem Mol Biol.* 2013;138C:267-272.
3. das Neves VJ, Tanno AP, Cunha TS, et al. Effects of nandrolone and resistance training on the blood pressure, cardiac electrophysiology, and expression of atrial β-adrenergic receptors. *Life Sci.* 2013;92:1029-1035.
4. Hassan AF, Kamal MM. Effect of exercise training and anabolic androgenic steroids on hemodynamics, glycogen content, angiogenesis and apoptosis of cardiac muscle in adult male rats. *Int J Health Sci (Qassim).* 2013;7:47-60.
5. Volterrani M, Rosano G, Iellamo F. Testosterone and heart failure. *Endocrine.* 2012;42:272-277.

Gonadal Steroids and Body Composition, Strength, and Sexual Function in Men

Finkelstein JS, Lee H, Burnett-Bowie S-AM, et al (Biostatistics Ctr, Rockville, MD)
N Engl J Med 369:1011-1022, 2013

Background.—Current approaches to diagnosing testosterone deficiency do not consider the physiological consequences of various testosterone levels or whether deficiencies of testosterone, estradiol, or both account for clinical manifestations.

Methods.—We provided 198 healthy men 20 to 50 years of age with goserelin acetate (to suppress endogenous testosterone and estradiol) and randomly assigned them to receive a placebo gel or 1.25 g, 2.5 g, 5 g, or 10 g of testosterone gel daily for 16 weeks. Another 202 healthy men received goserelin acetate, placebo gel or testosterone gel, and anastrozole (to suppress the conversion of testosterone to estradiol). Changes in the percentage of body fat and in lean mass were the primary outcomes. Subcutaneous- and intraabdominal-fat areas, thigh-muscle area and strength, and sexual function were also assessed.

Results.—The percentage of body fat increased in groups receiving placebo or 1.25 g or 2.5 g of testosterone daily without anastrozole (mean testosterone level, 44 ± 13 ng per deciliter, 191 ± 78 ng per deciliter, and 337 ± 173 ng per deciliter, respectively). Lean mass and thigh-muscle area decreased in men receiving placebo and in those receiving 1.25 g of testosterone daily without anastrozole. Leg-press strength fell only with placebo administration. In general, sexual desire declined as the testosterone dose was reduced.

Conclusions.—The amount of testosterone required to maintain lean mass, fat mass, strength, and sexual function varied widely in men. Androgen deficiency accounted for decreases in lean mass, muscle size, and strength; estrogen deficiency primarily accounted for increases in body fat; and both contributed to the decline in sexual function. Our findings support changes in the approach to evaluation and management of hypogonadism in men. (Funded by the National Institutes of Health and others; ClinicalTrials.gov number, NCT00114114.).

▶ Testosterone deficiency is increasingly diagnosed in men, and sales of testosterone to treat the deficiency have escalated. Many men are treated using testosterone based on symptoms that overlap with normal men. Testosterone is also a prehormone for dihydrotestosterone made in the prostate and hair follicles. These 2 potent androgens activate the androgen receptor, and estradiol stimulates the estrogen receptor, which has benefit for bone health also in men. Finkelstein et al conducted studies in men to determine the effects of gonadal steroids on body composition, strength, and sexual function in men under suppression of endogenous testosterone and estradiol. They confirmed that lean body mass, muscle size, and strength were expected, whereas body fat increases were estradiol dependent as expected. Sexual function was contributed to by both androgens and estrogens; it is somewhat unexpected that both classes of sex steroids participate in influencing sexual function. Further study is needed to unravel the degree of hypogonadism under which undesirable effects develop.[1-4]

A. W. Meikle, MD

References

1. Yassin A, Doros G. Testosterone therapy in hypogonadal men results in sustained and clinically meaningful weight loss. *Clin Obes*. 2013;3:73-83.
2. Kido Y, Sakazume S, Abe Y, et al. Testosterone replacement therapy to improve secondary sexual characteristics and body composition without adverse behavioral problems in adult male patients with Prader-Willi syndrome: an observational study. *Am J Med Genet A*. 2013;161:2167-2173.
3. Behre HM, Tammela TL, Arver S, et al. A randomized, double-blind, placebo-controlled trial of testosterone gel on body composition and health-related quality-of-life in men with hypogonadal to low-normal levels of serum testosterone and symptoms of androgen deficiency over 6 months with 12 months open-label follow-up. *Aging Male*. 2012;15:198-207.
4. Burney BO, Hayes TG, Smiechowska J, et al. Low testosterone levels and increased inflammatory markers in patients with cancer and relationship with cachexia. *J Clin Endocrinol Metab*. 2012;97:E700-E709.

Metabolic Syndrome

Independent Effects of Testosterone on Lipid Oxidation and VLDL-TG Production: A Randomized, Double-Blind, Placebo-Controlled, Crossover Study

Høst C, Gormsen LC, Christensen B, et al (Aarhus Univ Hosp, Denmark; et al)
Diabetes 62:1409-1416, 2013

Low testosterone (T) levels in men have been shown to predict development of the metabolic syndrome, but the effects of T on lipid metabolism are incompletely understood. In a randomized, double-blind, placebo-controlled, crossover study, 12 healthy, young males received gonadotropin-releasing hormone agonist treatment 1 month prior to 3 of 4 trial days to induce castrate levels of T. On trial days, T gel was applied to the body containing either high or low physiological T dose or placebo. On the 4th trial day, participants constituted their own eugonadal controls. Each study comprised a 5-h basal period and a 3-h hyper-insulinemic-euglycemic clamp. Short-term hypogonadism did not affect VLDL triglyceride (TG) secretion, nor did it affect VLDL-TG concentrations. It was, however, characterized by lower total lipid oxidation. In addition, acute rescue with high physiological T increased VLDL-TG secretion during both basal and clamp conditions. These data show that T can act through fast nongenomic pathways in the liver. In addition, the early hypogonadal state is characterized by decreased total lipid oxidation, but whether these changes represent early hypogonadal metabolic dysfunction warrants further investigations. T is not a major determinant of resting VLDL-TG kinetics in men (Fig 4).

▶ Low testosterone concentrations in men have been associated with cardiovascular morbidity and mortality.[1-4] Testosterone replacement therapy in hypogonadal men is associated with a reduction in fat mass and an increase in fat-free mass or muscle mass. The effects of testosterone on lipid metabolism

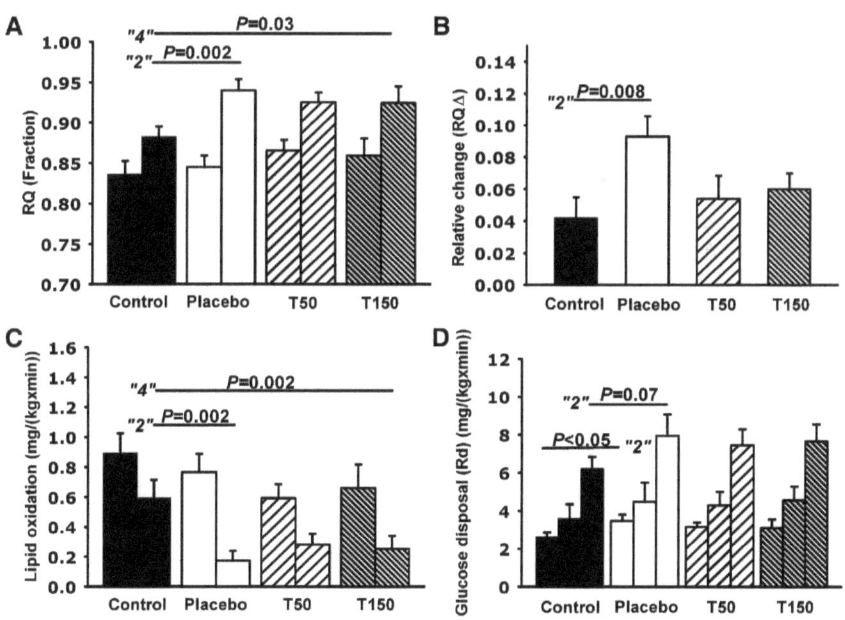

FIGURE 4.—RQ (*A*), change in RQ (DRQ) (*B*), lipid oxidation rates (*C*), and insulin-stimulated glucose disposal (columns represent oxidative glucose disposal, nonoxidative glucose disposal, and total glucose disposal) (*D*). *A* and *C*: Columns represent basal and clamp period, respectively. Data are mean ± SEM. (Copyright © 2013, American Diabetes Association from Diabetes. Høst C, Gormsen LC, Christensen B, et al. Independent effects of testosterone on lipid oxidation and VLDL-TG production: a randomized, double-blind, placebo-controlled, crossover study. *Diabetes*. 2013;62:1409-1416, pages reprinted with permission from The American Diabetes Association.)

to include lipids and triglycerides are less clear. Hypogonadal men are prone to develop the metabolic syndrome with insulin resistance and hypertriglyceridemia. If the hypogonadal men are overweight, they tend to store more meal-derived free fatty acids in fat stores. Høst et al observed that hypogonadal men have reduced total lipid oxidation, but testosterone is not a major determinant of resting very-low-density lipoprotein. These conclusions were based on short-term manipulation of testosterone concentration. The authors suggest that impaired oxidation before any signs of insulin resistance or changes in resting energy expenditure might be an early metabolic feature of male hypogonadism in which uninhibited peripheral lipoprotein lipase activity might lead to increased triglyceride uptake and storage. Long-term studies are needed to determine the impact of testosterone on these metabolic lipid alterations.

A. W. Meikle, MD

References

1. de Souza-Junior TP, Yamada AK, Simão R, et al. Supra-physiological doses of testosterone affect membrane oxidation of human neutrophils monitored by the fluorescent probe C_{11}-BODIPY$^{581/591}$. *Eur J Appl Physiol.* 2013;113:1241-1248.
2. Koutsari C, Ali AH, Nair KS, et al. Fatty acid metabolism in the elderly: effects of dehydroepiandrosterone and testosterone replacement in hormonally deficient men and women. *J Clin Endocrin Meta.* 2009;94:3414-3423.
3. Birzniece V, Meinhardt UJ, Handelsman DJ, Ho KK. Testosterone stimulates extra-hepatic but not hepatic fat oxidation (Fox): comparison of oral and transdermal testosterone administration in hypopituitary men. *Clinical Endocrinol.* 2009; 71:715-721.
4. Amaral S, Oliveira PJ, Ramalho-Santos J. Diabetes and the impairment of reproductive function: possible role of mitochondria and reactive oxygen species. *Curr Diabetes Rev.* 2008;4:46-54.

Aging and Sex Steroid Risk Factors

In Older Men an Optimal Plasma Testosterone Is Associated With Reduced All-Cause Mortality and Higher Dihydrotestosterone With Reduced Ischemic Heart Disease Mortality, While Estradiol Levels Do Not Predict Mortality

Yeap BB, Alfonso H, Chubb SAP, et al (Univ of Western Australia, Perth, Australia; et al)

J Clin Endocrinol Metab 99:E9-E18, 2014

Context.—Testosterone (T) levels decline with age and lower T has been associated with increased mortality in aging men. However, the associations of its metabolites, dihydrotestosterone (DHT) and estradiol (E_2), with mortality are poorly defined.

Objective.—We assessed associations of T, DHT, and E_2 with all-cause and ischemic heart disease (IHD) mortality in older men.

Participants.—Participants were community-dwelling men aged 70 to 89 years who were residing in Perth, Western Australia.

Main Outcome Measures.—Plasma total T, DHT, and E_2 were assayed using liquid chromatographytandem mass spectrometry in early morning samples collected in 2001 to 2004 from 3690 men. Deaths to December 2010 were ascertained by data linkage.

Results.—There were 974 deaths (26.4%), including 325 of IHD. Men who died had lower baseline T (12.8 ± 5.1 vs 13.2 ± 4.8 nmol/L [mean ± SD], $P = .013$), DHT (1.4 ± 0.7 vs 1.5 ± 0.7 nmol/L, $P = .002$), and E_2 (71.6 ± 29.3 vs 74.0 ± 29.0 pmol/L, $P = .022$). After allowance for other risk factors, T and DHT were associated with all-cause mortality (T: quartile [Q] Q2:Q1, adjusted hazard ratio [HR] = 0.82, $P = .033$; Q3:Q1, HR = 0.78, $P = .010$; Q4:Q1, HR = 0.86, $P > .05$; DHT: Q3:Q1, HR = 0.76, $P = .003$; Q4:Q1, HR = 0.84, $P > .05$). Higher DHT was associated with lower IHD mortality (Q3:Q1, HR = 0.58, $P = .002$; Q4:Q1, HR = 0.69, $P = .026$). E_2 was not associated with either all-cause or IHD mortality.

Conclusions.—Optimal androgen levels are a biomarker for survival because older men with midrange levels of T and DHT had the lowest death rates from any cause, whereas those with higher DHT had lower IHD mortality. Further investigations of the biological basis for these associations including randomized trials of T supplementation are needed.

► Serum testosterone is the main circulating androgen in adult men, but most is bound to sex hormone binding globulin (SHBG), whereas some is bound to albumin, with a lesser amount being free. There is a decline in serum testosterone concentrations as men age but SHBG concentrations increase, which modulates the total concentration and lowers the free testosterone. Whether serum testosterone concentrations are a risk factor for coronary artery disease and death is unresolved. Studies have associated lower testosterone values with poorer health outcomes, including cardiovascular disease (CVD) and mortality. However, men with normal values for testosterone also suffer from CVD and mortality. Correcting low testosterone in men has been associated with lower mortality during follow-up. It is not disputed that testosterone replacement increases lean body mass, lowers body fat, and improves bone health in men. Yeap and associates observed that older men with optimal plasma testosterone concentrations had reduced all-cause mortality and higher dihydrotestosterone (DHT). Ischemic heart disease mortality was also reduced. Estradiol was not a predictor of mortality. Older men with midrange values of testosterone and DHT had the lowest death rates from any cause.[1-7]

A. W. Meikle, MD

References

1. Magnani JW, Moser CB, Murabito JM, et al. Association of sex hormones, aging, and atrial fibrillation in men: the framingham heart study. *Circ Arrhythm Electrophysiol.* 2014;7:307-312.
2. Yeap BB, Flicker L. Hormones and cardiovascular disease in older men. *J Am Med Dir Assoc.* 2014 Feb 11 [Epub ahead of print].
3. Kaplan AL, Trinh QD, Sun M, et al. Testosterone replacement therapy following the diagnosis of prostate cancer: outcomes and utilization trends. *J Sex Med.* 2014; 11:1063-1070.
4. Hilbert-Walter A, Buttner R, Sieber C, Bollheimer C. Testosterone in old age: an up-date. *Dtsch Med Wochenschr.* 2012;137:2117-2122.

5. Yeap BB. Hormones and health outcomes in aging men. *Exp Gerontol.* 2013;48: 677-681.
6. Morris PD, Channer KS. Testosterone and cardiovascular disease in men. *Asian J Androl.* 2012;14:428-435.
7. Lerchbaum E, Pilz S, Boehm BO, Grammer TB, Obermayer-Pietsch B, März W. Combination of low free testosterone and low vitamin D predicts mortality in older men referred for coronary angiography. *Clin Endocrinol (Oxf).* 2012;77: 475-483.

Circulating Estrone Levels Are Associated Prospectively With Diabetes Risk in Men of the Framingham Heart Study

Jasuja GK, Travison TG, Davda M, et al (Boston Univ, MA; Boston Univ School of Medicine, MA; et al)
Diabetes Care 36:2591-2596, 2013

Objective.—In postmenopausal women and preclinical murine models, estrogen administration reduces diabetes risk; however, the relationship of estradiol and estrone to diabetes in men is poorly understood. We determined the relationship between circulating estradiol and estrone levels and diabetes risk in community-dwelling men of the Framingham Heart Study (FHS).

Research Design and Methods.—Cross-sectional relationships of estradiol and estrone levels with diabetes were assessed at examination 7 (1998–2001) in FHS generation 2 men (n = 1,458); prospective associations between hormone levels at examination 7 and incident diabetes were assessed 6.8 years later at examination 8. Type 2 diabetes mellitus was defined as fasting glucose >125 mg/dL, medication use, or both. Estradiol, estrone, and testosterone levels were measured with liquid chromatography–tandem mass spectrometry, and free estradiol and estrone were calculated.

Results.—In cross-sectional models, men with elevated estrone and estradiol had 40% and 62% increased likelihoods of existing diabetes per cross-sectional doubling of estrone and estradiol levels, respectively. Free estrone (cross-sectional odds ratio 1.28 [95% CI 1.02–1.62], $P = 0.04$) was associated with impaired fasting glucose at examination 7. There was an increase in risk of existing diabetes with increasing quartiles of total and free estrone and estradiol and an increase in risk of incident diabetes with increasing quartiles of estrone levels. In multivariate longitudinal analyses, a twofold increase in total or free estrone levels at examination 7 was associated with 77 and 93% increases, respectively, in odds of incident diabetes at examination 8.

Conclusions.—Although both estradiol and estrone exhibit cross-sectional associations with diabetes in men, in longitudinal analyses estrone is a more sensitive marker of diabetes risk than is estradiol.

▶ As men age, there is a decline in glucose tolerance and impaired glucose fasting, and an increase in type II diabetes. Endogenous sex hormones have been implicated in the development of type II diabetes, and the decline of serum testosterone concentrations has been associated with the increased risk of type II diabetes. The influence of estrogens on this relationship is less well studied. In women, clinical trials have suggested that estrogen therapy lowers the risk for type II diabetes and that reducing estrogen receptor α increases, susceptibility to diabetes in experimental animals. The report of Jasuja et al observed that estrone was a more robust marker for diabetes than estradiol when evaluated in a prospective study. The authors speculate that the differential actions of estrone and 17β-estradiol on estrogen receptor α and β bind both to the estrogen receptors, although 17β-estradiol has higher affinity. This study might stimulate additional study on the biologic effects of estrone in men.[1-5]

A. W. Meikle, MD

References

1. Travison TG, Zhuang WV, Lunetta KL, et al. The heritability of circulating testosterone, oestradiol, oestrone and sex hormone binding globulin concentrations in men: the Framingham Heart Study. *Clin Endocrinol (Oxf)*. 2014;80:277-282.
2. Jasuja GK, Travison TG, Davda M, et al. Age trends in estradiol and estrone levels measured using liquid chromatography tandem mass spectrometry in community-dwelling men of the Framingham Heart Study. *J Gerontol A Biol Sci Med Sci.* 2013;68:733-740.
3. Travison TG, Nguyen AH, Naganathan V, et al. Changes in reproductive hormone concentrations predict the prevalence and progression of the frailty syndrome in older men: the concord health and ageing in men project. *J Clin Endocrinol Metab.* 2011;96:2464-2474.
4. Fonda SJ, Bertrand R, O'Donnell A, Longcope C, McKinlay JB. Age, hormones, and cognitive functioning among middle-aged and elderly men: cross-sectional evidence from the Massachusetts Male Aging Study. *J Gerontol A Biol Sci Med Sci.* 2005;60:385-390.
5. Abdelrahaman E, Raghavan S, Baker L, Weinrich M, Winters SJ. Racial difference in circulating sex hormone-binding globulin levels in prepubertal boys. *Metabolism.* 2005;54:91-96.

Longitudinal Changes in Testosterone Over Five Years in Community-Dwelling Men

Shi Z, Araujo AB, Martin S, et al (Univ of Adelaide, South Australia, Australia; New England Res Insts, Inc, Watertown, MA; et al)
J Clin Endocrinol Metab 98:3289-3297, 2013

Context.—There are few population-based studies reporting longitudinal changes in total T, LH, FSH, and SHBG levels, and there is limited information on risk factors for their change.

Objective.—The objective of the study was to examine 5-year changes in serum T, LH, FSH, and SHBG levels among Australian men.

Design.—The study initially included a randomly selected, community-based cohort of 1588 men age 35 years or older at recruitment (mean age, 54 ± 11 y) with available data at 2 visits. Men on medications known to affect, or with established pathology of, the hypothalamo-pituitary-gonadal axis were excluded, leaving 1382 for analysis.

Results.—Mean baseline and follow-up T levels were 16.2 ± 1.4 and 15.6 ± 1.4 nmol/L, a change of −0.13 nmol/L/y. Annualized T changes were associated with obesity, being unmarried, and smoking at baseline, but not with diabetes, hypertension, or cardiovascular disease. T declined in men who had persistent depression or developed chronic disease, and it increased in men who were married, as compared to unmarried, at both time points. In the multivariate analysis, smoking cessation, development of central obesity (waist ≥100 cm), or generalized obesity (body mass index ≥30 kg/m^2) resulted in T decreases of 0.36, 0.25, and 0.20 nmol/L/y, respectively. Quitting smoking, developing obesity, and having persisting depression were inversely related to SHBG change.

Conclusions.—An age-related decline in T levels is not inevitable but is largely explained by smoking behavior and intercurrent changes in health status, particularly obesity and depression.

▶ Serum testosterone concentrations are determined by many factors, including hypothalamic-pituitary-testicular function, but are also affected by age, obesity, cardiovascular disease, type 2 diabetes, hypertension, depression, smoking, and insulin resistance. Treatment of men with low testosterone has been associated with a reduced risk of mortality over about 2 years. Shi et al did a longitudinal study in men over 5 years and quantitated serum testosterone concentration by mass spectrometry. They evaluated the influence of multiple factors to determine if the decline in testosterone was independent of aging and related to identifiably factors. Lifestyle factors and chronic conditions were found to contribute to the testosterone decline. The strength of the study was that it was a large randomly selected population with accurate measurement of serum testosterone. On the other hand, the study was limited to mainly urban-dwelling white men. Further investigation is required to determine whether reversal of the adverse factors would result in elevation of testosterone.[1-5]

A. W. Meikle, MD

References

1. Meldrum DR. Aging gonads, glands, and gametes: immutable or partially reversible changes? *Fertil Steril.* 2013;99:1-4.
2. Kim YS, Hong D, Lee DJ, Joo NS, Kim KM. Total testosterone may not decline with ageing in Korean men aged 40 years or older. *Clin Endocrinol (Oxf).* 2012; 77:296-301.
3. O'Connor DB, Lee DM, Corona G, et al. The relationships between sex hormones and sexual function in middle-aged and older European men. *J Clin Endocrinol Metab.* 2011;96:E1577-E1587.
4. Grossmann M. Low testosterone in men with type 2 diabetes: significance and treatment. *J Clin Endocrinol Metab.* 2011;96:2341-2353.
5. Bhasin S, Pencina M, Jasuja GK, et al. Reference ranges for testosterone in men generated using liquid chromatography tandem mass spectrometry in a community-based sample of healthy nonobese young men in the Framingham Heart Study and applied to three geographically distinct cohorts. *J Clin Endocrinol Metab.* 2011;96:2430-2439.

8 Neuroendocrinology

Pituitary - General

Non-functioning pituitary macro-incidentalomas benefit from early surgery before becoming symptomatic

Messerer M, Dubourg J, Raverot G, et al (Université de Lausanne, Switzerland; Hospices Civils de Lyon, Bron, France; et al)

Clin Neurol Neurosurg 115:2514-2520, 2013

Objective.—Pituitary incidentalomas (PIs) constitute an increasingly clinical problem. While the therapeutic management is well defined for symptomatic non-functioning PIs (NFPIs), a controversy still exists for asymptomatic macro-NFPIs between surgery and a "wait and see" approach. The aim of this study is to compare surgical results between symptomatic and asymptomatic macro-NFPIs.

Methods.—We conducted a retrospective study on 76 patients with newly diagnosed symptomatic and asymptomatic macro-NFPIs operated on between 2001 and 2010. We compared age, tumor size and surgical results between these two patient groups.

Results.—After the initial evaluation, 48 patients were found to be symptomatic. Gross total removal (GTR) rate was significantly higher in asymptomatic (82%) than in symptomatic patients (58%; $p = 0.03$). Gross total removal was strongly associated with Knosp's classification ($p = 0.01$). Postoperative endocrinological impairment was significantly associated with the existence of preoperative symptoms ($p = 0.03$). It was 10 times less frequent in the asymptomatic group. In symptomatic patients, postoperative visual and endocrinological impairment were present in 49% and 78% versus 0% and 14% in asymptomatic patients respectively.

Conclusions.—The endocrinological and visual outcome was better in those patients who underwent surgery for asymptomatic tumors. The extent of tumor resection was also significantly greater in smaller tumors. It would therefore be appropriate to offer surgery to patients with asymptomatic macro-NFPIs.

▶ Next to prolactinomas, nonfunctioning pituitary adenomas are the most frequent presentation of pituitary tumors. Whereas autonomous hormonal secretion almost always leads to either surgical or medical treatment in pituitary adenomas, the indication for treatment is less well established in nonfunctioning pituitary adenomas. Patients without any clear clinical symptoms (headache, visual field abnormalities, pituitary insufficiency) may be followed by a "wait and see" approach. The decision for surgery likely depends on an individual patient's wish and the endocrinologist's and neurosurgeon's experience. So far, it is unclear, whether the delay in surgery until development of clear clinical symptoms results in worsening of surgical outcome.

This study compared retrospectively the outcomes in patients with nonfunctioning pituitary adenomas operated in a symptomatic stage with those operated in a nonsymptomatic stage. The results clearly indicate that the outcome with respect to extent of tumor removal, pituitary insufficiency, and visual impairment was clearly better in those operated in an asymptomatic stage.

One may be inclined to use these results as an argument for earlier surgery in patients with nonfunctioning pituitary adenomas. However, until randomized studies comparing the outcome of surgery in asymptomatic stage versus during follow-up and development of symptoms become available, the evidence for any advice remains weak. Furthermore, other factors such as age of the patient and growth rate of the tumor may also be included in the advice to the patient. Whereas younger patients may eventually experience symptoms, older patients with slow-growing tumors may not.

S. Petersenn, MD

Prolactin

Mutant Prolactin Receptor and Familial Hyperprolactinemia

Newey PJ, Gorvin CM, Cleland SJ, et al (Univ of Oxford, UK)

N Engl J Med 369:2012-2020, 2013

Hyperprolactinemia that is not associated with gestation or the puerperium is usually due to tumors in the anterior pituitary gland and occurs occasionally in hereditary multiple endocrine neoplasia syndromes. Here, we report data from three sisters with hyperprolactinemia, two of whom presented with oligomenorrhea and one with infertility. These symptoms were not associated with pituitary tumors or multiple endocrine neoplasia but were due to a heterozygous mutation in the prolactin receptor gene, *PRLR*, resulting in an amino acid change from histidine to arginine at codon 188 (His188Arg). This substitution disrupted the high-affinity ligand-binding interface of the prolactin receptor, resulting in a loss of downstream signaling by Janus kinase 2 (JAK2) and signal transducer and activator of transcription 5 (STAT5). Thus, the familial hyperprolactinemia appears to be due to a germline, loss-of-function mutation in *PRLR*, resulting in prolactin insensitivity.

▶ Measurement of prolactin levels is routinely performed in patients with fertility issues as well as in women with menstrual irregularities or galactorrhea. Furthermore, all patients with pituitary tumors undergo prolactin investigation to exclude a prolactinoma, which would allow for medical treatment. Mild elevations of prolactin are also found with stress and hypothyroidism. However, the most frequent cause of hyperprolactinemia is treatment with various drugs, such as neuroleptics and antidepressants. Therefore, once hyperprolactinemia is established, the differential diagnosis may be difficult, leaving some patients with a diagnosis of idiopathic hyperprolactinemia, mostly of unknown significance.

This article describes a new cause of hyperprolactinemia in 3 sisters from 1 family. Careful molecular investigation of both the prolactin and the prolactin receptor molecule detected a heterozygous mutation in a very conserved amino acid of the prolactin receptor (Fig 1 in the original article). Structural modeling suggested that this mutation would result in a loss of the high-affinity binding site of the receptor, thereby interrupting dimerization. Indeed, elegant analysis of a cell culture model investigating various intracellular responses to prolactin binding confirmed loss of function due to the mutation, probably due to a dominant-negative effect of the mutated receptor on nonmutated receptor function. This would also explain the autosomal inheritance in the affected family.

This article allows for several interesting conclusions: First, a previously unknown cause of hyperprolactinemia was established, which is of special interest for families with hyperprolactinemia of unknown reason. Clinicians should be aware of this probably rare cause of hyperprolactinemia and initiate screening in affected families. Second, further characterization of the phenotype allows for a deeper understanding of the functional role of the prolactin molecule. Lack of function in the affected family members apparently did not result in an altered immune function, disputing somehow a major role of prolactin as a lymphopoietic hormone. On the other hand, affected family members did demonstrate some symptoms with either oligomenorrhea or infertility. This could be due to chance, an oversecretion of prolactin in relation to the receptor insensitivity, a lack of fine-tuning of prolactin receptor activation, or other prolactin receptor signal transduction pathways that are thus far unrecognized and differently affected by the receptor mutant. Third, because one of the affected women had normal ovulatory cycles but was infertile, prolactin action may be required for fertility.

Further characterization of the phenotype in other families with the same receptor mutation will shed some light on these questions. In addition, it remains to be established, through investigation of large cohorts, in which instances patients with hyperprolactinemia should be screened for the mutation established in this article.

S. Petersenn, MD

A Cross-Sectional Study of the Prevalence of Cardiac Valvular Abnormalities in Hyperprolactinemic Patients Treated With Ergot-Derived Dopamine Agonists

Drake WM, on behalf of the UK Dopamine Agonist Valvulopathy Group (St Bartholomew's Hosp, London, UK; et al)
J Clin Endocrinol Metab 99:90-96, 2014

Context.—Concern exists in the literature that the long-term use of ergot-derived dopamine agonist drugs for the treatment of hyperprolactinemia may be associated with clinically significant valvular heart disease.

Objective.—The aim of the study was to determine the prevalence of valvular heart abnormalities in patients taking dopamine agonists as treatment for lactotrope pituitary tumors and to explore any associations with the cumulative dose of drug used.

Design.—A cross-sectional echocardiographic study was performed in a large group of patients who were receiving dopamine agonist therapy for hyperprolactinemia. Studies were performed in accordance with the British Society of Echocardiography minimum dataset for a standard adult transthoracic echocardiogram. Poisson regression was used to calculate relative risks according to quartiles of dopamine agonist cumulative dose using the lowest cumulative dose quartile as the reference group.

Setting.—Twenty-eight centers of secondary/tertiary endocrine care across the United Kingdom participated in the study.

Results.—Data from 747 patients (251 males; median age, 42 y; interquartile range [IQR], 34–52 y) were collected. A total of 601 patients had taken cabergoline alone; 36 had been treated with bromocriptine alone; and 110 had received both drugs at some stage. The median cumulative dose for cabergoline was 152 mg (IQR, 50–348 mg), and for bromocriptine it was 7815 mg (IQR, 1764–20 477 mg). A total of 28 cases of moderate valvular stenosis or regurgitation were observed in 24 (3.2%) patients. No associations were observed between cumulative doses of dopamine agonist used and the age-corrected prevalence of any valvular abnormality.

Conclusion.—This large UK cross-sectional study does not support a clinically concerning association between the use of dopamine agonists for the treatment of hyperprolactinemia and cardiac valvulopathy.

▶ Surgery is considered the primary treatment option for many pituitary adenomas, offering the chance of cure. However, potential side effects include pituitary insufficiency and local complications. Furthermore, tumors extending into the lateral cavernous sinus may not be completely resectable even in the hands of the most experienced neurosurgeon. Interestingly, for prolactinoma, one of the most frequent entities of pituitary adenomas, medical treatment with a dopamine agonist has been well established. It offers both control of prolactin hypersecretion and tumor proliferation and is well tolerated by most patients. However, because treatment is lifelong in the majority of patients, some side effects may be recognized only after many years, as recently demonstrated for clinically significant valvular heart disease in patients treated with high doses of dopamine agonists for Parkinson disease.[1,2]

Those publications posed new questions with respect to the medical treatment of prolactinoma and whether surgery should be reconsidered in patients with resectable tumors. Although most studies did not find an increased risk for the lower doses of dopamine agonists used for prolactinoma, the underlying analyses may have had insufficient power to detect theses changes because of the relatively small number of patients and years of follow-up.

A recent large cohort study[3] from Denmark did not find any increased incidence of valve heart disease but relied on diagnosis encoded in the Danish

National Registry of Patients, without any sufficient information on both the frequency of echocardiography in these patients and clinically undetected valve disease.

The current study of 28 centers of endocrine care across the United Kingdom required a transthoracic echocardiogram in all patients. Again, no clear association was found between cumulative doses of bromocriptine and cabergoline and the prevalence of valvular abnormalities. These data may assure patients that treatment doses used for prolactinoma do not pose a significant risk for valvular heart disease. However, we probably have to wait for reports of longer treatment times because the follow-up times are still relatively short compared with the life expectancy of patients after diagnosis of prolactinoma. Furthermore, we need more information on other dopamine agonists; for example, quinagolide is thought not to cause valvular changes because of its receptor selectivity.

S. Petersenn, MD

References

1. Zanettini R, Antonini A, Gatto G, Gentile R, Tesei S, Pezzoli G. Valvular heart disease and the use of dopamine agonists for Parkinson's disease. *N Engl J Med.* 2007;356:39-46.
2. Schade R, Andersohn F, Suissa S, Haverkamp W, Garbe E. Dopamine agonists and the risk of cardiac-valve regurgitation. *N Engl J Med.* 2007;356:29-38.
3. Steffensen C, Maegbaek ML, Laurberg P, et al. Heart valve disease among patients with hyperprolactinemia: a nationwide population-based cohort study. *J Clin Endocrinol Metab.* 2012;97:1629-1634.

Outcome of prolactinoma after pregnancy and lactation: a study on 73 patients

Domingue M-E, Devuyst F, Alexopoulou O, et al (Université Catholique de Louvain, Brussels, Belgium; Université Libre de Bruxelles, Brussels, Belgium)
Clin Endocrinol 80:642-648, 2014

Context.—Prolactinoma is the most frequent pituitary tumour among women of child-bearing age. Only a few studies have addressed the outcome of prolactinoma after pregnancy.

Objective.—To study remission, defined as prolactin normalization without medical treatment, after pregnancy and lactation in women with prolactinoma.

Patients and Methods.—A retrospective study conducted in 2 Belgian academic centres including 73 patients (54 microprolactinomas and 19 macroprolactinomas) with 104 pregnancies continuing beyond first trimester. Dopamine agonists were stopped in early pregnancy in all treated cases. Prolactin level and adenoma size at pituitary magnetic resonance imaging (MRI) were recorded before pregnancy and throughout follow-up.

Results.—Thirty of 73 women (41%) were in remission after a median follow-up of 22 months after delivery or cessation of lactation. Adenoma size at diagnosis was smaller in women in remission (5 *vs* 8 mm). There was a nonsignificant higher rate of remission for microprolactinomas than for macroprolactinoma (46% *vs* 26%). The first pituitary MRI after pregnancy and lactation showed no tumour and a decreased adenoma size in 23% and 39% of women, respectively. MRI normalization was associated with remission. The number of pregnancies per woman as well as breastfeeding and its duration did not influence remission rate.

Conclusion.—More than 40% of women with previous diagnosis of prolactinoma have normal PRL level without medical treatment for a median follow-up of 22 months after pregnancy and lactation. The likelihood of remission is associated with a smaller initial adenoma size and normalization of pituitary MRI after pregnancy (Table 3).

▶ Next to cyclic irregularities, fertility issues are one of the main clinical situations in which a diagnosis of a prolactinoma is considered. Treatment then aims to restore fertility. Interestingly, considering the relative frequency of prolactinomas, few data are published on the outcome of pregnancy with respect to changes in tumor proliferation and autonomous hormone secretion. Several previous case reports and mostly small studies have indicated that prolactinomas

TABLE 3.—Clinical Characteristics in Women with and Without Remission After Pregnancy and Lactation

	All n = 73	Remission n = 30	Nonremission n = 43	*P**
Age at diagnosis (y)	28 [18–37]	29 [17–35]	27 [19–37]	NS
Microadenoma, *n* (%)	54	25 (46)	29 (54)	NS
Macroadenoma, *n* (%)	19	5 (26)	14 (74)	
Adenoma size at diagnosis (mm)	7·0 [2_5–17·5]	5·0 [2·4–13·2]	8·0 [4·0–17·0]	0·002
Adenoma size before pregnancy (mm)[†]	5·0 [1·6–14·4]	5·0 [1·6–11·0]	5·8 [3·9–9·0]	NS
PRL at diagnosis (×ULN)	3·2 [1·4–17·4]	2·6 [1·4–14·7]	3·5 [1·5–11·1]	NS
PRL under treatment (×ULN)	0·2 [0·1–0·9]	0·1 [0·1–0·9]	0·3 [0·1–1·0]	0·028
Previous neurosurgery, *n* (%)	11	4 (36)	7 (64)	NS
Treatment duration before pregnancy (months)	18 [4–80]	18 [4–77]	17 [4–75]	NS
Cabergoline dose at conception (mg/week)	0·5 [0·1–1·5]	0·3 [0·1–1·0]	0·5 [0·3–1·5]	0·009
Cabergoline cumulative dose (mg)	38 [6–291]	23 [8–120]	45 [7–325]	NS
Singleton pregnancies, *n* (%)[‡]	97	26 (27)	71 (73)	NS
Twin pregnancies, *n* (%)[‡]	7	4 (57)	3 (43)	
Breastfeeding duration (weeks)[‡]	20 [1–72]	18 [1–61]	20 [1–73]	NS
Duration of follow-up after last pregnancy (months)	22 [2–110]	14 [2–101]	27 [2–105]	NS
Adenoma size in post-partum (mm)	5·0 [0–12·0]	0 [0–7·5]	6·0 [0–12·0]	<0·001
Normal post-partum MRI, *n* (%)	15	12 (80)	3 (20)	<0·001
Adenoma size at last follow-up (mm)	4·4 [0–8.0]	3·0 [0–6·5]	5·0 [0–7·5]	0·008
Normal last follow-up MRI, *n* (%)	16	11 (73)	5 (31)	0·002

Results are expressed as *median [P5-95 range]*. Percentages are related to the total number of women or pregnancies (with and without remission) for the corresponding characteristic.

**P*-value for Mann–Whitney U-test and chi-Square/Fisher's exact test.

[†]Prepregnancy MRI available only for 31 subjects (18 in nonremission and 13 in remission).

[‡]These parameters are related to the 104 pregnancies.

may be cured during pregnancy, probably due to necrosis occurring with the usual enlargement of the pituitary during pregnancy.

This study investigated a large cohort of 73 pregnant patients despite previous diagnosis of prolactinoma. Interestingly, a relevant percentage of patients—more than 40%—did not require any treatment after delivery, for a median respectable follow-up time of 22 months (Table 3). Smaller size of the prolactinoma indicated a better chance for such a cure.

The results of this study, taken together with previous literature published on this issue, indicate that female patients should be offered a treatment pause after delivery to check for such a "cure," but this should be determined only after lactation.

S. Petersenn, MD

Growth Hormone

Progression of Vertebral Fractures Despite Long-Term Biochemical Control of Acromegaly: A Prospective Follow-up Study

Claessen KMJA, Kroon HM, Pereira AM, et al (Leiden Univ Med Ctr, The Netherlands)

J Clin Endocrinol Metab 98:4808-4815, 2013

Background.—In active acromegaly, pathologically elevated GH and IGF-1 levels are associated with increased bone turnover and a high bone mass, the latter being sustained after normalization of GH values. In a cross-sectional study design, we have previously reported a high prevalence of vertebral fractures (VFs) of about 60% in patients with controlled acromegaly, despite normal mean bone mineral density (BMD) values. Whether these fractures occur during the active acromegaly phase or after remission is achieved is not known.

Objective.—Our objective was to study the natural progression of VFs and contributing risk factors in patients with controlled acromegaly over a 2.5-year follow-up period.

Methods.—Forty-nine patients (mean age 61.3 ± 11.1 years, 37% female) with controlled acromegaly for ≥2 years after surgery, irradiation, and/or medical therapy and not using bisphosphonates were included in the study. Conventional spine radiographs including vertebrae Th4–L4 were assessed for VFs according to the Genant method. VF progression was defined as development of new/incident fractures and/or a minimum 1-point increase in the Genant scoring of preexisting VFs. BMD was assessed by dual-energy x-ray absorptiometry (Hologic 4500).

Results.—Prevalence of baseline VFs was 63%, being highest in men, and fractures were unrelated to baseline BMD. VF progression was documented in 20% of patients, especially in men and in case of ≥2 VFs at baseline. VF progression was not related to BMD values or BMD changes over time.

Conclusion.—Findings from this longitudinal study show that VFs progress in the long term in 20% of patients with biochemically controlled acromegaly in the absence of osteoporosis or osteopenia. These data suggest that an abnormal bone quality persists in these patients after remission, possibly related to pretreatment long-term exposure to high circulating levels of GH.

▶ Acromegaly is a devastating disease affecting many organs. Clinically relevant consequences include acral changes, metabolic disturbances, heart disease, sleep apnea syndrome, and tumor development. With respect to bone, it is still unclear whether development of osteoporosis in some patients is due to growth hormone excess or the presence of hypogonadism. Importantly, there appears to be a dissociation between bone mineral density usually used to screen for osteoporosis and real incidence of vertebral fractures. This study demonstrates vertebral fractures in nearly two-thirds of patients with controlled acromegaly (without any relation to bone mineral density), with additional fractures developing in 20% over a follow-up period of 2.5 years. Therefore, risk factors for vertebral fractures appear to persist even with long-term control of acromegaly, making bone changes one of the most debilitating long-term consequences of acromegaly.

Because assessment of bone mineral density was not able to predict the risk for bone fractures in those patients and other clear predictive parameters are not apparent, screening for vertebral fractures in patients with acromegaly by conventional spine radiographs should be included in the routine follow-up programs.

S. Petersenn, MD

Prevalence of Posttraumatic Growth Hormone Deficiency Is Highly Dependent on the Diagnostic Set-up: Results From The Danish National Study on Posttraumatic Hypopituitarism

Klose M, Stochholm K, Janukonyté J, et al (Copenhagen Univ Hosp, Denmark; Aarhus Univ Hosp, Denmark; et al)

J Clin Endocrinol Metab 99:101-110, 2014

Context.—Recent international guidelines suggest pituitary screening in patients with moderate and severe traumatic brain injury (TBI). Predominantly isolated GH deficiency (GHD) was reported in the literature, raising the question of potential methodological bias.

Objective.—Our objective was to assess the prevalence of GHD in patients admitted in 2008 with TBI, with concurrent assessment of methodological bias.

Design and Setting.—We conducted a nationwide population-based cohort study at tertiary referral university hospitals.

Participants.—Participants were Danish patients with a head trauma diagnosis from the Danish Board of Health diagnostic code registry; 439 patients and 124 healthy controls underwent dynamic assessment of GH secretion 2.5 years (median) after TBI.

Main Outcome.—We evaluated the prevalence of GHD given use of 1) local versus guideline cutoffs, 2) insulin tolerance test (ITT), pyridostigmine (PD)-GHRH or GHRH-arginine (arg) test, 3) single versus repeated testing, and 4) GH assessment by assays with different isoform specificities.

Results.—The prevalence of GHD was lower by local than by guideline cutoffs (12% vs 19% [PD-GHRH/GHRH-arg, $P < .001$]; 4.5% vs 5% [ITT, $P = .9$]), and by ITT than by PD-GHRH/GHRH-arg ($P = .006$ [local cutoffs]; $P < .001$ [guideline cutoffs]). Only 1% of patients had GHD according to 2 tests. GH assessment by the Immulite or iSYS assay caused no significant diagnostic differences.

Conclusions.—The study confirmed a high risk of bias in the management of pituitary testing of patients with TBI and stresses the importance of a proper control group and stringent GH testing including confirmatory testing in cohorts with low a priori likelihood of GHD such as in TBI. Our results question the evidence for newly introduced recommendations for routine pituitary assessment in TBI.

► Pituitary insufficiency may be due to various causes such as pituitary tumors, surgery and radiation in the sellar region, and traumatic brain injury, the last of which was most recently described. Whereas adrenal insufficiency, secondary hyperthyroidism, and secondary hypogonadism result in severe symptoms easily recognized by an experienced physician, the symptoms of growth hormone deficiency are much more difficult to establish. Changes in fat tissue and muscle mass, bone structure, and mood may all be due to growth hormone deficiency but are also found in a variety of other diseases and simply with aging. Biochemical testing is therefore the hallmark to define growth deficiency. Unfortunately, there is no clear gold standard, considering the variety of tests, assays, and cutoffs seen in the literature.

This study evaluated the outcome of testing in a large cohort of patients with a rather low likelihood of growth hormone deficiency. However, because of the high frequency of traumatic brain injury among the subjects, even a low percentage of patients affected by growth hormone deficiency could result in a relevant absolute number of patients potentially requiring growth hormone. Next to the potential benefits to the patients, this presents a significant cost burden for society.

Results presented in this study demonstrate a large variability in the diagnosis of growth hormone deficiency, ranging from 1% after dual testing and use of locally established cut-offs to 19% when a guideline cut-off was applied in patients tested only once (Fig 2 in the original article). This obviously presents an unacceptable outcome for a diagnostic procedure, demonstrating the relevant difficulties to establish a diagnosis only on the basis of biochemical tests.

One explanation proposed for the higher frequency of growth hormone deficiency when guideline cutoffs are applied relates to the trade-off between sensitivity and specificity for a diagnostic test. Because guideline cutoffs that offer high sensitivity so as not to overlook growth hormone deficiency may be chosen, this may be acceptable in patients with a high likelihood of disease, but not in patients with traumatic brain injury but lower likelihood of growth hormone deficiency. Furthermore, it has to be recognized that in pituitary disease, growth hormone deficiency usually occurs first, followed by insufficiency of other pituitary axes. In contrast, in traumatic brain injury, there is no clear order in the development of insufficiencies of the various pituitary axes. Therefore, when considering growth hormone substitution, the label requirement of additional pituitary insufficiencies certainly improves diagnostic accuracy in patients with pituitary disease but not in patients with traumatic brain injury.

The indications for testing and growth hormone substitution in traumatic brain injury should therefore be reconsidered, possibly requiring 2 positive test results before any therapeutic measures are taken, with careful reevaluation to establish benefit.

S. Petersenn, MD

ACTH

A Cellular and Molecular Basis for the Selective Desmopressin-Induced ACTH Release in Cushing Disease Patients: Key Role of AVPR1b Receptor and Potential Therapeutic Implications

Luque RM, Ibáñez-Costa A, López-Sánchez LM, et al (Univ of Córdoba, Spain; et al)

J Clin Endocrinol Metab 98:4160-4169, 2013

Context.—Desmopressin is a synthetic agonist of vasopressin receptors (AVPRs). The desmopressin stimulation test is used in the diagnosis and postsurgery prognosis of Cushing disease (CD). However, the cellular and molecular mechanisms underlying the desmopressin-induced ACTH increase in patients with CD are poorly understood.

Objective.—The objectives of this study were to determine, for the first time, whether desmopressin acts directly and exclusively on pituitary corticotropinoma cells to stimulate ACTH expression/release and to elucidate the cellular and molecular mechanisms involved in desmopressin-induced ACTH increase in CD.

Design.—A total of 8 normal pituitaries (NPs), 23 corticotropinomas, 14 nonfunctioning pituitary adenomas, 17 somatotropinomas, and 3 prolactinomas were analyzed for AVPR expression by quantitative real-time RT-PCR. Primary cultures derived from corticotropinomas, nonfunctioning pituitary adenomas, somatotropinomas, prolactinomas, and NPs were treated with desmopressin, and ACTH secretion/expression, $[Ca^{2+}]_i$ kinetics, and AVPR expression and/or proliferative response were evaluated. The relationship between AVPR expression and plasma adrenocorticotropin/cortisol levels obtained from desmopressin tests was assessed.

Results.—Desmopressin affects all functional parameters evaluated in corticotropinoma cells but not in NPs or other pituitary adenomas cells. These effects might be due to the dramatic elevation of AVPR1b expression levels found in corticotropinomas. In line with this notion, the use of an AVPR1b antagonist completely blocked desmopressin stimulatory effects. Remarkably, only AVPR1b expression was positively correlated with elevated plasma adrenocorticotropin levels in corticotropinomas.

Conclusions.—The present results provide a cellular and molecular basis to support the desmopressin stimulation test as a reliable, specific test for the diagnosis and postsurgery prognosis of CD. Furthermore, our data indicate that AVPR1b is responsible for the direct/exclusive desmopressin stimulatory pituitary effects observed in CD, thus opening the possibility of exploring AVPR1b antagonists as potential therapeutic tools for CD treatment.

▶ The differential diagnosis of adrenocorticotropic hormone (ACTH)-dependent Cushing syndrome may be challenging, requiring biochemical tests and sometimes inferior petrosal sinus sampling (IPSS). Because of limited availability and costs of corticotropin-releasing hormone (CRH), the desmopressin test has been advocated as an alternative. However, in contrast to CRH, the principles of desmopressin activation of the hypothalamic-pituitary-adrenal axis are unclear. This study demonstrates clear effects of desmopressin at the level of the corticotropic pituitary cell, possibly due to high expression of its receptor in ACTH-secreting pituitary cells. A receptor antagonist blocked desmopressin responses, supporting the notion of specific effects of desmopressin but also suggesting a potential new therapeutic approach for Cushing disease. The data support further studies of desmopressin to determine large cohort cutoffs for the differential diagnosis of Cushing syndrome during both biochemical testing and IPSS. Because the effects of medical therapy on Cushing syndrome are still limited, the use of desmopressin antagonists in models of Cushing disease are certainly of interest.

S. Petersenn, MD

Preoperative Normalization of Cortisol Levels in Cushing's Disease After Medical Treatment: Consequences for Somatostatin and Dopamine Receptor Subtype Expression and In Vitro Response to Somatostatin Analogs and Dopamine Agonists

van der Pas R, Feelders RA, Gatto F, et al (Erasmus Med Ctr, Rotterdam, The Netherlands; et al)

J Clin Endocrinol Metab 98:E1880-E1890, 2013

Context.—Corticotroph pituitary adenomas often highly express the dopamine 2 receptor (D_2R) and somatostatin receptor subtype 5 (sst_5). The sst_2 expression is relatively low, likely resulting from downregulating effects of high cortisol levels. This may explain why the sst_2-preferring somatostatin analog octreotide, compared with the multi-receptor-targeting somatostatin analog pasireotide, is generally ineffective in Cushing's disease.

Objective.—Our objective was to compare sst and D_2R expression levels between adenomas from patients with elevated and normalized preoperative urinary free cortisol excretion.

Patients and Design.—Corticotroph adenoma tissue was examined from patients from group 1 (n = 22; elevated preoperative urinary free cortisol) and group 2 (n = 11; mean duration of preoperative normocortisolism 10 weeks). Somatotroph adenoma tissue from 10 acromegalic patients was examined to compare receptor expression profiles.

Main Outcome Measures.—We evaluated receptor mRNA and protein expression levels and effects of octreotide, pasireotide, and cabergoline on ACTH secretion by cultured human corticotroph adenoma cells.

Results.—The sst_2 mRNA expression in group 2 was 10-fold higher than in group 1 ($P < .01$), even comparable to that in somatotroph adenomas. There were no statistically significant differences in sst_5 and D_2R mRNA expression or in sst_2, sst_5, and D_2R protein expression between both groups of corticotroph adenomas. In responders, octreotide (n = 2 out of 4; −30.5% ± 10.4%) was less potent than pasireotide (n = 5 out of 6; −47.0% ± 4.2%) and cabergoline (n = 3 out of 4; −41.9% ± 3.1%) with respect to inhibition of ACTH secretion by adenomas from group 2.

Conclusions.—After achieving normocortisolism induced by medical therapy, cortisol-mediated sst_2 downregulation on corticotroph adenomas appears to be a reversible process at the mRNA but not at the protein level. Octreotide remains less potent than pasireotide and cabergoline with respect to in vitro inhibition of ACTH secretion. Whether sustained normocortisolism induced by medical therapy induces re-expression of functional sst_2 protein in corticotroph adenomas and whether this increases the ACTH-lowering potency of octreotide remains to be established.

▶ Whereas surgery clearly remains the first-line treatment in Cushing disease, the therapeutic approach in remnant or recurrent disease is less well established. Potential options include radiation, bilateral adrenalectomy, and various forms of medical treatment. Classical somatostatin analogs like octreotide and lanreotide with a well-proven efficacy and side-effect profile in acromegaly did not show any efficacy in Cushing disease, the underlying reason being low levels of somatostatin receptor subtype 2 (sst_2) in those tumors. Several elegant studies have indicated that hypercortisolism may lead to a down-regulation of sst_2,[1] whereas sst_5 usually remains at high level. Therefore, the multisomatostatin receptor ligand pasireotide, with high-binding efficacy to sst_5, has been studied for the treatment of Cushing disease, showing efficacy in a relevant percentage of patients. This compound is currently licensed for patients in whom surgery failed or was refused. However, activation of sst_5 also leads to inhibition of insulin secretion and, therefore, hyperglycemia in some patients. It has been suggested that normalization of cortisol levels may allow for up-regulation of sst_2, thereby allowing sst_2 ligands like octreotide and lanreotide to become effective. This study analyzed mRNA levels of sst_2 in patients with normalization of cortisol levels before surgery compared with patients untreated before surgery. Indeed, sst_2 levels were higher in those patients pretreated but unfortunately still did not respond to treatment with octreotide in a cell culture model, possibly because of a lack of sst_2 protein. The authors wonder whether longer duration of treatment is necessary to allow for sufficient sst_2 protein expression. Until further information is available, medical treatment of Cushing disease will focus on sst_5 ligands, dopamine agonists, adrenal inhibitors, and glucocorticoid receptor antagonists.

S. Petersenn, MD

Reference

1. Colao A, Petersenn S, Newell-Price J, et al. Pasireotide B2305 Study Group. A 12-month phase 3 study of pasireotide in Cushing's disease. *N Engl J Med*. 2012;366: 914-924.

High variability in baseline urinary free cortisol values in patients with Cushing's disease

Petersenn S, Newell-Price J, Findling JW, et al (ENDOC Ctr for Endocrine Tumors, Hamburg, Germany; Univ of Sheffield, UK; Med College of Wisconsin, Milwaukee; et al)

Clin Endocrinol 80:261-269, 2014

Objective.—Twenty-four-hour urinary free cortisol (UFC) sampling is commonly used to evaluate Cushing's syndrome. Because there are few data on UFC variability in patients with active Cushing's disease, we analysed baseline UFC in a large patient cohort with moderate-to-severe Cushing's disease and assessed whether variability correlates with hypercortisolism severity. These data will help clinicians establish the minimum number of UFC samples required to obtain reliable data.

Design.—Observational study (enrolment phase of Phase III study).

Methods.—Patients (n = 152) with persistent/recurrent or *de novo* Cushing's disease and mean UFC (mUFC) $\geq 1 \cdot 5 \times$ULN (normal: 30–145 nmol/24 h) were included. Mean UFC level was calculated from four 24-h urine samples collected over 2 weeks.

Results.—Over 600 24-h UFC samples were analysed. The mUFC levels of samples 1 and 2 and samples 3 and 4 were 1000 nmol/24 h (SD 1872) and 940 nmol/24 h (SD 2148), respectively; intrapatient coefficient of variation (CV) was 38% for mUFC. The intrapatient CV using all four samples was 52% (95% CI: 48–56). The intrapatient CV was 51% (95% CI: 44–58) for samples 1 and 2, 49% (95% CI: 43–56) for samples 3 and 4 and 54% (95% CI: 49–59) for samples 1, 2 and 3. Variability in mUFC increased as UFC levels increased. There were no correlations between UFC and clinical features of hypercortisolism.

Conclusions.—There is intrapatient variability of approximately 50% in 24-h UFC measurements, which is relevant to targets set to estimate any treatment effect. Analysing more than two 24-h collection periods in individual patients does not result in a relevant decrease in variability. Interestingly, UFC levels did not correlate with hypercortisolism severity.

▶ Current guidelines recommend a combination of late-night cortisol, dexamethasone suppression testing, and urinary free cortisol for the screening of hypercortisolism. Each of these has its own advantages and disadvantages. With respect to urinary free cortisol, variations in assays as well as collection errors are among the major problems. Because urinary free cortisol is the only parameter widely accepted for the follow-up of Cushing syndrome during medical treatment, standardization of collection and establishment of reference ranges is of major interest.

This study analyzed variability of urinary free cortisol with repeated sampling in a large cohort of patients with confirmed Cushing disease. Interestingly, even four 24-hour urine collections demonstrated a relevant variability of approximately 50%, without any major improvement compared with 2 or 3 collection periods. Because of the relevant variability, only changes of more than 50% in urinary free cortisol may present real treatment effects outside of chance variability.

These results clearly indicate the need for better tools for assessment of disease activity in Cushing disease to allow for optimal management of therapy.

Another major finding relates to the lack of significant correlation between urinary free cortisol and various clinical indicators of hypercortisolism, calling into question the use of biochemical parameters alone to follow patients with Cushing disease.

S. Petersenn, MD

General

Diagnosis, Evaluation, and Treatment of Hyponatremia: Expert Panel Recommendations

Verbalis JG, Goldsmith SR, Greenberg A, et al (Georgetown Univ Med Ctr, Washington, DC; Univ of Minnesota, Minneapolis; Duke Univ Med Ctr, Durham, NC; et al)

Am J Med 126:S1-S42, 2013

Hyponatremia is a serious, but often overlooked, electrolyte imbalance that has been independently associated with a wide range of deleterious changes involving many different body systems. Untreated acute hyponatremia can cause substantial morbidity and mortality as a result of osmotically induced cerebral edema, and excessively rapid correction of chronic hyponatremia can cause severe neurologic impairment and death as a result of osmotic demyelination. The diverse etiologies and comorbidities associated with hyponatremia pose substantial challenges in managing this disorder. In 2007, a panel of experts in hyponatremia convened to develop the *Hyponatremia Treatment Guidelines 2007: Expert Panel Recommendations* that defined strategies for clinicians caring for patients with hyponatremia. In the 6 years since the publication of that document, the field has seen several notable developments, including new evidence on morbidities and complications associated with hyponatremia, the importance of treating mild to moderate hyponatremia, and the efficacy and safety of vasopressin receptor antagonist therapy for hyponatremic patients. Therefore, additional guidance was deemed necessary and a panel of hyponatremia experts (which included all of the original panel members) was convened to update the previous recommendations for optimal current management of this disorder. The updated expert panel recommendations in this document represent recommended approaches for multiple etiologies of hyponatremia that are based on both consensus opinions of experts in hyponatremia and the most recent published data in this field.

▶ The differential diagnosis and appropriate treatment of hyponatremia still remain a major challenge for the caring clinician. More importantly, hyponatremia is often overlooked and diagnosed only at an advanced stage. With implementation of patients' early discharge after surgery in many societies, outpatients should be regularly investigated in the initial postoperative phase. Neuroendocrinologists may become involved during postoperative care of patients after pituitary surgery or in patients with undiagnosed adrenal insufficiency.

The complex interplay between electrolytes and volume changes in the human body complicate the interpretation of biochemical testing. Even with an underlying endocrine disease, other potential factors aggravating hyponatremia need to be considered. Therefore, some practical guidance is of special importance and is given by the expert panel recommendations in this publication. Search strategies of the current literature, determination of level of evidence, and development of a consensus are clearly described in the Methods section. The relevance of plasma tonicity and patient's extracellular fluid volume status for the initial approach to the patient are emphasized. Because therapy depends on severity and duration of hyponatremia, treatment recommendations for each situation are summarized in boxes, including measures to avoid the life-threatening osmotic demyelination syndrome.

S. Petersenn, MD

9 Pediatric Endocrinology

Introduction

This year's article selections span a diverse set of topics that include novel discoveries in molecular genetics, advancements in clinical management, and important new observations based on population data. "Large-Scale Pooled Next-Generation Sequencing of 1077 Genes to Identify Genetic Causes of Short Stature" illustrates the potential power of cutting-edge genetic sequencing tools, which allow for an exhaustive search for new mutations through investigation of a multitude of different genes simultaneously. "Growth Hormone Therapy for Children and Adolescents with Prader-Willi Syndrome Is Associated With Improved Body Composition and Metabolic Status in Adulthood" adds to several earlier studies reporting possible beneficial long-term results of growth hormone therapy on body composition and metabolic status in individuals with Prader Willi syndrome. "Impact of Hydrocortisone on Adult Height in Congenital Adrenal Hyperplasia–The Minnesota Cohort" further refines the factors that have an adverse impact on adult height in patients with CAH. The next two studies "Central Precocious Puberty Caused by Mutations in the Imprinted Gene *MKRN3*" and "A Single Histrelin Implant Is Effective for 2 Years for Treatment of Central Precocious Puberty" both deal with central precocious puberty (CPP). The first reports a major breakthrough in identification of the genetic basis of familial CPP, while the second recounts an incremental but significant improvement in the therapeutic armamentarium of affected patients. "Urinary Phthalates From 168 Girls and Boys Measured Twice a Year During a 5-year Period: Associations With Adrenal Androgen Levels and Puberty" and "Onset of Breast Development in a Longitudinal Cohort" also pertain to puberty, but from distinctly different standpoints.

The first of this pair investigated the relationship between an endocrine disruptor, in this case urinary phthalates, and pubertal development in a cohort of boys and girls during a 5-year interval. The second study builds on a landmark 1997 paper reporting a secular trend of earlier onset of puberty in girls. In the case of this recent cohort, even earlier breast development was seen in overweight girls, while the timing of pubertal onset in the normal weight subset was equivalent to the 1997 study. "Delayed

Puberty and Estrogen Resistance in a Woman with Estrogen Receptor Alpha Variant" describes the first known case of estrogen resistance in a human female caused by a homozygous mutation in the estrogen receptor alpha. "Factors Associated With Hearing Impairment in Patients With Congenital Hypothyroidism Treated Since the Neonatal Period: A National Population-Based Study" represents an important contribution to our understanding of the risk of hearing impairment in congenital hypothyroidism and has the advantage of utilizing a National Registry of adults with that condition.

The next article relates to congenital adrenal hyperplasia (CAH). "Congenital Adrenal Hyperplasia and the Second Newborn Screen" details the very favorable experience that one state has had with implementation of a two-tiered newborn screening program for the disease within the past 10 years. The theme of the adrenal glands is continued with the following two articles. "Skeletal Maturation in Children with Cushing Syndrome Is Not Consistently Delayed: The Role of Corticotropin, Obesity, and Steroid Hormones, and the Effect of Surgical Cure" reports the surprising discovery that bone ages are often not delayed in children with Cushing syndrome, and "Increased Scalp Hair Cortisol Concentrations in Obese Children" finds higher scalp hair cortisol levels in exogenous obesity. Lastly, "Parathyroid Hormone as a Functional Indicator of Vitamin D Sufficiency in Children" is a straightforward, but elegant illumination of how parathyroid hormone concentration can be a valuable indicator of vitamin D sufficiency in the pediatric population.

In summary, the articles represented in this YEAR BOOK are an eclectic collection. However, they are a good reflection of the diversity of the field of Pediatric Endocrinology and will hopefully provide insights into the types of scientific and clinical questions that we encounter every day. It is my hope that they will be both informative and interesting!

Erica Eugster, MD

Growth/Growth Hormone

Large-Scale Pooled Next-Generation Sequencing of 1077 Genes to Identify Genetic Causes of Short Stature

Wang SR, Carmichael H, Andrew SF, et al (Harvard Med School, Boston, MA; Oregon Health and Science Univ, Portland)
J Clin Endocrinol Metab 98:E1428-E1437, 2013

Context.—The majority of patients presenting with short stature do not receive a definitive diagnosis. Advances in genetic sequencing allow for large-scale screening of candidate genes, potentially leading to genetic diagnoses.

Objectives.—The purpose of this study was to discover genetic variants that contribute to short stature in a cohort of children with no known genetic etiology.

Design.—This was a prospective cohort study of subjects with short stature.

Setting.—The setting was a pediatric endocrinology and genetics clinics at an academic center.

Patients.—A total of 192 children with short stature with no defined genetic etiology and 192 individuals of normal stature from the Framingham Heart Study were studied.

Intervention.—Pooled targeted sequencing using next-generation DNA sequencing technology of the exons of 1077 candidate genes was performed.

Main Outcome Measures.—The numbers of rare nonsynonymous genetic variants found in case patients but not in control subjects, known pathogenic variants in case patients, and potentially pathogenic variants in *IGF1R* were determined.

Results.—We identified 4928 genetic variants in 1077 genes that were present in case patients but not in control subjects. Of those, 1349 variants were novel (898 nonsynonymous). False-positive rates from pooled sequencing were 4% to 5%, and the false-negative rate was 0.1% in regions covered well by sequencing. We identified 3 individuals with known pathogenic variants in *PTPN11* causing undiagnosed Noonan syndrome. There were 9 rare potentially nonsynonymous variants in *IGF1R*, one of which is a novel, probably pathogenic, frameshift mutation. A previously reported pathogenic variant in *IGF1R* was present in a control subject.

Conclusions.—Large-scale sequencing efforts have the potential to rapidly identify genetic etiologies of short stature, but data interpretation is complex. Noonan syndrome may be an underdiagnosed cause of short stature.

► This study is an excellent illustration of the truly remarkable power of cutting-edge molecular sequencing techniques combined with the potentially small yield that may initially result from an exhaustive investigation of genetic variants thought to impact height. That thousands more variants were identified in children with short stature than in controls provides confirmation of the relevance of the chosen genes, and yet the contribution of each of them to an individual patient's stature is unclear. It is noteworthy that of 4 subjects found to have pathologic conditions, 3 of them had Noonan syndrome caused by mutations in *PTPN11*. This speaks to the extreme phenotypic heterogeneity of Noonan syndrome and the need to maintain a high index of suspicion when evaluating a child with short stature in the clinical setting. On the flip side, the authors demonstrate the critical importance of incorporating clinical information in the interpretation of genetic variants, as was shown by the inconsequential nature of all but one of the rare *IGF1R* variants found. Undoubtedly, it is at the intersection of large-scale gene sequencing endeavors such as this and old-fashioned clinical characterization of patients that new insights regarding the underpinnings of variations of growth will emerge.

E. Eugster, MD

Growth Hormone Therapy for Children and Adolescents with Prader-Willi Syndrome Is Associated With Improved Body Composition and Metabolic Status in Adulthood

Coupaye M, Lorenzini F, Lloret-Linares C, et al (Pitié-Salpêtriére Hospital, Paris, France; French Reference Centre for Prader-Willi Syndrome, Toulouse, France; et al)

J Clin Endocrinol Metab 98:E328-E335, 2013

Context.—Children with Prader-Willi syndrome (PWS) who receive GH treatment have improved growth and body composition; however, data are lacking for adults when treatment is discontinued after completion of growth.

Objectives.—Our aim was to compare body composition and metabolic status in adults with PWS according to GH treatment in childhood and adolescence.

Design.—64 adults (mean age: 25.4 years) with a genetic diagnosis of PWS were evaluated: 20 received GH in childhood (T), which had been discontinued at the time of this study, and 44 did not receive GH (C). Mean duration of treatment in the T group was 4.4 ± 2.7 years, age at baseline was 11.8 ± 2.7 years, mean time between the end of treatment and the current evaluation was 7.0 ± 4.4 years.

Main Outcomes Measures.—Dual-energy X-ray absorptiometry was used to assess body composition and fasting biological analyses evaluated metabolic status.

Results (mean ± SD).—Body mass index and percentage of fat mass were significantly lower in the T group (32.4 ± 10.3 vs 41.2 ± 11.1 kg/m^2, $P = 0.05$ and 44.0 ± 9.6 vs 50.1 ± 7.2%, $P = 0.02$, respectively). Insulinemia and HOMA-IR in non-diabetic subjects were significantly lower in the T group (5.8 ± 5.9 vs 13.9 ± 11.6 μUI/ml, $P = 0.03$, and 1.6 ± 1.3 vs 2.7 ± 2.1, $P = 0.04$, respectively). Non-diabetic and diabetic subjects from the T group had a significantly lower HbA1c. Lipid profiles were similar between groups.

Conclusions.—GH treatment in childhood and adolescence is associated with significantly decreased body mass index and improved body composition and metabolic status in adults with PWS at several years after discontinuing treatment.

► That growth hormone (GH) therapy improves body composition in children with Prader-Willi syndrome (PWS) has been well established. However, to what degree the observed decreases in body mass index and percentage of body fat achieved from GH therapy are maintained after treatment is discontinued is unclear. Unlike in a 2010 publication reporting long-term follow-up of PWS adults,[1] this study found statistically significant differences in body composition in a group of PWS adults who had received GH compared with a group who had not been treated. Surprisingly, and also in contrast to the earlier study, the height SDS was no different in the treatment and control groups, despite an average duration of GH of more than 4 years. Lest we feel overly troubled about these conflicting reports, it is important to remember that each only had a sample size of 20, and neither was a randomized, controlled trial. Thus, we must await further studies before a definitive conclusion can be reached.

E. Eugster, MD

Reference

1. Sipilä I, Sintonen H, Hietanen H, et al. Long-term effects of growth hormone therapy on patients with Prader-Willi syndrome. *Acta Paediatr.* 2010;99:1712-1718.

Impact of Hydrocortisone on Adult Height in Congenital Adrenal Hyperplasia—The Minnesota Cohort

Sarafoglou K, Addo OY, Turcotte L, et al (Univ of Minnesota Amplatz Children's Hosp, Minneapolis; Univ of Minnesota, Minneapolis; et al)
J Pediatr 2014 [Epub ahead of print]

Objective.—To estimate the impact of the average daily dose of hydrocortisone (HC) on the amount of growth attained in children with congenital adrenal hyperplasia (CAH). The effect of glucocorticoid therapy on adult height (AH) in children with CAH has yet to be elucidated.

Study Design.—Triple-logistic models estimating components of growth and maturation were fitted to longitudinal records of 104 patients with classic CAH from 3 pediatric medical centers in Minnesota between 1955 and 2012. A total of 3664 clinical encounters were examined. Random-effects longitudinal models with time-related covariates were used to estimate the effect of HC therapy on linear growth.

Results.—The predicted AH z-score (-0.7) was similar between the sexes and among CAH subtypes. The mean growth period HC dose was 18.9 ± 5.6 mg/m^2/day. In the final regression model, HC dose was negatively associated with predicted AH, with each mg/m^2/day increase in average growth period HC dose predicting a 0.37-cm decrease in AH ($P < .004$).

Conclusion.—This study has quantified the fractional reduction in predicted final AH with an incremental increase in HC dose. These findings have important clinical implications in the decision making balance between HC replacement dose and adrenal androgen suppression in children with CAH.

► A multitude of studies including 2 meta-analyses[1,2] have addressed the issue of adult height deficit in classical congenital adrenal hyperplasia (CAH). Although the finding of a modest height decrement in this population has been a consistent one, delineating the exact factors responsible has proved difficult. Several investigators have failed to find a clear association between specific treatment variables and adult height. This study employed sophisticated statistical modeling to summarize the subjects' longitudinal growth data and to explore the relationship between treatment factors and outcome in terms of height. The results are striking in that each milligram per square meter per day of hydrocortisone during the growth period was associated with a 0.37-cm decrease in adult height. This is the first study to quantify the deleterious effect of glucocorticoid therapy in such a precise fashion. Several questions do nevertheless come to mind. Although the study is touted as being ambidirectional, it is unclear which aspect of the protocol was in fact prospective. Another issue is the question of hydrocortisone equivalencies, which for prednisone has been estimated as anywhere between 5 to 1 and 20 to 1 in terms of relative potency. That the authors were unable to identify any dose at which a decrease in predicted or actual adult height did not occur suggests that some degree of height deficit is unavoidable given our current therapeutic armamentarium for CAH. However, the lack of dose-related effects during infancy is highly reassuring because glucocorticoid dose requirements during the first 2 years of life in patients with CAH are often high.

E. Eugster, MD

References

1. Eugster EA, Dimeglio LA, Wright JC, et al. Height outcome in congenital adrenal hyperplasia caused by 21-hydroxylase deficiency: a meta-analysis. *J Pediatr.* 2001; 138:26-32.
2. Muthusamy K, Elamin MB, Smushkin G, et al. Clinical review: Adult height in patients with congenital adrenal hyperplasia: a systematic review and metaanalysis. *J Clin Endocrinol Metab.* 2010;95:4161-4172.

Miscellaneous

Central Precocious Puberty Caused by Mutations in the Imprinted Gene *MKRN3*

Abreu AP, Dauber A, Macedo DB, et al (Brigham and Women's Hosp and Harvard Med School, Boston, MA; Boston Children's Hosp, MA; Faculdade de Medicina da Universidade de São Paulo, Brazil; et al)
N Engl J Med 368:2467-2475, 2013

Background.—The onset of puberty is first detected as an increase in pulsatile secretion of gonadotropin-releasing hormone (GnRH). Early activation of the hypothalamic–pituitary–gonadal axis results in central precocious puberty. The timing of pubertal development is driven in part by genetic factors, but only a few, rare molecular defects associated with central precocious puberty have been identified.

Methods.—We performed whole-exome sequencing in 40 members of 15 families with central precocious puberty. Candidate variants were confirmed with Sanger sequencing. We also performed quantitative real-time polymerase-chain-reaction assays to determine levels of messenger RNA (mRNA) in the hypothalami of mice at different ages.

Results.—We identified four novel heterozygous mutations in MKRN3, the gene encoding makorin RING-finger protein 3, in 5 of the 15 families; both sexes were affected. The mutations included three frameshift mutations, predicted to encode truncated proteins, and one missense mutation, predicted to disrupt protein function. *MKRN3* is a paternally expressed, imprinted gene located in the Prader–Willi syndrome critical region (chromosome 15q11–q13). All affected persons inherited the mutations from their fathers, a finding that indicates perfect segregation with the mode of inheritance expected for an imprinted gene. Levels of *Mkrn3* mRNA were high in the arcuate nucleus of prepubertal mice, decreased immediately before puberty, and remained low after puberty.

Conclusions.—Deficiency of MKRN3 causes central precocious puberty in humans. (Funded by the National Institutes of Health and others.)

▶ This study represents an exciting major breakthrough in determining the genetic basis of central precocious puberty (CPP). Despite intensive investigation by scientists around the world, only 2 previous genetic causes of CPP in 2 isolated patients have been identified. The first, published in *New England Journal of Medicine* in 2008,[1] described a gain-of-function mutation in *GPR54*, also known as the *KISS-1* receptor, in an 8-year-old adopted girl with idiopathic CPP. The second, published in 2010, reported an activating mutation in the *KISS-1* gene in a boy in whom CPP developed at 1 year of age.[2] Functionally, both mutations appear to exert their pathophysiologic effect through prolonged intracellular signaling caused by delayed degradation of the mutant protein. This study contains numerous notable features. Not only does it involve a system previously unknown to be involved in the H-P-G axis, but the investigators found 4 novel mutations and a stunning 33% hit rate among the affected families! Making this discovery even more intriguing is that the *MKRN3* gene is in the Prader-Willi syndrome critical region and is maternally imprinted. Thus, all affected cases inherited the mutation from their unaffected fathers, who, in turn, inherited the mutant allele from their mothers. Not only will this important scientific development spur additional research in children with CPP, but it will undoubtedly illuminate new aspects of human reproductive biology and contribute to the gradual unraveling of the mystery known as the "black box" of puberty!

E. Eugster, MD

References

1. Teles MG, Bianco SD, Brito VN, et al. A GPR54-activating mutation in a patient with central precocious puberty. *N Engl J Med.* 2008;358:709-715.
2. Silveira LG, Noel SD, Silveira-Neto AP, et al. Mutations of the KISS1 gene in disorders of puberty. *J Clin Endocrinol Metab.* 2010;95:2276-2280.

A Single Histrelin Implant Is Effective for 2 Years for Treatment of Central Precocious Puberty

Lewis KA, Goldyn AK, West KW, et al (Indiana Univ School of Medicine, Indianapolis)

J Pediatr 2013 [Epub ahead of print]

We investigated whether a "yearly" histrelin implant would provide pubertal suppression when left in place for 2 years. Equivalent suppression was observed when comparing 12 and 24 months in 33 children with central precocious puberty. A single implant for 2 years reduces cost and numbers of implant procedures.

▶ Sometimes advances in clinical medicine occur from relatively simple and straightforward hypotheses based on logical deductions. This study, which investigated effectiveness of the yearly histrelin implant for the treatment of central precocious puberty (CPP) if left in place for 2 years, is one such example. Knowing that a single implant contains 50 mg of the highly potent gonadotropin-releasing hormone analog (GnRHa), histrelin, and that the drug is released at a rate of approximately 65 μg/d, a simple calculation reveals that a single implant could theoretically last 769 days, or precisely 2 years. Because theory and practice are different, however, it was essential to show that one implant actually would result in complete hypothalamic-pituitary-gonadal suppression for a full 2 years. Although the study was a resounding success in this regard, a few caveats are worth noting. Although use of a single implant for 2 years would decrease costs and surgical procedures, the 39% rate of difficulty with explantation is sobering when one considers that the procedures were all performed by a single highly experienced pediatric surgeon at one site. It is certainly likely that even more difficulty would be encountered under less-ideal circumstances. In addition, the fact that implants were removed early in 2 girls because of clinical concerns of pubertal progression despite complete pubertal suppression on GnRHa stimulation tests reminds us that clinical and biochemical indices can sometimes be discrepant. Regardless, this study represents a minor but a welcome incremental improvement in the treatment of children with CPP.

E. Eugster, MD

Urinary Phthalates From 168 Girls and Boys Measured Twice a Year During a 5-year Period: Associations With Adrenal Androgen Levels and Puberty

Mouritsen A, Frederiksen H, Sørensen K, et al (Univ of Copenhagen, Denmark)
J Clin Endocrinol Metab 98:3755-3764, 2013

Background.—Little is known about the possible deleterious effects of phthalate exposure on endogenous sex steroid levels in children.

Objective.—Our objective was to investigate whether urinary phthalate metabolite levels are associated with circulating adrenal androgen levels and age at puberty.

Methods.—This was a longitudinal study of 168 healthy children (84 girls) examined every 6 months for 5 years. Serum levels of dehydroepiandrostenedione sulfate (DHEAS), Δ4-androstenedione, testosterone, and urinary morning excretion of 14 phthalate metabolites, corresponding to 7 different phthalate diesters were determined. A variation in urinary excretion of phthalates was evident in each child, which made a mean of repetitive samples more representative for long-term excretion than a single determination.

Results.—We found that girls with excretion of monobutyl phthalate isomers (MBP) and di(2-ethylhexyl) phthalate metabolites above the geometric group mean (795 and 730 ng/kg, respectively) had lower levels of DHEAS and Δ4-androstenedione, although statistically significant only at 13 years of age. In boys, we found that excretion of monobenzyl phthalate above the geometric group mean (346 ng/kg) was associated with lower levels of DHEAS at 11 years of age but higher levels of testosterone at 13 years of age. The same trend was observed for MBP excretion, albeit not statistically significant. A lower age at pubarche was observed in boys with excretion of MBP above the geometric group mean (11.0 vs 12.3 years, $P = 0.005$).

Conclusion.—Our data indicate that exposure to dibutyl phthalate isomers (DBP) (in girls) and butylbenzyl phthalate (in boys) are negatively associated with adrenal androgen levels and in boys positively associated with testosterone level at 13 years of age. High exposure to DBP was associated with earlier age at pubarche in boys. In girls, no associations between phthalate exposure and age at pubertal milestones were observed.

▶ The results of this study are representative of the cumulative literature regarding effects of phthalate exposure on human reproductive function in pediatric patients. Unique strengths of this study include its longitudinal design, serial measurements during a 5-year interval, and inclusion of both prepubertal and postpubertal boys and girls. That virtually all 14 phthalate metabolites were detectable in all 788 urine samples from the 168 subjects is a vivid demonstration of how ubiquitously these compounds have infiltrated our day-to-day life. What the authors found regarding the association of urinary phthalate metabolites and adrenal androgen levels and pubertal timing, however, was not nearly so clear. The inverse relationship between dehydroepiandrostenedione sulfate, Adione, and some of the phthalate metabolite isomers in 13-year-old girls is consistent with the proposed antiandrogenic action of these chemicals. However, the observed lack of an effect on the age of pubarche in the girls in the study is obviously not. In boys, higher levels of the same isomer were not associated with lower adrenal androgens, and the earlier age of pubic hair development in this group would seem to be directly opposite to the hypothesis that phthalates would delay pubarche. That the relationship between testosterone levels and concentrations of different phthalate metabolites among boys went in opposite directions and the lack of any perceived effect of these agents on markers of central puberty creates even more ambiguity. Thus, this study joins the ranks of several others with conflicting and inconclusive results. Clearly, more research is needed!

E. Eugster, MD

Onset of Breast Development in a Longitudinal Cohort

Biro FM, Greenspan LC, Galvez MP, et al (Cincinnati Children's Hosp Med Ctr, OH; Kaiser Permanente, San Francisco, CA; Mount Sinai School of Medicine, NY; et al)

Pediatrics 132:1019-1027, 2013

Background and Objectives.—There is growing evidence of pubertal maturation occurring at earlier ages, with many studies based on cross-sectional observations. This study examined age at onset of breast development (thelarche), and the impact of BMI and race/ethnicity, in the 3 puberty study sites of the Breast Cancer and the Environment Research Program, a prospective cohort of >1200 girls.

Methods.—Girls, 6 to 8 years at enrollment, were followed longitudinally at regular intervals from 2004 to 2011 in 3 geographic areas: the San Francisco Bay Area, Greater Cincinnati, and New York City. Sexual maturity assessment using Tanner staging was conducted by using standardized observation and palpation methods by trained and certified staff. Kaplan-Meier analyses were used to describe age at onset of breast maturation by covariates.

Results.—The age at onset of breast stage 2 varied by race/ethnicity, BMI at baseline, and site. Median age at onset of breast stage 2 was 8.8, 9.3, 9.7, and 9.7 years for African American, Hispanic, white non-Hispanic, and Asian participants, respectively. Girls with greater BMI reached breast stage 2 at younger ages. Age-specific and standardized prevalence of breast maturation was contrasted to observations in 2 large cross-sectional studies conducted 10 to 20 years earlier (Pediatric Research in Office Settings and National Health and Nutrition Examination Survey III) and found to have occurred earlier among white, non-Hispanic, but not African American girls.

Conclusions.—We observed the onset of thelarche at younger ages than previously documented, with important differences associated with race/ethnicity and BMI, confirming and extending patterns seen previously. These findings are consistent with temporal changes in BMI (Fig 1).

▶ This is yet another study from the Breast Cancer and the Environment Research Program that joins a squad of similar reports implicating an earlier onset of puberty in girls. Particular strengths of this project include its substantive sample size, prospective nature, and inclusion of subjects with a range of ethnicities, body mass indexes (BMIs), and geographical settings. One of the main aspects of this particular study, which investigated average age at thelarche in girls, was a comparison of the current findings with those reported from 2 previous cross-sectional studies of pubertal timing in girls, one of which was published more than 16 years ago. Although the authors tout their finding of overall earlier breast development in white girls as evidence for a continued secular trend, in fact, no difference was seen in this metric in girls with BMIs less than 85th percentile between the 2 studies, as seen in Fig 1. This observation, along with the finding of similar ages of Tanner II breast

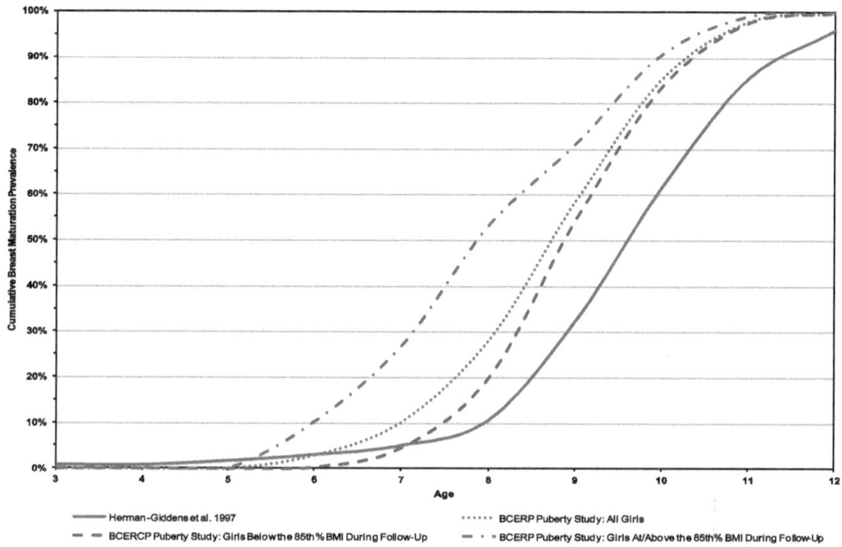

FIGURE 1.—Comparing the cumulative prevalence of Breast Stage 2+ for non-Hispanic white participants between the BCERP Puberty Study and PROS.[9] *Editor's Note*: Please refer to original journal article for full references. (Reproduced with permission from Pediatrics. Biro FM, Greenspan LC, Galvez MP, et al. Onset of breast development in a longitudinal cohort. *Pediatrics*. 2013;132:1019-1027, Copyright 2013, with permission from American Academy of Pediatrics.)

development in African-American girls in the current as well as the previous study, argues against any such trend. As has been noted in a plethora of similar reports, a higher BMI was statistically associated with earlier breast development, suggesting a direct relationship between the obesity epidemic and pubertal onset in girls. Whether this is caused by actual HPG axis activation or is occurring as a result of endocrine disrupting chemicals remains to be elucidated. An even more fundamental question, however, is whether the observed breast enlargement truly represents glandular breast tissue rather than adipose, particularly in the overweight cohort. Until studies such as this one incorporate objective biochemical markers such as kisspeptin, peak stimulated or random ultrasensitive luteinizing hormone, or pelvic ultrasound scans, it is likely premature to conclude that the controversy[1] regarding whether pubertal timing is continuing to decline is behind us!

E. Eugster, MD

Reference

1. Herman-Giddens ME. The enigmatic pursuit of puberty in girls. *Pediatrics*. 2013; 132:1125-1126.

Delayed Puberty and Estrogen Resistance in a Woman with Estrogen Receptor α variant

Quaynor SD, Stradtman EW Jr, Kim HG, et al (Georgia Regents Univ, Augusta; et al)

N Engl J Med 369:164-171, 2013

Although androgen resistance has been characterized in men with a normal chromosome complement and mutations in the androgen-receptor gene, a mutation in the gene encoding estrogen receptor α (*ESR1*) was previously described only in one man and not, to our knowledge, in a woman. We now describe an 18-year-old woman without breast development and with markedly elevated serum levels of estrogens and bilateral multicystic ovaries. She was found to have a homozygous loss-of-function *ESR1* mutation in a completely conserved residue that interferes with estrogen signaling. Her clinical presentation was similar to that in the mouse orthologue knockout. This case shows that disruption of *ESR1* causes profound estrogen resistance in women.

▶ Given the number of "mystery patients" that we encounter in the pediatric endocrine clinic, it is always exciting when a new genetic mutation is identified that solves a phenotypic puzzle. In this case, familiarity with the α-ERKO mouse model paved the way for the discovery of the first known case of estrogen resistance in a human female caused by a homozygous variant in estrogen receptor α. As is often found in these cases, the adopted woman's birth parents were likely second-degree relatives, and the affected residue is one that is highly conserved across species, including in the Sumatran orangutan and the African clawed frog! A few specific aspects of the case are worth contemplating. Although the patient's markedly enlarged multicystic ovaries are thought to have caused her abdominal pain, they seem out of proportion to the mildly elevated gonadotropins documented on several occasions. Given the apparent complete lack of response to exogenous estrogen, one can't help but wonder about the challenges of the clinical management in terms of bone mineral accrual and feminization. Finally, this case serves as a useful reminder to always keep an open mind when faced with a clinical conundrum. Had an estradiol level not been obtained (which many would have omitted in a patient with Tanner I breasts), this remarkable discovery may well have been missed.

E. Eugster, MD

Factors Associated With Hearing Impairment in Patients With Congenital Hypothyroidism Treated Since the Neonatal Period: A National Population-Based Study

Lichtenberger-Geslin L, Dos Santos S, Hassani Y, et al (Centre de Référence des Maladies Endocriniennes Rares de la Croissance, Paris, France; et al)

J Clin Endocrinol Metab 98:3644-3652, 2013

Context.—Untreated hypothyroidism is known to impair hearing, but little is known about the long-term hearing of patients treated for congenital hypothyroidism (CH) since the neonatal period.

Objective.—The purpose of this study was to assess hearing and its determinants in a population-based registry of young adult patients with CH.

Design, Setting, and Participants.—Self-declared hearing loss was evaluated in 1202 of the 1748 eligible patients with CH who completed a questionnaire on health status at a median age of 23.4 years. Audiograms were obtained for one third of the patients declaring hearing loss (37 of 107).

Main Outcome Measures.—Self-declared hearing loss and audiogram characteristics for patients reporting hearing impairment were measured.

Results.—These patients had a risk of self-declared hearing loss more than 3 times higher than that for the reference population (relative risk [RR] = 3.7; 95% confidence interval [CI], 2.9–4.7). Hearing impairment was diagnosed at a median age of 7.0 (25th–75th percentiles, 3.4–19.0) years, and 17% of affected patients required hearing support in early adulthood. Hearing loss was associated with the type of CH (patients with athyreosis and gland in situ were more frequently affected than those with an ectopic gland [RR = 2.61; 95% CI, 1.77–3.88]), with disease severity, as assessed by bone maturation delay at the time of diagnosis, with at least one knee epiphyseal ossification center absent in the most severe form (RR = 2.29; 95% CI, 1.39–3.79), and with other associated chronic diseases (RR = 3.64; 95% CI, 2.35–5.62). A trend for association with serum free T_4 concentration at diagnosis was also observed (RR = 1.47; 95% CI, 0.96–2.23). Hearing loss was mostly bilateral (90%), mild to moderate (96%), of the sensorineural type (76%), and concerned high or very high frequencies.

Conclusion.—Despite major improvements in prognosis, hearing loss remains a significant problem, particularly in patients with severe CH. Parents and primary care providers should be aware of this risk, because early diagnosis and intervention could improve the long-term prognosis in these patients.

▶ The association between congenital hypothyroidism (CH) and hearing impairment has long been recognized. However, to what extent this problem exists in adult patients with CH who were treated from early life has been unclear. A major strength of this study includes its sample size, which represents a national registry of patients with CH diagnosed in France in the decade after initiation of newborn screening. The greater than 3-fold relative risk of hearing loss in individuals with CH compared with the general population is concerning indeed. That the median age at diagnosis was 7 years highlights the need for pediatricians in particular to be aware of this risk. A few additional aspects of the study bear mention. It is somewhat counterintuitive that patients with anatomically normal thyroid glands were more likely to have hearing loss than those with ectopic thyroids, which typically result in CH that is intermediate in severity between athyreosis and dyshormonogenesis. The inclusion of subjects with poorly defined "other" conditions leads one to wonder if the hearing impairment in some of them could have been related to those other conditions rather than the CH. Lastly, one must always question the accuracy of self-reported data and a retrospective study design. Despite those flaws, the possibility of hearing problems in our young patients with CH should, at a minimum, be part of anticipatory guidance. Whether routine surveillance for hearing impairment should be implemented for these children is deserving of further study.

E. Eugster, MD

Congenital Adrenal Hyperplasia and the Second Newborn Screen

Chan CL, McFann K, Taylor L, et al (Children's Hosp Colorado and Univ of Colorado, Aurora; Univ of Colorado, Aurora; Colorado Dept of Public Health and Environment, Denver)

J Pediatr 2013, [Epub ahead of print]

Objective.—To evaluate the effectiveness of a second newborn screen for congenital adrenal hyperplasia (CAH) in the state of Colorado and report characteristics associated with cases identified on the first versus second screen.

Study Design.—Colorado implemented newborn screening for CAH with 17-hydroxyprogesterone beginning August 2000. The first screening is performed within 72 hours of life and the second between 8 and 14 days of life. We compared infants diagnosed on the basis of the first versus second newborn screen.

Results.—The first screen identified 29 cases of which 28 represented classical CAH. The incidence of classical CAH on the first screen was 1:24 766. The second screen identified 17 additional cases, of which 11 represented classical CAH. Combined, the incidence of classical CAH was 1:17 789. The sensitivity of the first screen was 71.79%. The false negative rate of the first screen was 28.2%. In the absence of a second screen, 1:47 824 infants would have been missed. Infants diagnosed on the first screen had higher 17-hydroxyprogesterone values compared with those diagnosed on the second screen ($P = .0008$).

Conclusions.—The use of a single newborn screen for CAH missed nearly 30% of classical CAH cases in Colorado. Addition of a second screen, therefore, can improve the operating characteristics of the newborn screening program.

▶ Newborn screening for congenital adrenal hyperplasia (CAH) has now been implemented in all 50 states and has clearly been a success. The importance of early detection, particularly for affected boys, has been shown by a decrease in apparent sudden infant death syndrome deaths in many states after the addition of CAH to the newborn screen. Despite these triumphs, occasional cases do get missed. One potential strategy that has been proposed to diminish this possibility is the adoption of a second screen. This study, which reports one state's experience with that model over a 10-year period, is a valuable contribution to the current debate. That nearly 30% of cases of classic CAH in Colorado were missed by the first screen certainly gives one pause. However, a universal second screen for CAH has been used by fewer than 20% of states thus far, illustrating that unanimity on whether the risk/benefit ratio of such an approach is favorable is lacking. Considering the potential downsides of a second screen is informative. One concern is that additional screening would almost certainly add to the burden of false-positive results in sick and preterm infants, which is already a considerable one. Another is the possible increase in the number of cases of nonclassic CAH detected, the optimal clinical management of which is often unclear. Finally, states must balance costs of expanded screening with the benefits of detecting additional cases and risks of delayed diagnosis, which, in the era of an ever-increasing number and complexity of disorders screened for, is no simple task. At a minimum, clinicians need to be aware that newborn screening is never perfect and to be familiar with the signs and symptoms of CAH during infancy and beyond.

E. Eugster, MD

Skeletal Maturation in Children with Cushing Syndrome Is Not Consistently Delayed: The Role of Corticotropin, Obesity, and Steroid Hormones, and the Effect of Surgical Cure

Lodish MB, Gourgari E, Sinaii N, et al (Natl Insts of Health, Bethesda, MD; Natl Insts of Health Clinical Ctr, Bethesda, MD; et al)

J Pediatr 164:801-806, 2014

Objective.—To assess skeletal maturity by measuring bone age (BA) in children with Cushing syndrome (CS) before and 1-year after transsphenoidal surgery or adrenalectomy, and to correlate BA with hormone levels and other measurements.

Study Design.—This case series conducted at the National Institutes of Health Clinical Center included 93 children with Cushing disease (CD) (43 females; mean age, 12.3 ± 2.9 years) and 31 children with adrenocorticotropic hormone–independent CS (AICS) (22 females, mean age 10.3 ± 4.5 years). BA was obtained before surgery and at follow-up. Outcome measures were comparison of BA in CD vs AICS and analysis of the effects of hypercortisolism, insulin excess, body mass index, and androgen excess on BA.

Results.—Twenty-six of the 124 children (21.0%) had advanced BA, compared with the expected general population prevalence of 2.5% ($P < .0001$). Only 4 of 124 (3.2%) had delayed BA. The majority of children (76%) had normal BA. The average BA z-score was similar in the children with CD and those with AICS (0.6 ± 1.4 vs 0.5 ± 1.8; $P = .8865$). Body mass index SDS and normalized values of dehydroepiandrosterone, dehydroepiandrosterone sulfate, androsteonedione, estradiol, and testosterone were all significantly higher in the children with advanced BA vs those with normal or delayed BA. Fifty-nine children who remained in remission from CD had follow-up BA 1.2 ± 0.3 years after transsphenoidal surgery, demonstrating decreased BA z-score (1.0 ± 1.6 vs 0.3 ± 1.4; $P < .0001$).

Conclusion.—Contrary to common belief, endogenous CS in children appears to be associated with normal or even advanced skeletal maturation. When present, BA advancement in CS is related to obesity, insulin resistance, and elevated adrenal androgen levels and aromatization. This finding may have significant implications for treatment decisions and final height predictions in these children.

▶ Evaluation of skeletal maturation through assessment of bone age x-ray is an integral part of the diagnostic armamentarium of pediatric endocrinologists. In general, a normal bone age is considered reassuring because it argues against a pathologic process being present. The endocrinopathies that result in linear growth arrest (ie, hypothyroidism, growth hormone deficiency, and hypercortisolism) are invariably presumed to result in a significant delay in skeletal maturation. This study reminds us that it is not so simple! Contrary to conventional wisdom, the majority of the 124 children with Cushing syndrome (CS) in this report had a normal bone age, whereas 21% actually had advanced skeletal maturation regardless of whether they had Cushing disease or adrenocorticotropic hormone–independent CS. Factors associated with an advanced bone age were the same ones that we see in other clinical situations, including obesity, insulin resistance, and hyperandrogenism. Although this information is undeniably useful, endogenous CS is extremely rare in pediatric patients. Far more common, however, is iatrogenic CS due to the pharmacologic use of glucocorticoids for a number of medical conditions. One would certainly expect that a delayed bone age would be more ubiquitous in that group of patients. A study similar to this one comparing skeletal maturation in endogenous and exogenous CS could help to support or refute this presumption.

E. Eugster, MD

Increased Scalp Hair Cortisol Concentrations in Obese Children

Veldhorst MAB, Noppe G, Jongejan MHTM, et al (Erasmus Med Ctr (MC), Rotterdam, The Netherlands; Sint Franciscus Gasthuis, PM Rotterdam, The Netherlands)

J Clin Endocrinol Metab 99:285-290, 2014

Context.—Pathologically increased cortisol exposure induces obesity, but it is not known whether relatively high cortisol within the physiological range is related to childhood obesity.

Objective.—The aim of the study was to compare hair cortisol concentrations between obese and normal-weight children.

Design.—We performed an observational case-control study.

Participants.—Twenty obese children (body mass index-SD score [BMI-SDS] > 2.3) and 20 age- and sex-matched normal-weight children (BMI-SDS < 1.1) aged 8–12 years were recruited.

Main Outcome Measures.—Scalp hair samples from the posterior vertex were collected, and hair cortisol concentrations were measured using ELISA. Body weight, height, and waist circumference were measured. From the obese children, additional data on blood pressure and blood lipid concentrations were collected.

Results.—In both groups, five boys and 15 girls were included; their mean age was 10.8 ± 1.3 vs 10.8 ± 1.2 years (obese vs normal weight; not significant). Body weight, BMI, BMI-SDS, and waist circumference were higher in the obese children compared with the normal-weight children (69.8 ± 17.2 vs 35.5 ± 7.2 kg; 29.6 ± 4.9 vs 16.4 ± 1.6 kg/m^2; 3.4 ± 0.5 vs −0.2 ± 0.8 SDS; 94 ± 13 vs 62 ± 6 cm; $P < .001$ all). Hair cortisol concentration was higher in obese than normal-weight children (median [interquartile range], 25 [17, 32] vs 17 [13, 21] pg/mg; $P < .05$).

Conclusions.—Hair cortisol concentration, a measure for long-term cortisol exposure, was higher in obese children than normal-weight children. This suggests long-term activation of the hypothalamus-pituitary-adrenal axis in obese children and may provide a novel target for treatment of obesity in children.

► Multiple studies have investigated whether exogenous obesity is associated with alterations in the hypothalamic-pituitary-adrenal (HPA) axis, and the results have been decidedly mixed. Although some investigators have found higher cortisol production and clearance rates in obese individuals, others have found normal or even lower values than those seen in normal-weight controls. This is an interesting study that utilizes a novel measure of chronic cortisol exposure and is the first such exploration in pediatric patients. Interestingly, scalp hair cortisol was significantly higher in the obese cohort, and significant correlations between log hair cortisol concentrations and both body mass index—SD score and waist circumference were also seen. This observation, although not particularly surprising, leaves one with the proverbial chicken-and-egg question. Longitudinal studies will be needed to answer it! In the meantime, whether the HPA axis could be a therapeutic target in the quest for effective intervention in the development of obesity is a tantalizing suggestion.

E. Eugster, MD

Bone/Calcium

Parathyroid Hormone as a Functional Indicator of Vitamin D Sufficiency in Children

Maguire JL, Birken C, Thorpe KE, et al (Univ of Toronto, Ontario, Canada; et al)
JAMA Pediatr 2014 [Epub ahead of print]

There has been debate on what constitutes physiologically normal 25-hydroxyvitamin D serum levels in children. The Institute of Medicine and the American Academy of Pediatrics have recommended that 25-hydroxyvitamin D levels in children be more than 50 nmol/L. The Canadian Paediatric Society has suggested that 25-hydroxyvitamin D levels be more than 75 nmol/L. Given the long time course for the development of chronic health outcomes that may be related to low vitamin D levels in children, physiological indicators of vitamin D sufficiency would be helpful.

One physiological indicator of bone health is parathyroid hormone (PTH). Studies of adults have identified that PTH levels cease to decline at 25-hydroxyvitamin D levels typically more than 75 nmol/L, suggesting physiological vitamin D sufficiency. In children, identifying such a plateau has been elusive. To address this, we conducted a study of healthy young

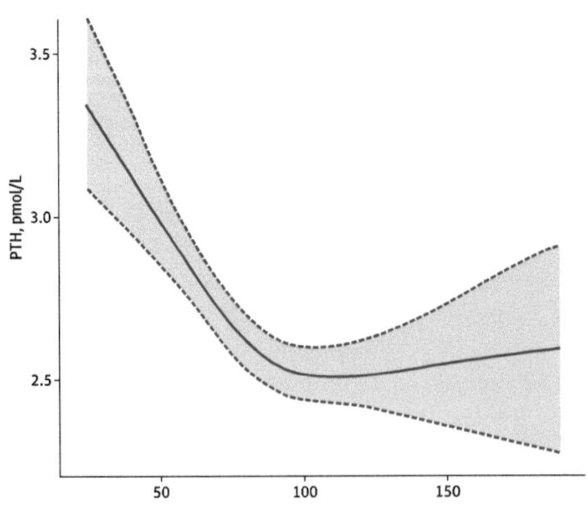

FIGURE.—Plot of the Regression Model for 25-Hydroxyvitamin D and Parathyroid Hormone (PTH). Shaded areas inside the dashed lines represent 95% confidence intervals. (Reprinted from Maguire JL, Birken C, Thorpe KE, et al. Parathyroid hormone as a functional indicator of vitamin D sufficiency in children. *JAMA Pediatr.* 2014;[Epub ahead of print], with permission from American Medical Association.)

children to determine whether a 25-hydroxyvitamin D plateau exists above which serum PTH is minimized (Fig).

► A potential deleterious effect of vitamin D insufficiency on human health has been a hot topic for quite a long time. This is hardly surprising when one considers the multitude of conditions for which insufficient vitamin D has been implicated as a risk factor. These have included everything from type 1 diabetes to schizophrenia to numerous cancers to multiple sclerosis to an earlier age of menarche in girls! Although these observations do not establish causality, the sheer magnitude of the evidence linking low serum vitamin D concentrations to adverse outcomes highlights that ensuring vitamin D sufficiency in children is paramount. Despite general unanimity on this issue, defining the precise level that signifies that 25-hydroxy vitamin D stores are replete has been enigmatic. Thus, this report represents an important contribution to this area. Particular strengths include the large sample size, the inclusion of subjects on vitamin D supplementation, and the young age of the participants. As seen in the figure, the inflection point for parathyroid hormone occurred at an approximate vitamin D concentration of 100 nmol/L (40 ng/dL). Not surprisingly, this is considerably higher than has been observed in adults. Additional studies such as this in older children and adolescents would be wonderful. In the meantime, this study finally provides concrete guidance to pediatricians regarding target serum vitamin D concentrations in our young patients.

E. Eugster, MD

Article Index

Chapter 1: Diabetes

Chapter 2: Lipoproteins and Atherosclerosis

Chapter 3: Obesity

Chapter 4: Thyroid

Chapter 5: Calcium and Bone Metabolism

Chapter 6: Adrenal Cortex

Chapter 8: Neuroendocrinology

Chapter 9: Pediatric Endocrinology

Author Index

A

B

C

D

E

F

G

H

I

J

K

L

M

N

O

P

Q

R

S

T

V

W

X

Y

Z

FSC
www.fsc.org
MIX
Papier | Fördert gute Waldnutzung
FSC® C083411

Kolibri 360 GmbH
Ferdinand-Jühlke-Straße 7
99095 Erfurt, Deutschland
produktsicherheit@kolibri360.de